Archaeopress Roman Archaeology 117

Thermalism in the Roman Provinces

The Role of Medicinal Mineral Waters across the Empire

Edited by

Silvia González Soutelo
Universidad Autónoma de Madrid/MIAS

Archaeopress Archaeology

ARCHAEOPRESS PUBLISHING LTD
Summertown Pavilion
18-24 Middle Way
Summertown
Oxford OX2 7LG
www.archaeopress.com

ISBN 978-1-80327-775-2
ISBN 978-1-80327-776-9 (e-Pdf)

'Tomás y Valiente' fellowship: Healing spas in Antiquity (MIAS/UAM).
Project of the Spanish Ministry of Science, Innovation and Universities 'THERMASCAPE: El paisaje termal en Hispania. El papel de los recursos termales en la península Ibérica desde época romana' (PID2022-138809NB-I00)

Thermalism in the Roman Provinces. The Role of Medicinal Mineral Waters across the Empire

Contents

3. Healing Spas and Ancient Roads. Pilgrims and visitors to thermal sites.

List of Authors

AUGUSTIN-ROLLAND, Lise. Université Clermont Auvergne (UAR 3550; ArAr, UMR 5138) / Ingénieure d'études, 4 rue Ledru, 63000 Clermont-Ferrand, France. lise.augustin@uca.fr

AVRAMOVA, Mariya. National Archaeological Institute with Museum – Bulgarian Academy of Sciences. avramova.m@gmail.com

BASSANI, Maddalena. Iuav University of Venice, Department of Architecture and Arts. Associate Professor of Classical Archaeology. Palazzo Badoer, San Polo 2468, 30125 Venezia (Italy). mbassani@iuav.it

BERNARDO, Helena. Museu Municipal de Penafiel y CITCEM. helena.bernardo@cm-penafiel.pt

CARNEIRO, Sérgio. UNIARQ – Centre for Archaeology. School of Arts and Humanities. University of Lisbon. Alameda da Universidade, 1600-214 Lisboa, Portugal; CCDR-LVT - Commission for Regional Development and Coordination of Lisbon and Tagus Valley, Department of Culture. sergio.carneiro@ccdr-lvt.pt

COSTA, Laurent. Research Engineer at the French National Centre for Scientific Research (CNRS) – PhD, The Huma-num Paris Time Machine (PTM) Consortium MSH Mondes, 21, allée de l'Université, 92023 Nanterre Cedex. laurent.costa@cnrs.fr

DARTEVELLE, Hélène. French Ministery of Cuture (ArAr, UMR 5138; ArScAn, UMR 7041) / Ingénieure d'études, Service régional de l'archéologie d'Auvergne-Rhône-Alpes, 4 rue Pascal, 63000 Clermont-Ferrand, France. helene.dartevelle@culture.gouv.fr

DI LUCA, Gioconda. Università degli Studi di Roma 'Tor Vergata'. latericium@hotmail.com

DOUSTEYSSIER, Bertrand. Université Clermont Auvergne (UAR 3550) / Ingénieur de recherche, 4 rue Ledru, 63000 Clermont-Ferrand, France. bertrand.dousteyssier@uca.fr

FÉNYES, Gabriella. Aquincum Museum of the Budapest History Museum. fenyes.gabriella@btm.hu

FOVET, Élise. CNRS, Université Clermont Auvergne (UAR 3550) / Ingénieure de recherche, 4 rue Ledru, 63000 Clermont-Ferrand, France. elise.fovet@uca.fr

GONZÁLEZ SOUTELO, Silvia. Universidad Autónoma de Madrid (UAM) and Madrid Institute for Advanced Studies (MIAS). Campus Cantoblanco. Faculty of Filosofía y Letras, Dep. Prehistory and Archaeology. silvia.gonzalezs@uam.es

KUŠAN ŠPALJ, Dora. Archaeological Museum in Zagreb. Zagreb, Croatia. dkusan@amz.hr

MARCATO, Matteo. Independent researcher. matteo.marcato.87@gmail.com

MARIOTTI, Emanuele. Università per Stranieri di Siena. emanuele.mariotti@unistrasi.it

NECTOUX, Élise. French Ministery of Cuture (ArAr, UMR 5138; ArScAn, UMR 7041) / Conservatrice du patrimoine, Service régional de l'archéologie d'Auvergne-Rhône-Alpes, 4 rue Pascal, 63000 Clermont-Ferrand, France. elise.nectoux@culture.gouv.fr

NIEBERLE, Matthias. Universität zu Köln, Archäologisches Institut, Albertus-Magnus-Platz 1, 5931 Köln. nieberlematthias@gmail.com

PEROK, Nikoleta. Archaeological Museum in Zagreb. Zagreb, Croatia. nperok@amz.hr

ROCQUE, Gabriel. Service d'archéologie préventive du département de l'Allier (Citeres, UMR 7324) / Operation manager, 1 avenue Victor Hugo BP 1669, 03000 Moulins, France. rocque.g@allier.fr

SABATIER, Richard. Government-accredited Architect (DPLG), Chairman of the Observatory for Archaeology and Heritage in Haute-Bigorre (OAPHB), 6, rue Gambetta, 65200 Bagnères-de-Bigorre. oaphb65.gmail.com

SAMPAIO, Jorge. Área Arqueológica do Freixo - Património Cultural I.P. jorgesampaio@patrimoniocultural.gov.pt

SCHAER, Andrea. Independent researcher. andrea.schaer@archaeokontor.ch

SEKULOV, Vane P. NI Institute for protection of cultural monuments and the Museum of Strumica. v.p.sekulov@gmail.com

SOEIRO, Teresa. CITCEM-Faculty of Letters. University of Porto (FLUP). teresasoeiro@sapo.pt

TABOLLI, Jacopo. Università per Stranieri di Siena. jacopo.tabolli@unistrasi.it

TURCHETTO, Jacopo. Department of Cultural Heritage, University of Padova / Research fellow, piazza Capitaniato, 7. 35139 Padova (Italy). jacopo.turchetto@unipd.it

ÜSKÜPLÜ AKGÜL, Gamze. Research Assistant, Trakya University, Faculty of Letters, Department of Archaeology, TR-22100 Edirne/Turkey. gamzeuskuplu@trakya.edu.tr

YARAŞ, Ahmet. Prof. Dr., Trakya University, Faculty of Letters, Department of Archaeology, TR-22100 Edirne/Turkey. ahmetyaras@trakya.edu.tr

ZANOVELLO, Paola. Department of Cultural Heritage, University of Padova / Associate professor, piazza Capitaniato, 7. 35139 Padova (Italy). paola.zanovello.1@unipd.it

Introduction

Silvia González Soutelo

Throughout history, mineral and thermal waters have been a source of health and a remedy for numerous ailments and diseases. Before the development of pharmacology, which occurred essentially from the mid-20th century onwards, this natural resource was a fundamental element for all those who, beset by various illnesses, travelled to the most highly valued thermal springs in order to undergo various treatments associated with their waters.

Based on the local population's empirical knowledge of their salutary properties, which had both religious and medical associations, the various types of water present in these natural springs were identified in accordance with their temperature, flow, colour, odour or flavour, which could be used to heal or alleviate certain physical problems. Given the importance the Romans placed on these waters in the process of expanding their Empire, this resource became a highly valued natural asset from multiple perspectives, including both strategic and functional considerations.

Indeed, the geology of Italic areas such as Etruria, Campania or Lazio formed a sort of laboratory in which the abundance of thermal springs, mainly hyperthermal, provided a breeding ground for the use of natural spaces (caves, crevices, pools, etc.), which were gradually copied and integrated through the creation of baths used not only for curative purposes (in the case of mineral-medicinal waters), but which also played a hygienic, social and cultural role (in the case of common water) that was easy to replicate in all settlements during the Roman period.

This is supported, for example, by physician Antyllus in Oribasius (X, 1, 6 and X, 3, 1) who writes in his first book on *Methods of Treatment and on Natural Mineral Baths* that "regarding the baths, some are composed of fresh water of poor quality, whilst others are impregnated with a certain quality and endowed with efficient and manifest properties (...). The action of *natural mineral baths* is far more efficient and energetic than that of *artificial baths*. Indeed, there are a large number of types of mineral waters, determined by the properties of the soils they pass through (...)"[1].

Thanks to this perception, which was shared by classical authors, the construction of sanctuaries and bathing houses may well have commenced in an Italian setting. Indeed, more and more specialised building solutions and infrastructures would gradually emerge of an increasingly monumental nature that would spread to the new provinces that made up the Empire.

In this sense, together with the steady expansion of hygienic baths, a new model of healing baths appeared that included spaces for immersion and ablutions, with pools and/or bathtubs, as well as the use of mud and *pediluvia*. The fact is, that from the Roman period at least, buildings and thermal complexes were built that made maximum use of these mineral waters, with attention being paid to the engineering difficulties involved in capturing those springs, as well as adapting the baths to the topography of the terrain and the myriad aspects that could affect these springs.

Gradually, many of these thermal sites would feature buildings and services that would allow widely varying settlements to be established around the waters. They included the construction of authentic spa towns, as well as individual facilities, dependent on cities or settlements of diverse nature, where ritual and salutary functions would play a major role in their layout.

However, much remains to be discovered. Despite pioneering work addressing the question of these waters aimed at pinpointing possible differences between baths with mineral and thermal water, very little research has been carried out that centres on the global nature of Roman thermalism, a phenomenon with numerous aspects that are still unknown to us.

That is the objective of this book. Starting from the hypothesis that the buildings that employed mineral-medicinal waters differed from the classic hygienic baths we all know, it features an interesting collection of thermal and archaeological sites located throughout the ancient Roman Empire and which evidence the complexities involved in their interpretation, reflected

[1] For a more detailed translation and study of this text and other works of classical authors who dealt with different topics on thermalism, see the project website www.healingspasinantiquity.es (in progress). This study on classical sources for the study of healing spas is also described in S. González Soutelo and S. Romano 2023. Sources for the study of ancient thermalism: a new proposal for editing and translation. *MonTI. Monografías de Traducción e Interpretación* 15: 179-205. DOI: 10.6035/MonTI.2023.15.06.

in the multiple physical and chemical determinants of these waters.

Indeed, the modern phenomenon of thermalism is that of a thermal-healing model associated with wellness spaces that today have spread beyond Europe, standing directly on sites that are hydrogeologically rich in thermal mineral waters. Yet in order to discover their origins and principles, we must go back to the Etruscan, Hellenistic and Roman worlds to obtain an insight into the plethora of cultural, social, political and economic phenomena that allowed this natural therapy to be put to use.

Furthermore, moving beyond this idea, we consider that the various baths that were constructed from the Hellenistic period onwards were essentially an attempt to imitate the natural sites where these waters emerged spontaneously and naturally. Consequently, the study of baths dating back to the Roman period also allows a far clearer insight into the origin and development of the various types of thermal and salutary complexes associated with each type of water. Many of them would therefore imitate the generation of steam and high temperatures these buildings were capable of through the use of boilers and complex hypocaust and heating systems.

In this sense, this volume addresses various questions of interest in order to understand this phenomenon. To what extent does thermalism display differences and similarities in each of the provinces the Roman Empire was divided into? What are the specific characteristics of each territory? Is this a singular or local occurrence, or can we find elements that are common to all thermal facilities?

In order to delve deeper into these and other aspects, this monograph includes a large number of studies, organised into various sections, featuring some of the most representative and internationally most studied sites and the leading specialists in each. Together, we seek to identify the various construction and functional solutions for thermal spas through the creation of a research network into ancient thermalism that provides a forum for the exchange of ideas and experiences in this field.

Therefore, and under the generic title *Thermal spas in the Roman Provinces: the role of medicinal mineral waters across the Empire*, and in the awareness that thermal waters were a much valued natural resource in antiquity, various authors attempt to respond to a series of questions that have arisen during the course of their research:

Addressing adaptation to topographical and geological conditions, we understand that the bath buildings that exploited mineral-medicinal waters had to be in keeping with the places where these waters emerged, overcoming the challenges of rivers, hills, or filtrations of different types, which undoubtedly made their construction difficult, as well as their maintenance and subsequent study. An exceptional example of this phenomenon is provided by **D. Kušan Špalj and N. Perok** from the Museum of Varaždinske Toplice (Croatia), in their description of the complex process of excavation and study of a unique thermal complex, whose ancient toponym (*Aquae Iasae*) reflects the value that has been attributed to these waters since ancient times. The same is true of the thermal sites of the French Massif Central, studied by the team of archaeologists formed by **L. Augustin-Rolland, B. Dousteyssier, E. Fovet, E. Nectoux, G. Rocque and H. Dartevelle.** Their combined efforts constitute an outstanding example of integration, collaboration and communication, highlighting exceptional sites and benchmarks in European thermalism that were in danger of falling into oblivion.

Likewise, the combination of nature and technical development during the Roman period is exemplified perfectly in the thermal site of Baia (Italy), the object of an in-depth study by **M. Nieberle** analysing the construction of one of the most elaborate thermal sites of entire Empire and a social, cultural, architectural and economic benchmark of the Roman period, located in the famous Bay of Naples. This combination is also reflected in the outstanding examples of adaptation and preparation of complex collection systems in the French sites studied by **M. Marcatto and S. González Soutelo**, which are still in use today at a considerable number of thermal sites. Further examples in Eastern Europe and Turkey are presented by **G. Fenyes** in the military context of the Roman limes with *Aquincum* (Budapest, Hungary) through the origins, singularity and thermal tradition of one of Europe's major thermal spa capitals; or in the architectural and monumental testimonies in the Anatolian peninsula by **A. Yaraş** and **G. Üsküplü Akgül**, focused mainly on the western area of modern-day Turkey, where local and Greco-Roman traditions come together in a territory with a longstanding thermal trajectory that extends to the current day.

Turning to the role Roman spas played in the landscape (the object of our ongoing RDI project "*THERMASCAPE: El paisaje termal en Hispania. El papel de los recursos termales en la península Ibérica desde época romana*" PID2022-138809NB-I00), the monograph includes an insight into the site at Bansko (Strumica), an exceptional thermal building and sanctuary situated in the countryside of what is today the Republic of North Macedonia, analysed by **V.P. Sekulov,** the site curator. Similar interest can be found in Italy, both in the research conducted by **M. Bassani**, at the thermal site of Montegrotto Terme (*Aquae Patavinae*, just outside Padua); and again in Baia (Italy), where the built and functional entity continued until the Late Antique period, thanks to **G. di Lucca**'s fascinating observations into this Mediterranean site associated with the city of Cumas; or in the magnificent example of the Etruscan-Roman sanctuary and healing site of *Bagno Grande* in San Casciano dei Bagni, also in Italy, presented by **J. Tabolli and E. Mariotti,** which in the last few years has generated a wealth of new and valuable information as well as highlighting the phenomenon of thermalism from the Etruscan period onwards.

Joining these contributions are the recent results of archaeological investigations conducted in highly significant sites such as *Aquae Helveticae* (Baden, Switzerland), by the archaeologist **A. Schaer,** who offers an intriguing diachronic vision of the thermal phenomenon in this Central-European spa town. The same is true of Bagnères-de-Bigorre in the French Pyrenees, studied by **L. Costa and R. Sabatier,** who address the role of these waters in these high mountains up until the current day. This same proposal is posited by the international team comprising **T. Soeiro, S. González Soutelo, H. Bernardo and J. Sampaio** regarding the Roman site of Termas de São Vicente (Penafiel) for the analysis of this spa within its historical and territorial context (between the 1st and 5th centuries AD). Similarly, the work of archaeologist **S. Carneiro** describes the exceptional testimony of the Roman spa of *Aquae Flaviae* (Chaves) and its surrounding area, as particularly topical case studies located within Portuguese territory.

This volume of studies would not be complete without a small section discussing the role of thermalism in shaping of the axes of communication in the Roman period and the role these waters may have played in the creation, emergence and development of new settlements in very diverse geographical areas. This section includes a case study of the Roman province of Thracia (in present-day Bulgaria), the work of **M. Avramova,** who analyses the road network laid out between some of the main thermal sites in the eastern part of the Empire. North Africa is also addressed thanks to the update on research into road layouts and thermal enclaves in the different African provinces from **P. Zanovello and J. Turchetto**.

As has been very briefly set out in this introduction, together, these examples form a tour of the Mediterranean that will enable us to begin to trace a global vision of thermalism from antiquity to the present day. Looking beyond the more traditional studies of these sites conducted in previous centuries, we can observe a change of mentality among researchers, and the unanimous perception of a new direction in research addressing this phenomenon, in keeping with the singularities required by the study of a natural resource that has been highly valued since antiquity.

1. Adaptations to Topographical and Geological Conditions. Healing Spas Over the Territory

The Roman Thermal Spa of *Aquae Iasae*, Varaždinske Toplice (Croatia)

Dora KUŠAN ŠPALJ
Archaeological Museum in Zagreb. Zagreb, Croatia
dkusan@amz.hr

Nikoleta PEROK
Archaeological Museum in Zagreb. Zagreb, Croatia
nperok@amz.hr

Abstract: The present-day town of Varaždinske Toplice (Northwest Croatia) was the site of the Roman settlement *Aquae Iasae*, famous as a thermal spa centre. It developed between the 1st and 4th centuries at the site of the therapeutic thermal springs. The main spring is located on the highest terrace (in the present-day park) and the Romans built the sanctuary around it and a bath complex to the south. As early as the 1st century, they organised the area around the thermal spring as a sanctuary giving the natural phenomenon a 'sacred spring' ambience. At the same time, they managed to 'control' the spring and used the thermal water in the baths and this was especially so after the construction of the spring reservoir in the 2nd century when a very complex and carefully planned hydraulic system was created. The beginning of the 4th century was the time frame of the renovation of the sanctuary and spring reservoir when numerous older inscriptions, reliefs, and even sculptures were used as construction material. The main feature of the *Aquae Iasae* sanctuary was the powerful cult of the nymphs but also the worship of various deities associated with the power of healing. Finds related to Apollo and the geological situation around the thermal spring suggest that it could have also been a place of oracles.

Keywords: thermal water, spring reservoir, nymphs, *Aquae Iasae*, Pannonia

Introduction

The Roman settlement of *Aquae Iasae* developed between the 1st and 4th centuries as a thermal spa centre at the site of the therapeutic thermal springs in the area of the present-day town of Varaždinske Toplice (Northwest Croatia). It extended onto the slopes and at the foot of a hill whose specific terraced configuration with travertine layers is the result of the long-term deposition of thermal waters.[1] The main spring is located on the highest terrace (in the present-day park) and the thermal water constantly flows out at 20 litres per second (nearly 2 million litres per day) at a temperature of 58°C[2] (Figure 1). The spring is located at the apex of an anticlinal structure, and the Upper Triassic layers are the main carriers of the thermal water. Most of the water that flows out at Varaždinske Toplice accumulates on the northern slopes of the Kalnik mountain, where the altitude is up to 350m higher than the spring in Varaždinske Toplice. The height difference is important because of the hydrostatic pressure, which, along with the permeability of the rocks, is essential for moving water on the principle of connected vessels (Šimunić 1988). On its way through the ground, the water dissolves the rocks it passes through,[3] and in order to warm up to 58°C, it must descend to approximately 1300m (Šimunić 1988: 29). The age of water is estimated at more than 40,000 years (Marković *et al.* 2020: 89).

It is very likely that a large amount of hot water flowing from the ground that evaporates and fills the space with a specific smell has attracted people since ancient times, arousing admiration and awe. Although numerous prehistoric artefacts from the Palaeolithic to the Iron Age have been found in the area of Varaždinske Toplice (Čabrian *et al.* 1973: 4–5; Malez 1979: 261–262; Bekić 2006: 21–30, 265–268, 271–272), besides the two prehistoric axes (Kušan Špalj and Nemeth-Ehrlich 2012: Fig. 25 y 26), there are no traces of activity around the spring before the Roman period. Regardless of the lack of findings, the assumption is that this natural phenomenon and the mystical space surrounding it were considered a holy place in ancient times, whether it was visited solely by individuals (sorcerers and priests) or it was accessible to ordinary worshipers as well. It was in the 1st millennium BC when this area was inhabited by the Pannonian tribe the Iasi (Mócsy 1968; Schejbal 2003: 395) and they were, as the meaning of

[1] In Varaždinske Toplice is the largest amount of travertine in Croatia formed as the result of long-term flow of thermal water, very likely since the beginning of the Pleistocene (Marković *et al.* 2020: 86).

[2] Until 1962, only the water that naturally springs out at the surface was used, however, since then it has been pumped up from deeper layers (via a borehole).

[3] The water belongs to a $NaCaMg\text{-}HCCO_3SO_4$ mixed type of water (Marković *et al.* 2015: 74).

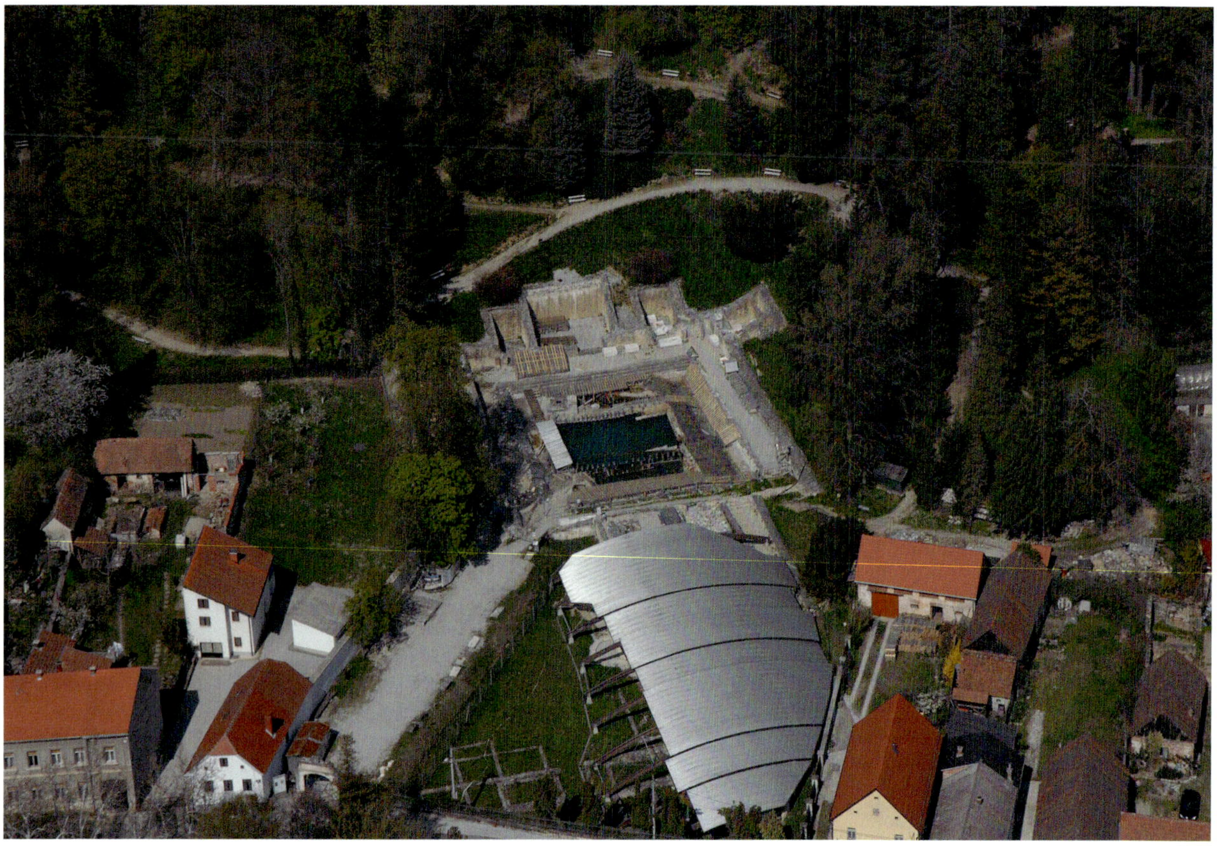

Figure 1. The complex of Roman public architecture in the park in Varaždinske Toplice, after the 2012 excavations (aerial photo by Vektra, Varaždin).

their name indicates,[4] most likely well acquainted with the healing properties of the thermal waters. The name given to the Roman settlement – *Aquae Iasae* – also confirms that they were living in the area and using the thermal water. It is assumed that in the pre-Roman period, the Iasi inhabited the area abundant with hot springs between the Sava and Drava rivers (present-day Northwest Croatia)[5] and that after the Roman conquest, it was integrated into the framework of the province of *Pannonia*, and from the beginning of the 2nd century it belonged to Upper *Pannonia*. During the 1st century, *Pannonia* was divided into several administrative units, which were named after the native tribes. It is very likely that the *civitas Iasorum* occupied the area between *Aquae Iasae* in the west and *Aquae Balissae* (today's Daruvar) in the east, both towns developed by the thermal springs (Schejbal 2003: 395).

In that period military administration was introduced over the conquered communities, that is, they were governed by prefects who were also military officers. This is confirmed by a marble pedestal for a statue found in the 2011 excavation of the *Aquae Iasae* sanctuary, which has an inscription made in honour of *Quintus Gavius Fronto* who was a centurion of *Legio XIII Gemina* and *praefectus civitatium Scordiscorum et Breucorum et Iasorum* (*HD*075016; Kušan Špalj 2022b: 60-61). He obviously governed a very large area between the Sava and Drava rivers, stretching all the way to the eastern border of southern Pannonia (Kušan Špalj 2014; 2015: 50-54). Most likely no later than 71 AD, this large area was divided into smaller units and military rule was substituted by the civilian administration of representatives of the local aristocracy. This is confirmed by a military diploma, dated to the year 71, in which as the witnesses the *principes Breoucorum, Boiorum, Antizitium and Iasorum* are mentioned.[6] There were obviously members of the elite among their communities and *Titus Flavius Serenus* who was the *princeps Iasorum* was even rewarded with citizenship slightly earlier (Migotti *et al.* 2018: 237).

The centre of *civitas Iasorum* was *Aquae Balissae*, also known from literary and epigraphic sources as *res publica Iasorum* and *Municipium Iasorum* (present-day Daruvar) (Migotti *et al.* 2018: 225). The town developed alongside the thermal springs, but unfortunately, apart from about 30 inscriptions, due to the lack of archaeological

[4] *Iasi* – 'healers' – a tribe living near the healing hot springs (Schejbal 2003: 397).

[5] Plin. *NH* III. 25, 147–148; Ptol. II; Mócsy 1968; Schejbal 2003: 395; Domić Kunić 2006: 76.

[6] AE 2002, 1771 = AE 2004, 89 = AE 2007, 93; Grbić 2014: 252–253, cat. 170; Migotti *et al.* 2018: 226, 237.

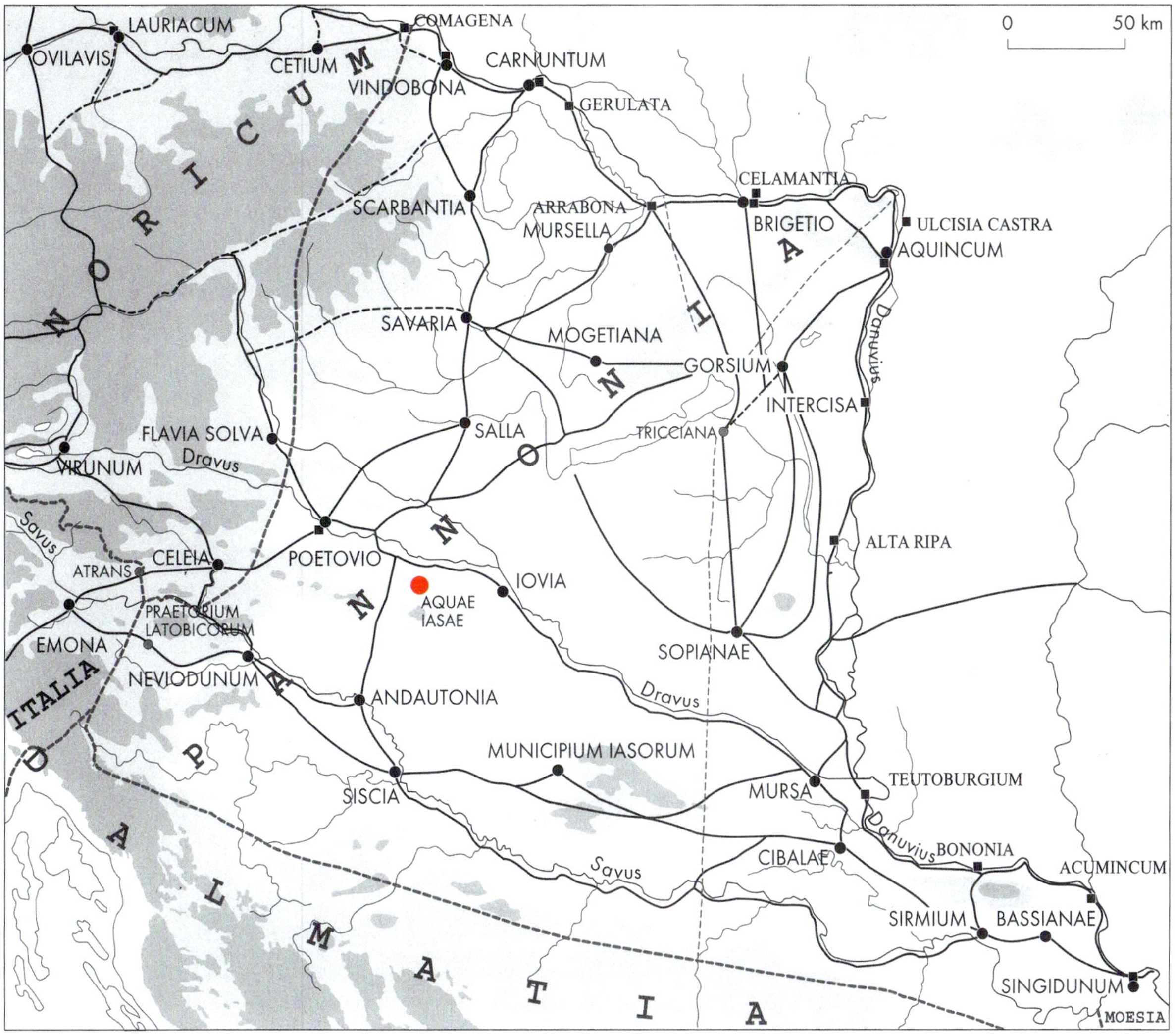

Map 1. Position of *Aquae Iasae* in Roman Pannonia (after: Šašel and Scherrer 2004).

excavations, there is not much information about its development and urban topography (Schejbal 2004; Migotti *et al.* 2018). During the reign of Hadrian, the town presumably received municipal status, while until then, *civitas Iasorum* was probably headed by a princeps from the local aristocracy. *Aquae Iasae*, which was in the western part of the Iasi territory, seems to have had a slightly different fate than the rest of the civitas, as it was very likely included in the territory of the Poetovio during the time of the Flavians (Horvat *et al.* 2003: 106; Ragolić 2014: 335–336; Migotti *et al.* 2018: 130, 134). After the administrative division of Pannonia in the 4th century, when under Diocletian's reform Poetovio was included in the province of Noricum, the settlement of *Aquae Iasae* remained in Upper Pannonia. During this period, *Aquae Iasae* probably became part of the territory of a town located on the site of present-day Ludbreg (*civitas Iovia*) (Gregl and Migotti 2004: 131–143; Migotti *et al.* 2018: 134). (Map 1)

The Roman settlement of *Aquae Iasae* – history of the research

Accidental finds in the area of Varaždinske Toplice

Even before the beginning of systematic archaeological research over the Varaždinske Toplice area, there were numerous accidental finds in the past centuries indicating the existence of an important Roman thermal spa (Bedeković 1752; Katančić 1795; Tkalčić 1869: Mommsen 1873; Ljubić 1879). Although most of those finds have not been preserved, mainly stone monuments have survived, which, according to the trends of the 18th and 19th centuries were used as decorations in various building structures (*CIL* III 04117–04121, 10891–10893). Among them is a monumental inscription, the so-called plaque of Emperor Constantine that was probably found as early as the late 17th century (*CIL* III 04121). Based on that inscription, it was M. P. Katančić who established in 1795 that the settlement was called *Aquae Iasae* (Katančić 1795: 221–223). Although this thesis is not confirmed in other literary or epigraphic sources, it is accepted in expert circles.

A very significant accidental discovery of several stone monuments occurred in 1843 (*CIL* III 4117; *HD*09301; *lupa* 5346, 5311, 5312, 5390, 22795, 5386) and 1846 (*lupa* 5331–5337) during excavations for the foundations of a building near the entrance to the town's park.[7] Some of these monuments had already been built into the gate of the park in 1865[8] while a group of large marble slabs (depicting Nereids, Eros, etc. *lupa* 5331–5337; Gorenc 1971) were placed as the frame of a thermal well.[9] There were other accidental finds of stone monuments later, in the 19th and 20th centuries (Tkalčić 1869; Ljubić 1879; Brunšmid 1907; *CIL* III 10890, 10891, 10893, etc), as well as finds of Roman architecture and various objects (Ljubić 1879: 35–36). The discovery of a pottery kiln in the 1960s at the foot of the hill provides information about the location of the workshop, but unfortunately, no precise documentation about the appearance of the kiln has been preserved (Vikić-Belančić 1975: 33, 36).

Written documents from the first half of the 19th century[10] mention the existence of the Roman water supply system and the Roman tunnel catchment on the hill above the thermal spring.[11] The tunnel (made of bricks) is built into the hill with the function of collecting fresh water from the spring and is still preserved to a length of about 10m. The Roman water supply system was in use in Varaždinske Toplice until 1974 and was renovated several times in the 19th century when stone pipes were discovered in several positions (Filipan 2002: 75–76, Fig. 1).

Archaeological excavations in the area of Varaždinske Toplice

The first archaeological excavations in Varaždinske Toplice were carried out in 1844 in the park,[12] in the area of the northern part of the 4th-century baths, which were later systematically investigated in the period from 1956 to 1959 (Vikić-Belančić and Gorenc 1961). The literature mentions the research conducted in 1867, but neither the documentation nor the findings have been preserved (Tkalčić 1869: 23; Solter 2016: 28). It is only known that the research was conducted opposite the entrance to the park where the inscription dedicated to nymphs was found (and unfortunately lost) (Tkalčić 1869: 23; Ljubić 1879: 41) and in several places around Varaždinske Toplice.[13]

The first systematic archaeological research began in 1953 when experts from the Archaeological Museum in Zagreb (M. Gorenc, B. Vikić, V. Damevski) began work on the upper terrace (present-day town park), where the thermal spring is located. (Figure 1) Research was conducted continuously until 1982, resumed in 1992 and has continued to the present day.[14] It revealed a complex of Roman public architecture (sanctuary and baths), over an area of 6,000 m^2, built around the thermal spring in the period from the 1st to 4th centuries. Parallel to the research, conservation work on the complex was also conducted from the beginning and is ongoing with the goal of a final museological presentation.

From 1959 to 1961, experts from the Zagreb Archaeological Museum also conducted investigations at the foot of Toplice Hill, where several buildings built from the 1st to the 4th centuries were discovered (Vikić-Belančić 1972). The earliest phase (1st-2nd century) is characterised by wooden structures that the researchers assumed were most likely small workshops or stores. The later phase at this site includes stone structures dating between the late 3rd and late 4th centuries that appear to have been a fair hall (Vikić-Belančić 1996: 29). Trade was a logical activity considering the large number of people who visited the spa and the inscription of Emperor Constantine (*CIL* III 04121) mentions that the Emperor introduced fairs once a week throughout the year.

Valuable information about the Roman settlement and its surroundings was also obtained through the archaeological rescue excavations and a survey being carried out since the 1950s (Vikić-Belančić 1972: 75; 1996: 12; Bekić 2006; Vlahović 2020). It contributed significantly to a clearer picture of the appearance and spatial distribution of the Roman settlement (Kušan Špalj 2024: 449-453).

The conditions for the specific arrangement of the Roman settlement were primarily subject to the location of the main thermal spring and the

[7] The stones were found at depth of 2 m but there is no other information about the circumstances of their discovery (Tkalčić 1869: 15).

[8] Where they are still today (*lupa* 5390; *CIL* III 4117; *HD*09301).

[9] They were transferred to the Toplice Museum after it was founded in 1937.

[10] From the documents of I. Kukuljević Sakcinski (dating back to 1836), on whose property the tunnel was located, the gathered information shows that he led his guests under torch light through the tunnel to enjoy the excellent water from the spring (Filipan 2002: 74–75).

[11] It is located on the hill above the sanctuary area with the thermal spring, about 1000m north, a height difference of about 100m.

[12] Thanks to a sketch made by M. Sabljar during his visit to Varaždinske Toplice in 1854-1856 the exact location can be determined (Solter 2016: 28).

[13] The excavation was performed under the leadership of I. Kukuljević Sakcinski and Count MacDonell, in a field called Gromača and in the village of Tuhovec (Tkalčić 1869: 24).

[14] The research was resumed thanks to D. Nemeth-Ehrlich who conducted the work until 2012, and since then the work has been led by D. Kušan Špalj and N. Perok.

geographical relief containing natural terraces and plains at the foot of the hill. Thus, it can be assumed that the narrowest part of the settlement extended on the slopes and foothills of Toplice Hill, mostly below the present houses of the modern town. Thus, on the highest terrace around the hot spring, there were the main public buildings, including a sanctuary area and a bathing complex. Residential buildings and visitor accommodation facilities were probably on the terraced slopes. At the foot of the hill were stores, workshops, magazines, and perhaps visitor facilities (e.g. *tabernae*), conveniently located near the roads that crossed the valley of Bednja River. At least two roads passed to the south of the settlement, one leading to the east, towards Iovia (Ludbreg), and the other approaching the settlement from the south. Part of that road was discovered in 2002, about 50m west of the current road.[15] There was probably a necropolis right next to this road, but unfortunately, it has not been confirmed in recent research (Bekić 2006). However, the discovery of graves in the area is mentioned and relates to the excavations that took place in 1867 (Tkalčić 1869: 24).[16] There are remains of Roman architecture found at several locations outside the modern town indicating locations of production and handicrafts facilities (Bekić 2006: 5, 31–66, 273–276). In two locations in the valley of the Bednja River, the existence of Roman villas is presumed,[17] however, this still needs to be confirmed by future archaeological excavations.

Since systematic research has only been carried out in the area around the thermal spring, that is, the sanctuary and the baths, and only small areas have been explored in other locations, it is hoped that future research will contribute to a more complete picture of the appearance and development of the Roman settlement.

The complex of Roman public architecture in the town park

Archaeological excavations of the sanctuary and baths area

The result of 70 years of archaeological excavations and other work in the park at Varaždinske Toplice is the museologically presented public area of the thermal spa *Aquae Iasae*. The complex was used from the 1st to the 4th centuries, and in all phases, there was the sanctuary area built around the thermal spring and the baths and the basilica to the south. Systematic archaeological excavations of the baths area began back in 1953, and by 1982 the baths' facilities that had been hidden for centuries under travertine sediments deposited by flowing thermal water were brought to light (Vikić-Belančić and Gorenc 1958, 1961, 1970; Gorenc and Vikić-Belančić 1980). The best-preserved structures are those of the 4th century, with walls up to 3m high, well-preserved wall paintings, plastered floors, a hypocaust system, etc. (Figure 2) Archaeological excavation of the sanctuary area was carried out in the period from 1962-1982, where temples, porticoes, canals, numerous altars and other stone monuments were found (Vikić-Belančić and Gorenc 1970; Gorenc and Vikić-Belančić 1980). Only the central part, in which the natural spring was located, remained unexplored since the active installations that supplied thermal water for the health resort were still active. The pinnacle of the explorations conducted at that time was the discovery of a sculpture of the goddess Minerva with a pedestal, found in the western temple in 1967 and 1968, which represents one of the finest examples of Norico-Pannonian sculpture.[18] The second phase of work on the site was restarted in the early 1990s, and it has continued to the present day. At first, various restorations, drainage and other works were carried out on the Roman structures, and since 1997, the archaeological research has continued. Particularly challenging was the excavation around the natural thermal spring, an area unexplored until 1998, where various post-Roman installations were located.[19] After the walls of the 13.5 x 8m structure began to appear in 1998, it became clear that it had been built to capture the spring (Kušan Špalj 1999). The finds of post-Roman installations and the layers deposited after the Roman period suggest that for a long period after the Roman buildings were abandoned, the thermal spring was not in use. After the collapse of the Roman catchment, the water overflowed uncontrollably, as witnessed by the thick layers of travertine above the ruined bath buildings (Aljinović *et al.* 2005). The reuse of the spring probably occurred no earlier than the 12th century[20] however, there is no evidence of the installations before the 18th century when the well was used to collect water.[21] The same method was likely used in earlier times, obviously without any knowledge of the Roman water catchment. The research of the spring area continued in 2006 when the walls of the spring reservoir were excavated down

[15] The road was found at the location called 'Gromače 1' during the archaeological rescue excavation before the construction work on the new Varaždinske Toplice bypass road (Bekić 2006: 5–20).

[16] Unfortunately, the exact position of the location excavated in 1867 has not been determined yet, since the name Gromače refers to a wider area of the valley south of Toplice.

[17] Site of village Tuhovec (Tkalčić 1869: 24; Bekić 2006: 278–280), and Gromače 3 (Bekić 2006: 268–271).

[18] ILJug-02, 01169; AE 1979, 00468; AE 1983, 00774, *lupa* 5388; Gorenc 1984.

[19] Before beginning the excavations in 1998, the Austro-Hungarian canals and the well had to be removed, including the facility for supplying thermal water to the spa after 1962, when borehole was used to extract water from deeper layers. The same borehole is still in function.

[20] The first written mention of Toplice dates to the 12th century (Čabrian *et al.* 1973: 16).

[21] Wooden pylons under the channels are dated using the C14 method (Lab. No. - Beta 435088, calibrated date AD 1780 to 1795 (Cal BP 170 to 155).

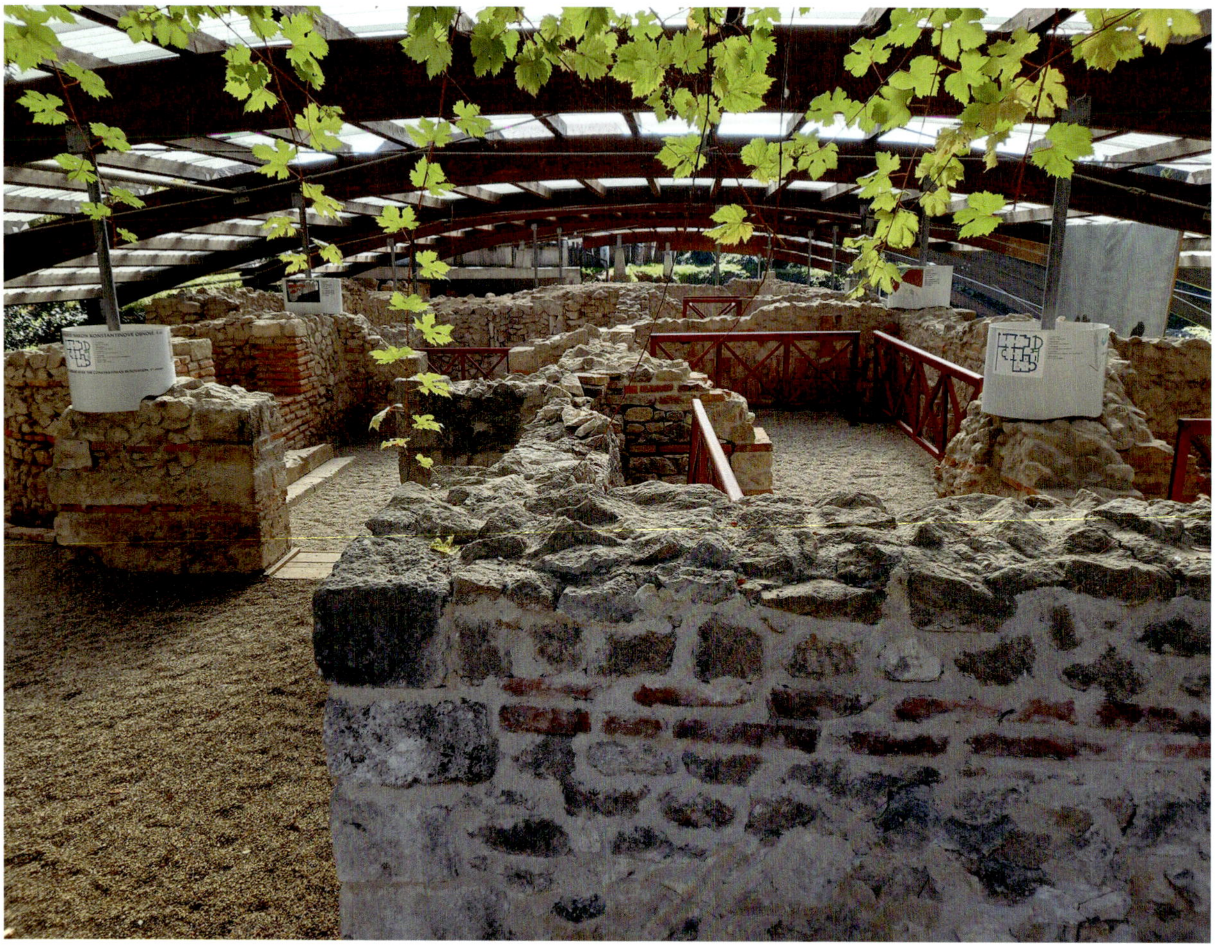

Figure 2. The 4th century baths looking south (photo by D. Kušan Špalj)

to the foundation level, confirming that from the 2nd century onwards the Romans had been capturing the thermal spring, inside a rectangular pool, with walls about 2 metres high (Nemeth-Ehrlich and Kušan Špalj 2011; Kušan Špalj and Nemeth Ehrlich 2012).

The excavation carried out around the thermal spring was a very complex and challenging task due to the presence of toxic gases[22] and the continuously gushing hot spring water. Several pumps had to be used to make the work and digging possible (Nemeth-Ehrlich and Kušan Špalj 2011; Nemeth-Ehrlich and Kušan Špalj 2014; 2015: 28–32, 42–45). Once the work was finished and the pumps used during excavation were turned off, the thermal water poured back into the reservoir for the first time since Roman times. It took about 24 hours for the water to completely fill the reservoir, which has a volume of about 220m3. At the same time, the entire space was filled with steam and a strong smell, so the atmosphere of the Roman sanctuary 'came to life.'

Work continued from 2011 to 2017, exploring the deeper layers and the area around the reservoir, leading to new and unexpected discoveries.[23] It turned out that the renovation of the reservoir took place at the beginning of the 4th century and that the earlier inscriptions, reliefs and even sculptures had been used as building material.

Approximately 18,000 Roman coins were found in the mud layers inside the spring reservoir (Bilić 2014; 2015), testifying to the large number of visitors who threw votive offerings into the 'sacred spring.'[24]

As the southern and northern walls of the spring reservoir were found in a very damaged state it is obvious that due to instability and the constant inflow

[22] The presence of carbon monoxide (CO) and hydrogen sulphide (H2S) was ascertained. The volume of gas emissions had to be continually measured and when the amount exceeded the allowed level, the work inside the reservoir was halted and ventilators were used.

[23] Nemeth-Ehrlich and Kušan Špalj 2014; 2015; Kušan Špalj 2017a; 2020a; 2020b; 2022b; 2024; Kušan Špalj *et al.* 2019.

[24] The reservoir was filled with a layer of extremely greasy mud that, after removal, was rinsed out on specially made platforms equipped with sieves (Kušan Špalj *et al.* 2014; 2015: Cat. no. 90–145).

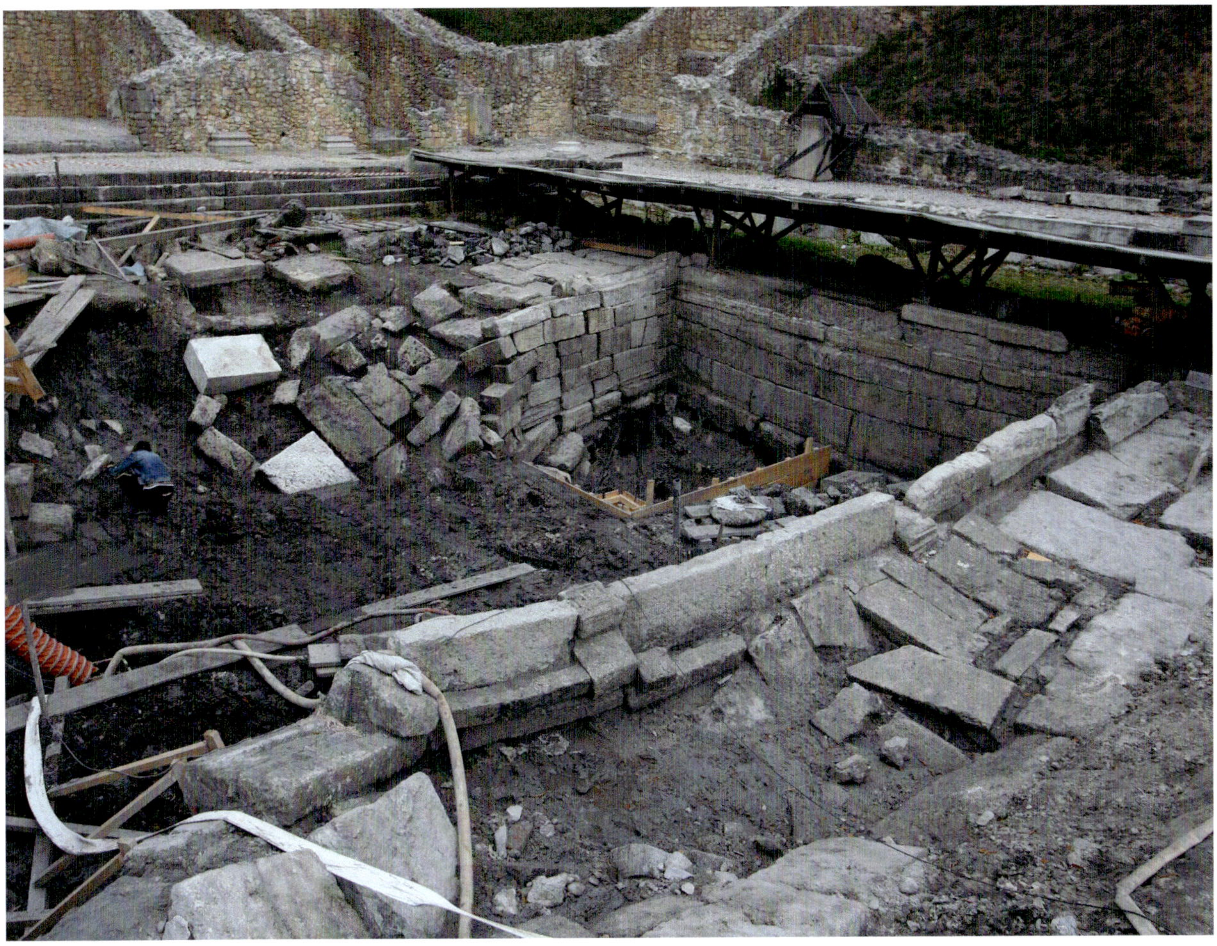

Figure 3. Roman spring reservoir during the 2011 excavations looking north-east (photo by D. Nemeth-Ehrlich).

of water, the ground collapsed again, probably at some time after the Roman period. The central part of the northern wall was found to have collapsed (along with the pavement behind it) while the southern wall simply moved toward the centre of the reservoir, 'taking with it' the pavement of the southern part. (Figure 3)

The sanctuary and baths area – construction phases

The sanctuary and baths area in the 1st century

It is very likely that the Romans, as early as the second half of the 1st century BC while conquering the area between the Sava and Drava rivers (Domić Kunić 2006: 97), became aware of the exceptional therapeutic properties of the thermal water in the area of present-day Varaždinske Toplice. Probably, at the very beginning, the healing benefits of the water may have been exploited without the undertaking of any major construction around the spring. It can be assumed that the well-planned capture of the spring and the construction of the surrounding area was most likely carried out by the early 1st century when the findings of the first bathing facilitates can be also dated (Vikić-Belančić 1996: 14–15).

The capture of the spring was a very demanding and carefully planned construction project in the area where the thermal water continuously bubbles up. Since archaeological excavations have not confirmed any building activity around the spring in the pre-Roman period, it is difficult to imagine what the Romans found around the spring and what the site looked like. The thermal spring is located on a terrace, bordered on three sides by slopes with layers of solid clay that slope obliquely towards the spring. The area is open to the south and its soil is very unstable and muddy. Therefore, it can be assumed that in pre-Roman times the thermal water spilled out towards the south. This indicates that, as a precondition for capturing the spring and as the first intervention in the area, the Romans put up a 'dam' on the south side of the area, designated for the sanctuary. The remains of oak pylons were found,[25] connected by planks between which there

[25] The wood was dated using the C14 method (Lab. No. - Beta 435090, calibrated date 75-55 BC / Cal BP 2025-2005).

was firmly packed clay. In this way, the area south of the natural spring was strengthened (about 200 m^2), which enabled thermal water to be 'retained' in a narrower area, on a higher terrace (Kušan Špalj 2022b: 56; 2024: 454, Fig. 6). The fact that the dam was a precondition for capturing the spring, as well as for using the water in a controlled manner, by draining it through canals (in free fall) into the bathing area confirms that it was a part of well-planned construction of an entire complex with sanctuary and baths. The strength of the dam made it possible to keep the water inside the spring reservoir with the water level higher than that of the baths' floors. The precise height of the water level in the reservoir could have been determined by the height of the overflow channel, as is confirmed by the wooden overflow channel found in the southwest corner of the spring area (Kušan Špalj 2022b: 57).

Since the walls of the 1st-century reservoir that 'enclosed' the thermal spring were destroyed in a later construction, it is possible that they were made of stone, or there was a wooden structure that surrounded the natural pit.[26] As the results of the 2012-2015 excavation have shown, the reservoir was surrounded by the sanctuary walls containing niches and by a temple to the north, most likely dedicated to the nymphs.[27] In front of the temple was a stepped wooden and plastered stone structure, while in front of the walls, there were probably porches. The described appearance of the sanctuary most likely did not change much since the early 1st century, when some of the structures can be dated (phase 1a). It seems that in the mid-1st century, the sanctuary was renovated, but the concept of the space remained. This is suggested by the remains of some walls that lie below or next to the walls of the later 1st century (phase 1b). The remains of the rectangular niche on the west side also belong to phase 1a, as it was demolished on purpose when a semi-circular one was built next to it in the mid-1st century. It is clear that in both phases, the sanctuary was designed as a relatively enclosed space where visitors moved through porches and toured the 'sacred spring' into which they inserted votive gifts (primarily coins) in the hope of healing.

The remains of the 1st-century bath facilities, located in the southwestern part of the complex, show the same construction phases as the sanctuary area. Some fragmentarily preserved walls and remains of floors are dated to the first half of the 1st century while the better-preserved building is dated to the mid-1st century. Two rectangular pools, several rooms, and supply and drainage channels have been preserved from that period (Vikić-Belančić and Gorenc 1958: 1961, 1970; Vikić-Belančić 1996: 14-15). The large *basilica thermarum* located in the southeast part of the complex was probably also built in the mid-1st century and was connected to the baths at that time by a door on the western wall. (Figure 4)

The sanctuary and baths area in the 2nd and 3rd centuries

The bath facilities built in the 1st century remained in use until the first half of the 2nd century when they were demolished, the terrain was levelled and new baths were built further north, between the sanctuary and the basilica. (Figure 4) Not much is preserved of the 2nd-century baths, while the 4th-century bath building was built on top of them, retaining the same orientation. There are some walls and semicircular pools (with hypocaust) still visible on the west and north sides, while other walls were demolished or incorporated into later structures. There was a door in the centre of the north wall of the basilica, used as entrance to the 2nd-century baths (Vikić-Belančić and Gorenc 1970; Vikić-Belančić 1996: 15).

The construction of new baths in the first half of the 2nd century was part of a major building project in which the new and grander sanctuary was built. This seems to be a consequence of the growing popularity of this thermal spa, the increased number of visitors, as well as the introduction of new cults, attributed to the power of healing. The source of significant investment was probably the town of Poetovio (Kušan Špalj 2022a), which became a colony at the time, and *Aquae Iasae* was very likely the main thermal spa centre in its territory (Horvat *et al.* 2003: 106; Ragolić 2014: 335-336). It can be inferred from the epigraphic monuments, especially those erected by the entire *res publica Poetovionensis* (*CIL* III 4117; *HD*069301; Kušan Špalj 2022b: 62, 63) that *Aquae Iasae* most likely had the patronage of Poetovio in its building activities.

In this phase of the sanctuary, the area around the spring was designed as an open paved courtyard with elevated porticoes around it, while there were three temples on the north side. The temples and two side rooms (probably also used as the temples) were dug into the slope, and the whole construction was additionally reinforced by massive retaining walls on the east and west sides (Nemeth-Ehrlich and Kušan Špalj 2014; 2015: 33-34, 47-49; Kušan Špalj *et al.* 2019: 176 -183). (Figure 4) The complete reconstruction of the spring catchment shows that it was an extensive and well-thought-out construction project, based on good knowledge of the soil and natural conditions. In this phase, the water was captured by the large 13.5 x 8m pool-shaped reservoir with walls 2m high. This was followed by the construction of a new canal

[26] It is possible that two well-preserved upright oak piles connected with boards (found south of the spring), belonged to the 1st century reservoir The wood was dated using the C14 method (Lab. No. - Beta 435087, calibrated date 10 BC to AD 0 / Cal BP 1960 to 1950).

[27] Inscriptions dating to the 1st century are dedicated to the nymphs (*CIL* III, 04118; *CIL* III, 10893)

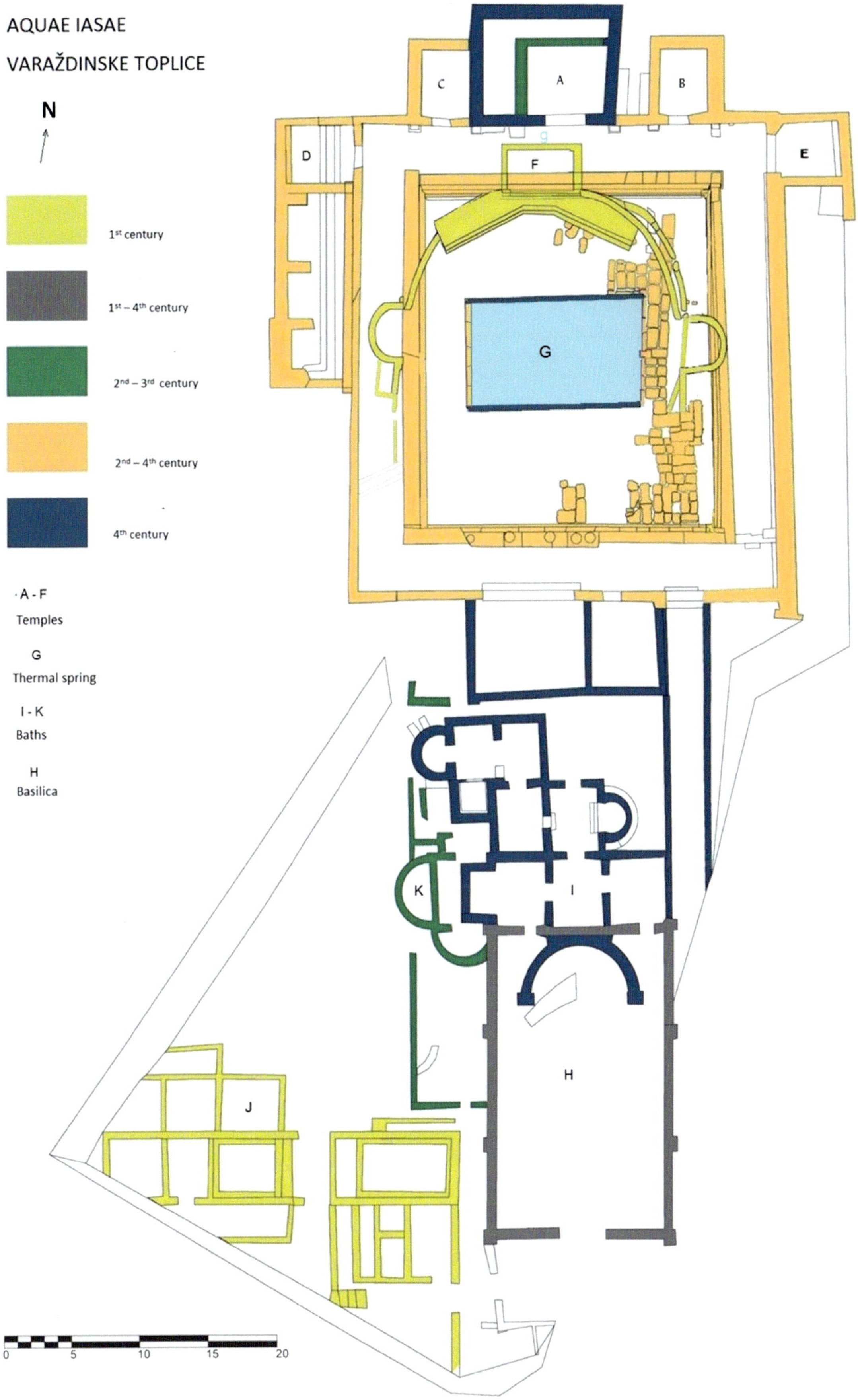

Figure 4. Plan of the sanctuary and baths area – construction phases (made by Studio Kušan)

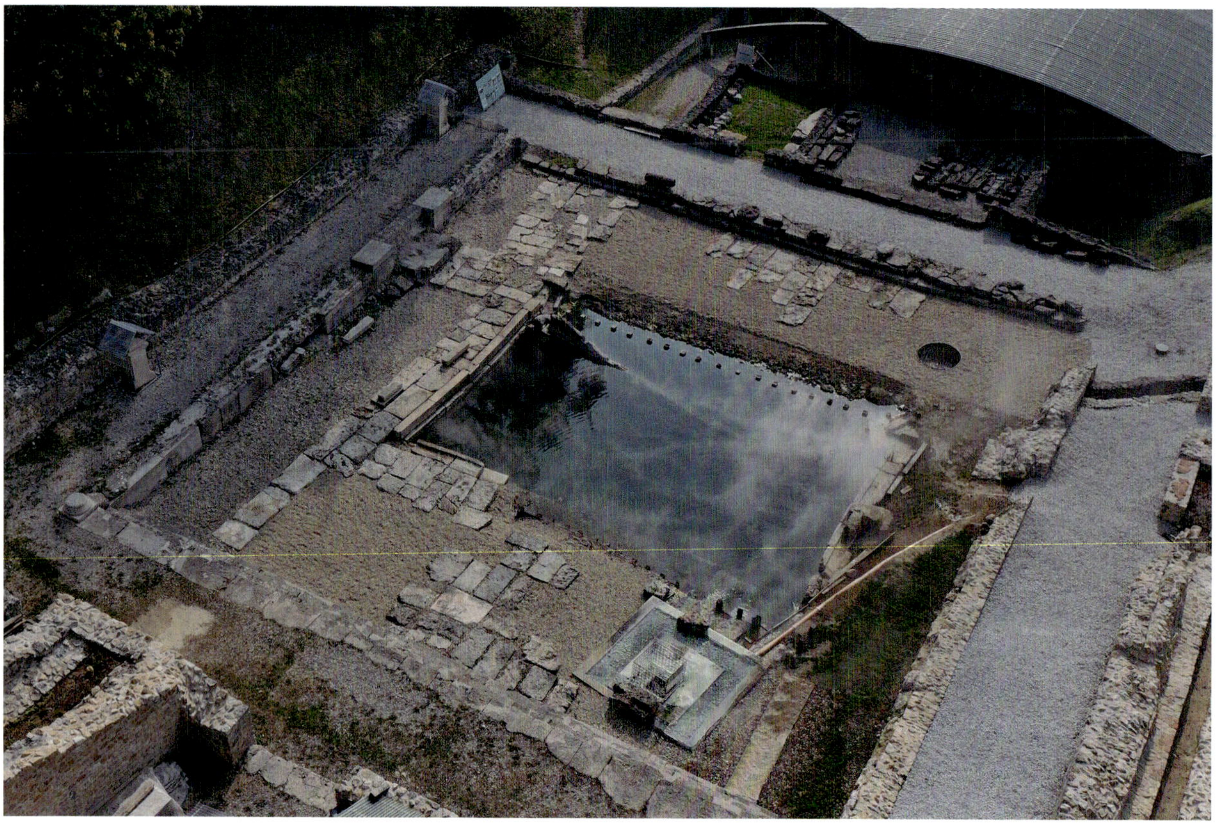

Figure 5. The sanctuary area with Roman spring reservoir, after conservation work in 2022, looking south-east (photo by M. Vuković).

system, which carried thermal water to the new baths and excess water to the sewers. The relatively unusual position of the reservoir, not centred in the 2nd-century sanctuary area but slightly shifted westward, reveals that it probably followed the location of an earlier one, as its position fits better in relation to the 1st-century temple (and stairs in front of it).

The construction of the spring reservoir was a very complex and demanding process preceded by the discharge of water, which enabled the reservoir to be built on dry ground. South of the reservoir is a channel, deeper than the bottom level of the reservoir, probably used for cleaning purposes or during the construction of the reservoir.[28] At the same time, a very complex soil consolidation procedure was carried out in order to create stable ground for the construction of the walls (Kušan Špalj 2017b: Fig. 7). These consisted of oak pylons arranged very densely in a system with wooden planks and compacted clay. The well-preserved elements of this construction have been found under the foundations and behind the walls as well as inside the reservoir (Kušan Špalj 2017b: Fig. 7). (Figure 3) The preserved eastern and western walls of the spring reservoir have provided us with information about how the reservoir was built in the 2nd century (Nemeth-Ehrlich and Kušan Špalj 2014; 2015: 26–32, 40–45; Kušan Špalj 2024: 456-460). After the consolidation of the ground, the foundation rows (composed of large limestone blocks and smaller stones underneath) were laid. The upper part of the wall consists of three rows built using the *opus quadratum* technique, that is, with blocks arranged in alternating headers and stretchers. These blocks were made of very dense, but soft, fine-grained *biomicrite* limestone that could be worked with great precision to make the blocks fit together.[29] Layers of clay behind the walls were added so that it was a watertight structure. The top row consists of stone slabs made of less dense *biomicrite* limestone, with central grooves on the upper surface that served as beds for the guard-rail. The rail was about 70cm high and made also of *biomicrite* limestone elements - beams and the connecting stones, of which some parts are still preserved.

During the construction of the spring reservoir, work on the pavement around the reservoir was also carried out; the paving laid in the 2nd century is preserved in

[28] Two deep wooden canals (dated to the 1st and 4th centuries) were also found south of the reservoir most probably used for same purposes in the 1st and 4th-century phases (Kušan Špalj 2017b: Fig. 6).

[29] The stone was obviously processed on the site so that it could fit better into the wall structure because the remains of stone processing have been found behind the walls.

the eastern part of the sanctuary and is constructively connected to the reservoir structure with connecting stones (Figure 5).

The sanctuary and baths area in the 4th century

According to the results of archaeological excavation, at the beginning of the 4th century, the restoration of the sanctuary and the construction of new baths took place. This is the period that corresponds to the assumed restoration phase of *Aquae Iasae* (after it had been destroyed by fire) as mentioned on the 'inscription of Emperor Constantine' (*CIL* III, 04121). Typical of this phase is the frequent use of already processed stone (inscriptions, altars, etc.) for renovation of different building structures. This was commonly done in the 4th century and reflects the state's efforts to rationalize costs and invest more in renovation than new construction (Kušan Špalj 2017a). This kind of construction is most visible in the restoration of the spring reservoir, which dates from this phase. Although the Romans fortified the grounds during construction in the 2nd century, by the end of the 3rd or beginning of the 4th century, the northern and southern walls of the spring reservoir were severely damaged due to the nature of the soil and continuous bubbling up of the water. On both walls, the original parts from the 2nd century remained in the corners, while the central parts were repaired and on that occasion, more than 50 various inscriptions, altars, reliefs, and other processed stones were used as building material (Nemeth-Ehrlich and Kušan Špalj 2014; 2015: 26–32, 40–45). Based on the appearance of the walls, it is evident that an attempt was made to imitate the method of building walls in the 2nd century, that is, by combining large blocks as stretchers and headers. Since the available, already processed stone blocks, such as limestone and marble altars were used, the regularity of the structure was lost, and the rows became much more irregular. (Figure 3) Both walls were renovated from the foundation level, so that parallel with the construction of the walls, the space behind was filled with larger or smaller stones and clay. In these layers behind the northern wall parts of sculptures were even found (Apollo/Sol, Diana/Luna) (*lupa*, 30106; 30107; Kušan Špalj 2017a: 280-285), along with various inscriptions, reliefs and other processed stones (Figure 7). After the construction of the walls was completed, the pavement was renewed, in which several monuments were also utilised as secondary paving material (such as large marble reliefs and pedestals) (*HD*075016; *HD*075022; *HD*075019; Kušan Špalj 2022b; 58, 59). (Figure 3, 8)

The work carried out at that time in the sanctuary area did not cause major changes in its appearance while apart from the renovation of the spring reservoir, the central temple was enlarged and some structures (pillars, roofs, etc.) were restored (Vikić-Belančić and Gorenc 1970). New baths were built over the earlier bath building, from which numerous walls were incorporated into the new rooms as were the fragments of various monuments used in the building of the walls (Vikić-Belančić and Gorenc 1970; Vikić-Belančić 1996: 16) (Figure 2) At the same time, the existing *basilica thermarum* was renovated, so the entire bath complex was provided with a hypocaust system and decorated in the same style as the wall paintings. The installation of the apse in the basilica should be dated to this phase, which confirms the same style of wall painting as in the baths and other walls of the basilica (fields with tendrils and vine leaves in the lower part, and above red-framed fields with geometric representations, rosettes or imitation marble) (Vikić-Belančić and Gorenc 1961: 198-201; Kušan Špalj 2022a: 309). Entry to the complex was from the south through the basilica, from which, through two side rooms to the east and west of the apse, one passed to the baths, first in the *apodyterium*, then in the *frigidarium*, and the *caldarium*. (Figure 4)

There were some changes in the second half of the 4th century when part of the complex was already being used for Christian ceremonies. At that time, the *basilica thermarum* was converted into a Christian basilica, in which two construction phases during the 4th century related to the early Christian horizon are noticeable (Kušan Špalj 2020a). As for the continuation of the 'life' of the sanctuary in the later 4th century, interesting information was revealed by the votive gifts found in the spring, which shows that the cult of the 'sacred spring' was still relevant at the time. Hence, several rings with a Christogram motif (Kušan Špalj *et al.* 2014; 2015: Cat. no. 107, 108) testify not only to the coexistence of Christianity and the Roman cult but also to the inclusion of members of the Christian community into the centuries-old rituals of the pagan sanctuary.

Cults in the Aquae Iasae sanctuary

The Nymphs

Based on the numerous epigraphic monuments found in the area of Varaždinske Toplice so far, it can be assumed that a very complex religious life took place in the sanctuary. While the stone monuments testify to the visit of the upper classes of society and wealthier visitors, the 18,000 coins and other votive gifts found in the spring reservoir speak of numerous individuals who came to *Aquae Iasae* hoping for healing and recovery. The offerings were most frequently addressed to the nymphs because about 45 inscriptions and several reliefs dedicated to them have been found so far. As the nymphs have been associated with springs since Greek times, considered to provide and take care of the water in the springs (*Od.* 13, 109; 17, 205-211), it is not

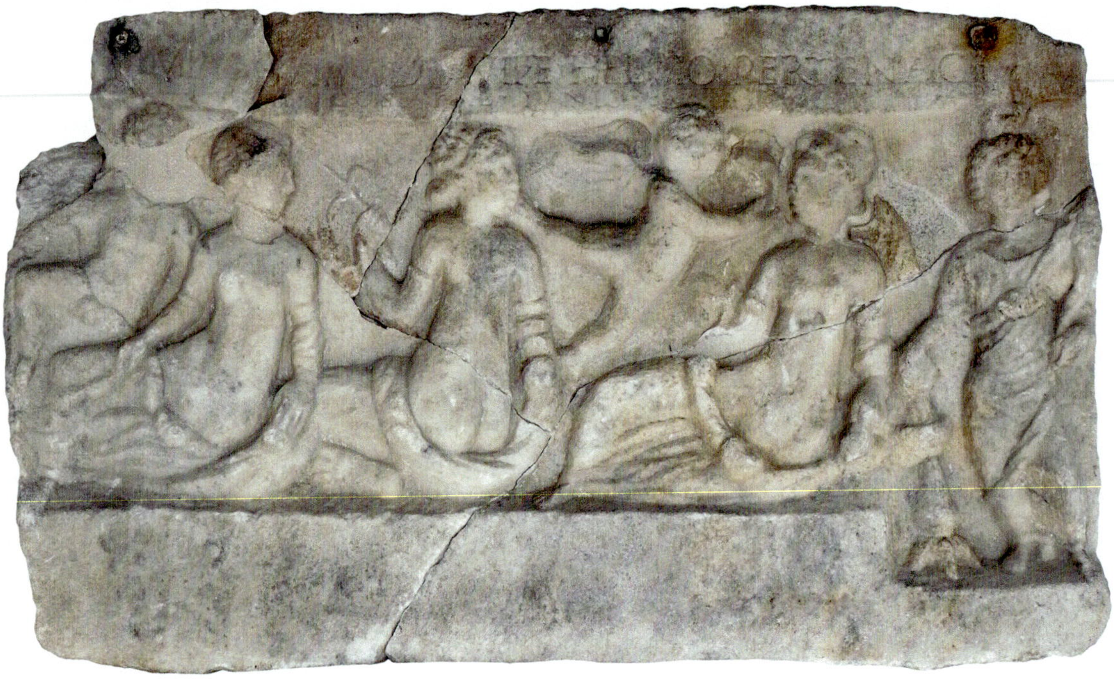

Figure 6. A relief with a depiction of female divinites (Isis Fortuna, Venus and three nymphs) and a dated inscription, erected on the occasion of a festival on 1st June, 192 (photo by Zottmann Gmbh)

surprising that prayers, votive gifts and sacrifices were also offered to them in the *Aquae Iasae* sanctuary built around the spring of thermal water (Kušan Špalj 2014; 2015: 58-66, 84-92).

On the reliefs found in Varaždinske Toplice nymphs are depicted as three young, naked girls with attributes marking them as spring nymphs. Compositionally they are depicted in two ways, in a standing or seated (semi-seated) position (Kušan Špalj 2014; 2015: 84-86; Kušan Špalj 2022a: 101-103). Observing the way that these reliefs were made, it can be concluded that they are the product of local workshops although made in accordance with well-known iconographic depictions from the Roman period, that follow Hellenistic models associated with the goddess Aphrodite. The depiction of nymphs in the manner of Aphrodite can be traced in Roman art from the 1st century BC, and both types (the sitting and the standing nymphs) appear at the same time.[30] The close link between the iconographic depictions of nymphs and Aphrodite/Venus is confirmed by the relief from Varaždinske Toplice, where there are four semi-nude female figures represented in a seated position (Kušan Špalj 2014, 2015: Cat. no. 74; Kušan Špalj 2017a: 294-297). All four are depicted and dressed in the same manner, but as one has Amor next to her, it signifies her as being Venus, most likely here in the function of the goddess of fertility and life. (Figure 6)

Besides eight reliefs (some of which also contain an inscription),[31] 47 votive inscriptions dedicated to the nymphs have been found in Varaždinske Toplice so far,[32] testifying that the worship of the nymphs, as protectors of the spring, was the main feature of the *Aquae Iasae* sanctuary. The epithet *Iasae* that appears on three inscriptions found so far (AE 1985, 00714; ILJug-02, 1171; Kušan Špalj 2022a: Cat. no. 9, 10) confirms that the worshipers were addressing the nymphs of the very spring of *Aquae Iasae*. There are several other epithets connected with the nymphs documented on the inscriptions, like *salutares* (*CIL* III 108931; 108932, etc.) and *augustae* (*CIL* III 4117; 4119, etc.), as the most common but there are also *peone* (*paeonae*) (Kušan Špalj 2020b: 177; Kušan Špalj 2022b: Cat. no. 8) and *sanctae*

[30] In the house of Romulus and Remus in Pompeii, one fresco depicts two nymphs standing and between them, one is in a semi-lying position (Bieber 1955: Fig. 636).

[31] A total of eight reliefs and five more fragments were found (*lupa* 5329, 5390+22795, 16735; Kušan Špalj *et al.* 2014, 2015: 56-66, 82-92, Cat. no. 2, 4, 74, 77, 78, 80, 82-88).

[32] This refers to 20 inscriptions found up until 1982 (Rendić-Miočević 1992; Rendić-Miočević and Šegvić 1998; Lučić 2013; Cvetko 2022) and 27 inscriptions found in the 2011-2015 excavations (Kušan Špalj 2017a; 2022a; 2023). Among the mentioned inscriptions there are six on which nymphs are mentioned together with other deities. There is a total of 61 monuments erected in the honour of nymphs (Kušan Špalj 2023, T.-1.)

(*lupa* 25465). Very often there is also a combination of several epithets on a single inscription, but there are also examples where they are absent. On a recently found inscription, there is in four cases a dedication in the form of *numini nympharum*.[33]

One interesting object provides information about the importance of the cult of the nymphs as well as about the functioning and organisation of the sanctuary itself. It is a *thesaurus* – a kind of money receptacle ('a money box') – for the offerings made in the form of coins (Kušan Špalj 2014; 2015: 65-66; Kušan Špalj 2022a: 104-105, Fig. 31). The marble *thesaurus* found in the *Aquae Iasae* sanctuary in 2006 and 2011 in the rubble of the northern spring reservoir wall, belongs to the group of the two-part types and the semicircular upper part, a lid with a slot for dropping the coins into has been preserved. It bears the inscription *sacrum nymphis*, so the offerings were consecrated to the nymphs. It is known that in the sanctuaries, the pilgrims would drop their offerings into a *thesaurus*, and the money thus collected would be used to address the needs of the sanctuary (Kaminski 1991: 63-181). Something very similar likely happened in the *Aquae Iasae* sanctuary, where the money collected in the *thesaurus* was used for the temples' operating expenses or sacrificial offerings to the nymphs.

The earliest inscriptions dedicated to the nymphs date from the 1st century (*CIL* III 04118, 10893) when most likely the entire sanctuary was dedicated to them, while the finds of numerous monuments erected in their honour in the 2nd and 3rd centuries testify the importance of their cult in the second phase of the sanctuary.[34] From the 2nd century, the votive offerings were also addressed to other deities related to health and healing, and in several cases together with the nymphs. It certainly indicates the coexistence of various cults in this sanctuary, as well as their 'fitting' into the local cult of the spring. There are inscriptions dedicated to the nymphs and Apollo[35] i.e. Sol (Kušan Špalj 2022a: Cat. no. 8), and one together with Apollo and Diana (*HD*075031, *lupa* 30108). There is also an inscription mentioning the nymphs with Minerva, Juno (Regina) and Apollo (*HD*075033), as is one that has a dedication to the nymphs and Serapis (AE 2014 1049; *HD*074973). Particularly interesting is the inscription dedicated to the nymphs and Fortuna *Iasoniana* (*HD*075021; Kušan Špalj *et al.* 2014; 2015: 70, 95, Cat. no. 76). The toponym *Iasoniana* used for naming the goddess signifies her importance as well as the inclusion of her cult in this very sanctuary. There are several other monuments erected in her honour[36] among which is an example where the goddess is associated with Isis, in typical Roman syncretistic form (Kušan Špalj 2014; 2015: Cat. no. 74; Kušan Špalj 2017: 294-297). It is an already mentioned relief representing three nymphs and Venus (with Amor) where on the right side is the goddess Isis/Fortuna in a dress (with the Knot of Isis tied at the front) and a characteristic headdress (horns and Sun disc). She is holding a *patera* in her right hand and pouring an offering above a smaller burning altar. The *cornucopia* that she holds in her left hand implies that this is Isis/Fortuna. Above the relief is an inscription, which actually represents a date and allows the accurate dating of the plaque to 1st June 192, that is, to the reign of Emperor Commodus (whose name was subsequently removed, an example of *damnatio memoriae*):

IMP (eratore) [[Commodo]] VII ET HELVIO PERTENACI/
II CO(n)S(ulibus) KAL(endis) IVNIS.

Based on the preserved inscription and the depiction on the relief, we can assume that the plaque was placed in the sanctuary during a festivity (or perhaps a mystery) in honour of the goddess Isis/Fortuna (and other female deities). (Figure 6)

Other cults

Especially prominent among the cults practised at *Aquae Iasae* from the 2nd century onwards was the one dedicated to Minerva, who was worshipped as the goddess of healing and health. The statue of the goddess Minerva (dated in the middle of the 2nd century) testifies to the temples being furnished with works of art of utmost quality (Gorenc 1984). The fragments of statue and the pedestal (ILJug-02 01169; AE 1979, 00468; AE 1983, 00774; *HD*000496; *lupa* 5388, etc) were found in excavations in 1967 and 1968 in the western temple (and in front of it). The mentioning of Minerva on several other inscriptions[37] testify to the popularity of her cult as a goddess of healing and health as well as being worshipped by different social classes (Kušan Špalj 2014; 2015: 92-93; Kušan Špalj 2017: 287-288).

In the sanctuary of *Aquae Iasae*, fragments of another two sculptures that might have also stood in one of the temples were found in recent excavations. These are sculptures of Apollo/Sol and Diana/Luna, the divine

[33] Inscriptions were found in the 2011 excavation of the spring reservoir (Kušan Špalj 2023, Cat. no 11, 12, 13, 14).

[34] It is most likely that the nymphs had the role of protectors of the spring during the 4th century as well (Kušan Špalj 2018: 312-313), which might be indicated by the votive gifts in the spring most probably dedicated to them (4th century coins and rings) and an inscription that possibly dates back to that period (AIJ 470; Lučić 2013: 213-214).

[35] Inscription was found in the 2011 excavation of the spring reservoir (Kušan Špalj 2023: Cat. no. 3).

[36] An altar dedicated to Fortuna (*HD*012321, *lupa* 5321, Rendić-Miočević 1975), a pedestal dedicated to Juno (Regina) and Fortuna (ILJug-02, 01168; *HD*034992; *lupa* 5324), a smaller pedestal with a dedication to Fortuna sancta (Kušan Špalj 2022b: 64-65, Fig. 10).

[37] There are two altars dedicated to Minerva (*HD*075017; *lupa* 30298; *HD*075018; *lupa* 30297) and an altar dedicated to Juno, Minerva, Apollo and the nymphs (*HD*075033).

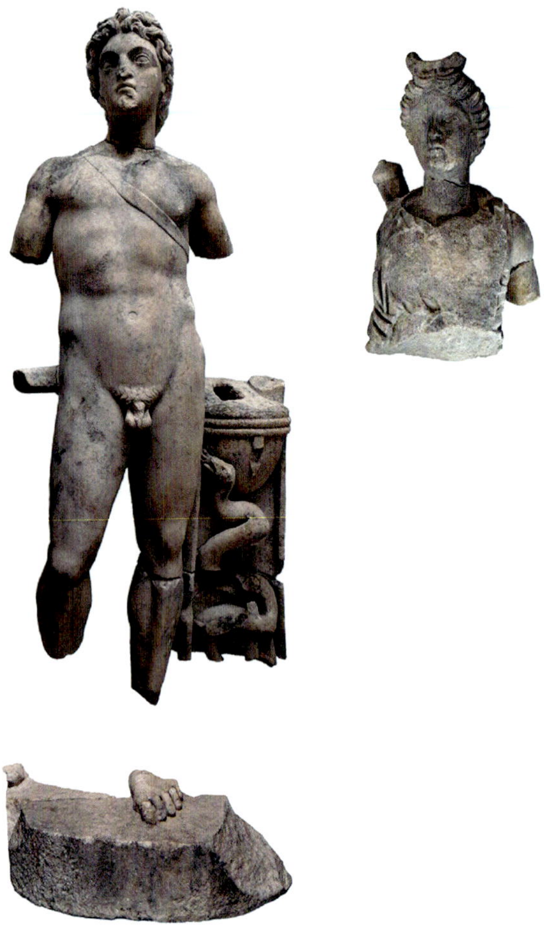

Figure 7. Sculptures of Apollo/Sol and Diana/Luna, early 3rd century (photo by Zottmann Gmbh)

twins, found in 2011 in the construction of the spring reservoir (Kušan Špalj 2014; 2015: 101-102; Kušan Špalj 2017: 280-284). (Figure 7) The statue of Apollo/Sol depicts a young god, with a crown of sunbeams (with 12 rays), leaning on a tripod around which a snake has wrapped itself (as Pythian Apollo) (Kušan Špalj 2017a: 280-282; *lupa* 30106). It is no surprise that Apollo as the god of healing was worshipped at this type of sanctuary, however, the statue indicates that he was worshipped also as the god of the Sun and of prophecy. The sculpture of Diana/Luna, of which the upper part is preserved, is depicted in accordance with Greek iconography, as Artemis, the goddess of the hunt, to whom a crescent moon has been added (Kušan Špalj 2017a: 282-283; lupa 30107). Her facial features are very similar to those of Apollo, which correlates with the concept of the sculptures as divine twins. The identification of Apollo with the solar deity Helios and Artemis with Selene is known from Greek mythology, and the Romans adopted these cults and associated Apollo with Sol and Diana with the goddess of the moon, Luna (Ando 2005: 49). These cults grew especially popular in the era of the Severan Dynasty, but most of all it was characteristic of the official religion in Caracalla's time when even the emperor himself was depicted with a crown of sunbeams (Mráv 2000: 85-9). The importance of the cults of Apollo, Sol and Diana in the sanctuary of *Aquae Iasae* in the 2nd and 3rd centuries is confirmed by numerous other inscriptions dedicated to them,[38] but the syncretistic form in which the sculptures are presented certainly places the peak of the worship of these cults to the Severian period. The statues of Apollo/Sol and Diana/Luna have to, therefore, be considered within the context of that period and their precise dating can be made considering the stylistic similarities in comparison with a relief depicting healing deities also found in 2011. This is a marble slab with a relief and inscription based on which the monument can be precisely dated in the period of Caracalla's reign (212-214).[39] (Figure 8) The relief depicts Aesculapius, his daughter Salus (*Hygeia*),[40] and his son Telesphorus who is believed to grant recovery from illness. The inscription that is visible above and below the relief reveals the official character of the dedication to the emperor's health and victory (*pro salute et victoriis*). It was donated by *Lucius Alfenus Avitianus*, governor (*praeses*) of the province of Arabia and legate of the *Legio X*, therefore a prominent personality in the service of the state and the emperor himself, most probably from the close circle of the emperor's most trusted men. The relief is of exquisite quality and it is obviously the work of a master craftsman, and the fact that the marble from which the relief was made came from the Alps, locates its production to the Norico-Pannonian circle. The figure of Aesculapius who is shown as a strong, young man, quite unlike the established depiction of an older figure is particularly interesting. Even more surprising is the representation of his face that shows characteristics of Caracalla's portraits from the beginning of his autonomous reign (in 212), featuring an accentuated emotionality typical of the portrayals of that time. This is why it can be concluded that the relief represents Emperor Caracalla himself and together with a dedication which attributes him divine characteristics (the emperor's *numen*) it is a reflection of the worship of the cult of the emperor. Literary sources mentioned that Caracalla fell ill after having his brother Geta murdered, and in his despair, he appealed to Apollo, Asclepius and Serapis for good health. He

[38] There are inscriptions dedicated to Apollo, Diana and the nymphs (*HD*075031; *lupa* 30108), to Apollo with Minerva, Juno and the nymphs (*HD*075033), to Apollo (Sol) and the nymphs (Kušan Špalj 2022a: Cat. no. 8; 2024: Cat. no. 3), to Sol (AE 2013, 1207; *HD*049105). There are accidental finds of inscriptions dedicated to Diana (AIJ 459; AE 2013,1207; *HD*069293; *lupa* 5341) and Diana and the nymphs (AIJ 460; *HD*022299; *lupa* 5340) found in the 1930s.

[39] *HD*075019; *lupa* 30105; Kušan Špalj 2014; 2015: 96-99, Cat. no. 69; Kušan Špalj 2017a: 271-280.

[40] There is one fragment of an altar dedicated to Asclepius and Hygeia found during the 2001 excavation in the sanctuary area (Nemeth-Ehrlich and Kušan Špalj 2012: 112: Kušan Špalj 2014; 2015: 96).

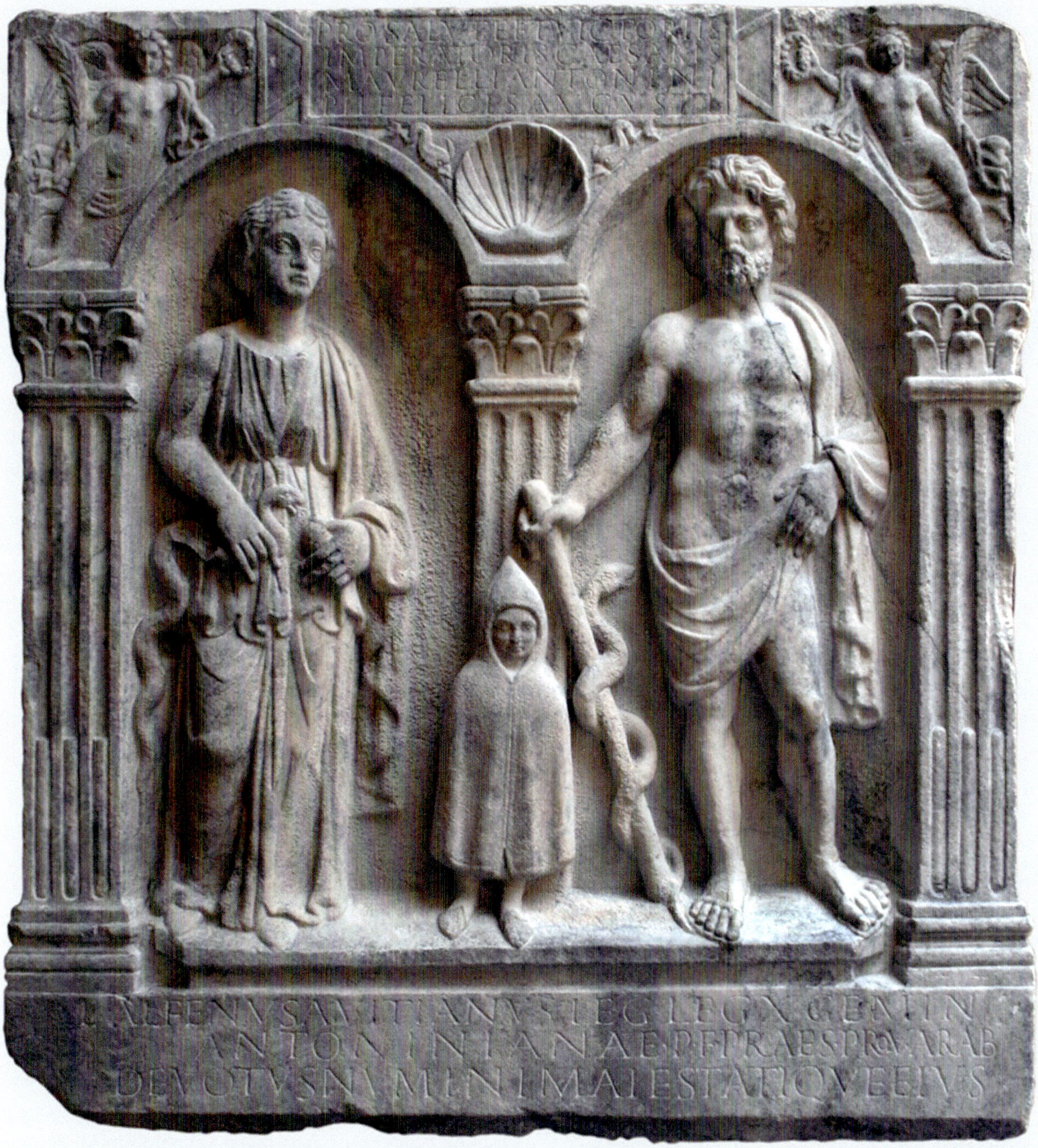

Figure 8. A relief with a depiction of Aesculapius, Hygeia and Telesphorus and an inscription for the health and victories of the emperor Caracalla (photo by Zottmann Gmbh).

would send his delegates with votive offerings to these deities at various sanctuaries or would visit them in person in the hope of recovery (*Cass. Dio* 78, 5-7). Although the visit to *Aquae Iasae* is not recorded in literary sources, according to the mentioned relief, it is very likely that the emperor sent his delegation or even visited the sanctuary by himself, seeking healing or the oracle's advice (Mráv 2000: 86). This seems quite likely, as it was the only, known so far, sanctuary in Pannonia where all three deities - Apollo, Asclepius and Serapis were worshipped.

The inscriptions found in recent excavations of the spring reservoir testify to the worship of Serapis, along with the nymphs in the context of the local cult (AE 2014, 1049; *HD*074973; Kušan Špalj 2017a: 292-294), as well as a divine couple with Isis (AE 2014, 01048; *HD*074972; lupa 30299; Kušan Špalj 2014; 2015: 94, Cat. no. 73; 2017a: 290-292). The spread of the cult of Isis and Serapis in Pannonia can be traced back to the 1st century, however, its full development was at the end of the 2nd century and especially at the beginning of the 3rd century, when Serapis acquired a special role and was included in the state cult along with Isis (Selem 1997: 17-43). This is the period when the cults also became popular in *Aquae Iasae*, obviously due to their divine functions associated with healing. Their presence in the sanctuary should be linked to their popularity in nearby Poetovio, one of the most important centres of eastern cults in this part of the Empire (Jerala 2011: 75-86; Selem 1997: 127). It is therefore logical to conclude that the visitors from Poetovio, such as *Valerius Priscus* who was *Augustalis* in Poetovio and who dedicated an altar to Isis and Serapis (AE 2014, 01048; *HD*074972; lupa 30299; Kušan Špalj 2014; 2015: 94, Cat. no. 73; 2017a: 290-292), had an important role in spreading new cults in the *Aquae Iasae* sanctuary.

The worship of Egyptian deities in the sanctuary of *Aquae Iasae* possibly had the form of some special rituals like the practice of *incubatio* ('temple sleep'), mysteries or certain festivities. The already mentioned relief depicting Isis/Fortuna, the nymphs and Venus, probably represents a scene from such a festivity that might been performed in the sanctuary (Kušan Špalj 2014; 2015: 94-95; Kušan Špalj 2017a: 294-297). It reveals the complexity of the cults in this sanctuary, closely linked to the natural phenomenon of the healing powers of thermal water.

The presence of female donors and their dedications to feminine cults indicate that the water was used in relation to women's illnesses and fertility. Three inscriptions dedicated by female donors to local deities the Silvanae (AIJ 467, 468a, 468b; *HD*071772, *HD*071773; *lupa* 5343, 5344) could be interpreted in this way. Although votive inscriptions do not indicate the reasons for individuals' visits, it can be assumed that among donors from the military ranks, many came to treat their wounds. All these reveal that the Romans were well acquainted with the characteristics and healing power of thermal water, which has, as it is well known today, therapeutic properties in treating various disorders, such as bone and articular damage, as well as skin and gynaecological diseases.

The Temples

The appearance of the sanctuary in the 1st century, as well as the preserved inscriptions, indicate that the temple and whole sanctuary were dedicated to the nymphs. However, for the sanctuary built in the 2nd century, in which numerous deities related to healing were worshipped, there are many unknowns as to which deities the temples were dedicated. In that period the area of the sanctuary was designed with three temples on the north side, but there were also two lateral rooms that might have had the same purpose. Before the recent excavations, it was assumed, according to the discovery of the statue of the goddess Minerva and pedestal of Juno Regina (and Fortuna), that three temples were dedicated to the cult of the supreme divine Triad in a Capitolium. In the context of recent excavations and the character of stone monuments, among which not a single one dedicated to Jupiter was found, it seems completely logical that this is a type of sanctuary where only deities related to healing were worshipped. This is why Juno and Minerva were presumably worshipped in their healing capacity and not as components of a classical Triad. So, the already mentioned inscription dedicated to Apollo, Minerva, the nymphs and Juno (Regina) might give valuable information about the main cults in the sanctuary. The sacred spring itself was certainly dedicated to the nymphs, however, some rituals may have also been performed in some other areas. Based on the findings, it can only be established that Minerva was worshipped in the western temple, while the finding of the pedestal of Juno (Regina) and Fortuna may indicate that it was originally located in the eastern temple, in accordance with the custom to jointly worship several deities in common temples. We can presume that as a result of the very dynamic life in the *Aquae Iasae* sanctuary, the changes in the temples occurred over the centuries, as the result of the introduction of new cults or even in relation to the changes in the official imperial religion. In this context, it can be assumed that the statues of Apollo/Sol and Diana/Luna were placed at the beginning of the 3rd century in one of the temples and according to the epigraphic evidence in the same period the importance of Egyptian cults as well Asclepius was quite certain. These findings document that at the beginning of the 3rd century, the worship of the three favourite deities of Emperor Caracalla – Apollo, Asclepius and Serapis existed in *Aquae Iasae* sanctuary, which implies the influence of the official religion as well as its involvement in the local cult of the spring.

It is quite certain that the specificity of the sanctuary with its several temples and the mystical atmosphere of the space must have been reflected in all the cults and rituals, linking them to the specific cult of the holy spring characteristic for the *Aquae Iasae* sanctuary.

Conclusion

The exceptional therapeutic properties of the thermal water were undoubtedly the main reason for the popularity of *Aquae Iasae* as a thermal spa, however, the development of the settlement was also due to its strategic location, favourable climate, availability of sources of drinking water, the gentle, fertile valley of the Bednja River as well as the nearby slopes providing pastures and forests.

Based mainly on the results of the research of the sanctuary and bathing area in the town's park, we

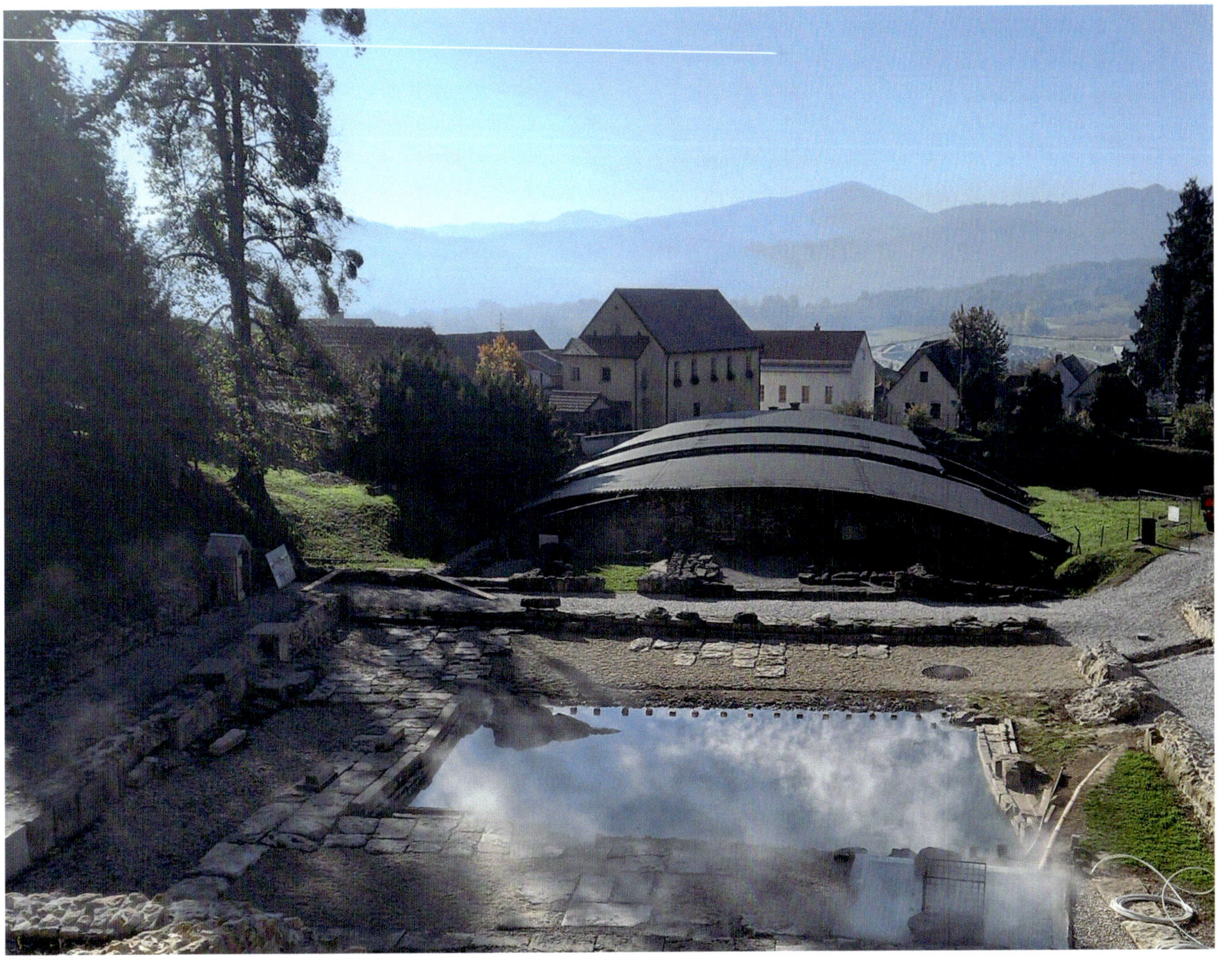

Figure 9. The sanctuary and baths' area looking south (photo by D. Kušan Špalj)

can assume that the settlement experienced its most significant growth and peaked in popularity in the 2nd and first half of the 3rd century when visitors came from various parts of the Empire (among them probably the emperors themselves). This assumption is confirmed by the existence of numerous epigraphic monuments from that period, while Emperor Constantine's investment in its reconstruction after the fire, documented in the inscription (*CIL* III, 04121), indicates the importance of the settlement in the 4th century.

Just as other sites with hot springs throughout the Roman Empire, the *Aquae Iasae* hot spring was honoured as a divine place and votive offerings were dedicated to the gods. As early as the 1st century, the Romans organised the area around the thermal spring as a sanctuary giving the natural phenomenon a 'sacred spring' ambience. At the same time, they managed to 'control' the spring and used the thermal water in the baths and this was especially so after the construction of the spring reservoir in the 2nd century when a very complex and carefully planned hydraulic system was created. After the renovation in the 4th century, the same system was used right up until the end of the complex, which confirms a good understanding of the local characteristics of the spring as well as the knowledge of its maintenance over many centuries. The system for capturing the continually emerging water included the system of canals and the spring reservoir in the shape of a large pool that collected water directly on the site where the hot spring rises, in a similar way known to have existed in *Aquae Sulis* (Cunliffe and Davenport 1985; Davenport 2021).

If we analyse the organisation of the sanctuary area, even in different building phases, we can conclude that the similar concept of space organisation was always applied, with the spring in the centre, the porticoes surrounding it, and the temple/temples to the north. This fact may have depended on the continuity of certain rituals that were part of the religious practice in this particular sanctuary. It was a place of worship and sacrifice where ceremonies took place. Visitors probably moved through the arcades, perhaps in some ritual procession, and approached the sacred spring in the middle, into which they threw votive offerings in the hope of receiving healing.

The main feature of the *Aquae Iasae* sanctuary was the powerful cult of the nymphs but also the worship of various deities associated with the power of healing throughout the 2nd and 3rd centuries. Finds related to Apollo and the geological situation around the thermal spring suggest that it could have also been a place of oracles (Kušan Špalj 2014; 2015: 101; Kušan Špalj 2017a: 282).

Most of the preserved epigraphic monuments confirm the private nature of religious worship, even when their dedicators were military or civil officials, while most of their stays in the spa were for personal reasons, due to illness and hope for recovery. The best evidence of the predominately private nature of the religion is recognisable through the votive offerings, 18,000 coins and several jewellery objects (Kušan Špalj *et al.* 2014; 2015), in the spring reservoir, behind which lie the many destinies of the people who were hoping to recover.

Although there is no evidence of votive inscriptions from the site dating back to the 4th century (probably removed from the sanctuary in a later period), the discovery of the statue of the goddess Minerva in her temple suggests that the worship of some pagan cults was practised until the complex ceased functioning.[41] What happened in the late 4th or even early 5th century, before the buildings were abandoned, we can only guess. The role of the basilica with Christian rites probably dominated the complex at that time, but considering the numerous 4th-century coins and the aforementioned rings with a Christogram found in the spring, it must be assumed that the pagan sanctuary functioned at that time as well. The main reason for this specific situation was the thermal spring and the mysticism of healing in this sanctuary over several centuries.

The smell and evaporation of the thermal water constantly bubbling up from under the ground, rippling and changing colour within the Roman spring reservoir, today still offers an unforgettable experience of encountering a natural phenomenon that only the Romans were able to use with unique skill and respect. (Figure 9)

[41] There are only fragments of three monumental metric inscriptions (mystical texts written in dactylic hexameter and iamb, in the glory of water, sun and nature) that are dated in the first half of the 4th century (Kuntić Makvić *et al.* 2012).

Bibliography

Aljinović, D., U. Barudžija, D. Kušan Špalj and D. Nemeth-Ehrlich 2005. *Mixed thermal and ambient water travertines of ancient Roman spa-Aquae Iasae, Croatia,* in: M. Özkul, S. Yagiz and B. Jones (eds) *Proceedings of 1st International Symposium on travertine – Denizli*: 71–74. Ankara: Kozan ofset Matbaacilik San Ve Tic. Ltd.

Ando, C. 2005. Interpretatio Romana. *Classical Philology* 100 (1): 41–51.

Bedeković, J. 1752. *Natale solum magni ecclesiae doctoris sancti Hyeronymi in ruderibus stridonis occultatum probatorum nihilominus historicorum at geographicorum opinionisbus.* Neostadii Austriae: Ex typographeo Mulleriano.

Bekić, L. 2006. *Zaštitna arheologija u okolici Varaždina: arheološka istraživanja na autocesti Zagreb - Goričan i njezinim prilaznim cestama/ Rescue Archaeology in the Varaždin Environs, Archaeological Research on the Zagreb Goričan Highway and its Access Roads.* Zagreb: Ministery of Culture RH.

Bieber, M. 1955. *The Sculpture of the Hellenistic Age.* New York: Columbia University Press.

Bilić, T. 2014. Numizmatične najdbe iz izvirskega bazena v Varaždinskih Toplicah / Numismatic Finds in the Spring Pool at Varaždinske Toplice, in N. Pirnat Spahić (ed.) *Aquae Iasae - Najnovejše rimske najdbe na območju Varaždinskih Toplic / Aquae Iasae - Recent Discoveries of Roman Remains in the Region of Varaždinske Toplice*: 120–125. Ljubljana: Cankarjev dom.

Bilić, T. 2015. Numizmatički nalazi iz izvorišnog bazena u Varaždinskim Toplicama / Numismatic Finds in the Spring Pool at Varaždinske Toplice, in N. Pirnat Spahić (ed.) *Aquae Iasae- Nova otkrića iz rimskog razdoblja na području Varaždinskih Toplica/ Aquae Iasae- Recent Discoveries of Roman Remains in the Region of Varaždinske Toplice:* 120–125. Zagreb: Arheološki muzej u Zagrebu.

Brunšmid, J. 1905. Kameni spomenici Hrvatskoga narodnoga muzeja u Zagrebu. *Vjesnik Arheološkog muzeja u Zagrebu* 8 (1): 37–104.

Cunliffe, B. and P. Davenport 1985, *The Temple of Sulis Minerva at Bath - Volume (1), The site.* Monograph 7. Oxford: Oxford University Commitee for Archaeology.

Cvetko, M. 2022. *Rimski zavjetni žrtvenici s područja Hrvatske.* Zagreb: FF Press.

Čabrian, J., M. Gorenc and B. Vikić 1973. *Pregled povijesti Varaždinskih Toplica.* Varaždinske Toplice: Turističko društvo i muzej.

Davenport, P. 2021. *Roman Bath, a New History and Archaeology of Aquae Sulis.*Gloucestershire: The History Press.

Domić-Kunić, A. 2006. Bellum Pannonicum (12-11. pr. Kr.) posljednja faza osvajanja Južne Panonije, (Bellum Pannonicum (12-11 B.C.). *Vjesnik Arheološkog muzeja u Zagrebu* 3 (39): 59–164.

Filipan, B. 2002. Rimski vodovod u funkciji razvoja kupališta u Varaždinskim Toplicama, in: B. Filipan (ed.) *Kukuljevićevi dani u Varaždinskim Toplicama, Zbornik radova znanstveno-stručnih skupova Matice hrvatske 1995-2000:* 73–88. Varaždinske Toplice: Matica Hrvatske.

Gorenc, M. 1984. Minerva iz Varaždinskih Toplica i njezin majstor. *Vjesnik Arheološkog muzeja u Zagrebu* 3 (16-17): 95–108.

Grbić, D. 2014. *Tribal Communities in Illyricum. Preurban Administration Structures in the Roman Provinces between the Adriatic and Danube (First-Third Centuries).* Belgrade: Institut for Balkan Studies of the Serbian Academy of Sciences and Arts.

Gregl, Z. and B. Migotti 2004. Civitas Iovia (Botivo), in M. Šašel Kos and P. Scherrer (eds) *The Autonomous Towns of Noricum and Pannonia, Pannonia II (Situla 42)*: 131–143. Ljubljana: Narodni muzej Slovenije.

Horvat, J., M. Lovenjak, A. Dolenc Vičič, M. Lubšina-Tušek, M. Tomanič-Jevremov and Z. Šubic 2003. Poetovio, Development and Topography, in M. Šašel Kos and P. Scherrer (eds) *The Autonomous Towns of Noricum and Pannonia, Pannonia I (Situla 41)*: 153–189. Ljubljana: Narodni muzej Slovenije.

Jerala, M. 2011. The topography of ritual monuments in Poetovio, in I. Lazar (ed.) *Religion in public and private sphere, Acta of the 4th International Colloquium, The Autonomous Towns of Noricum and Pannonia, Annales Mediterranei:* 7–86. Koper: Univerza na Primorskem.

Kaminski, G. 1991. Thesauros.Untersuchungen zum antiken Opferstock. *Jahrbuch des Deutchen Archaeologischen Instituts* 106: 63–181.

Katančić, M.P. 1795. *Specimen philologiae et geographiae Pannoniorum, in quo de origine lingua et literatura Croatorum, simul de Sisciae Andautonii Nevioduni Poetovionis urbium in Pannonia olim celebrium et his interiectarum via militari mansionum situ disseritur.* Zagreb: Typis episcopalibus.

Kuntić Makvić, B., A. Rendić-Miočević, M. Šegvić and I. Krajcar 2012. Intergracija i vizualna prezentacija ulomaka monumentalnog metričkog natpisa iz Varaždinskih Toplica), in J. Balen, M. and Šimek (eds) *Arheologija varaždinskog kraja i srednjeg Podravlja.* Izdanja Hrvatskog arheološkog društva 28: 285–295. Zagreb: Hrvatsko arheološko društvo.

Kušan, D. 1999. Forum rimskog naselja *Aquae Iasae*-njegov razvoj i značaj tijekom stoljeća (The Roman Forum in Varaždinske Toplice-its development and significance through the centuries). *Histria Antiqua* 5: 109–120.

Kušan Špalj, D. 2014. Zgodovina rimske naselbine *Aquae Iasae*; *Aquae Iasae* – zdraviliško, kultno in preroško svetišče; Rekonstrukcija prostora okoli naravnega izvira termalne vode – rituali in uporaba / History of the Roman Settlement *Aquae Iasae*; *Aquae Iasae* -a Center of Health, Cult and Oracle: Reconstruction of the Area Around the Natural Thermal Spring-Rituals and Utilization, in N. Pirnat Spahić (ed.) *Aquae Iasae - Najnovejše rimske najdbe na območju Varaždinskih Toplic/ Aquae Iasae - Recent Discoveries of Roman Remains in the Region of Varaždinske Toplice* : 50–119. Ljubljana: Cankarjev dom.

Kušan Špalj, D. 2015. Povijest rimskog naselja *Aquae Iasae*; *Aquae Iasae*- lječilišni, kultni i proročki centar; Rekonstrukcija prostora oko prirodnog izvora termalne vode-rituali i namjena / History of the Roman Settlement *Aquae Iasae*; *Aquae Iasae* -a Center of Health, Cult and Oracle; Reconstruction of the Area Around the Natural Thermal Spring-Rituals and Utilization, in N. Pirnat Spahić (ed.) *Aquae Iasae- Nova otkrića iz rimskog razdoblja na području Varaždinskih Toplica/ Aquae Iasae- Recent Discoveries of Roman Remains in the Region of Varaždinske Toplice:* Zagreb: 50–119. Arheološki muzej u Zagrebu.

Kušan Špalj, D. 2017a. *Aquae Iasae* - new Discoveries in the Roman Sanctuary – with special regard to the cults of Apollo, Asclepius, and Serapis. *Vjesnik Arheološkog muzeja u Zagrebu* 50: 255–304.

Kušan Špalj, D. 2017b. Rimsko naselje *Aquae Iasae* (Varaždinske Toplice), primjer recikliranja građevinskog materijala, in I. Miloglav. A. Kudelić and J. Balen (eds) *Recikliraj, ideje iz prošlosti:* 163–180. Zagreb: Arheološki muzej u Zagrebu, Filozofski fakultet, Institut za arheologiju.

Kušan Špalj, D. 2020a. *Aquae Iasae* (Varaždinske Toplice) – ranokršćanski horizont, in M. Sanader, D. Tončinić, I. Kaić, and V. Matijević (eds) *Zbornik I. skupa hrvatske ranokršćanske arheologije:*303–320. Zagreb: Arheološki zavod Odsjeka za arheologiju Filozofskog fakulteta Sveučilišta u Zagrebu.

Kušan Špalj, D. 2020b. Roman settlement Aquae *Iasae*-recent discoveries in the sanctuary area, in V. Sekulov (ed.) *Vth International Symposium on Archaeology „Cult, Myth, Religion',* Acta Musei Tiberiopolitani 3: 171–184. Strumica: Institute for Protection of the Monuments of Culture and Museum Strumica.

Kušan Špalj, D. 2022a. *Aquae Iasae*- novi spomenici posvećeni nimfama iz rimskog svetišta-I. dio / *Aquae Iasae* - new Monuments dedicated to nymphs from the Roman Sanctuary-part I, *Vjesnik Arheološkog muzeja u Zagrebu* 55: 73–114.

Kušan Špalj, D. 2022b. Sanctuary area in the Roman Settlement *Aquae Iasae*, in M. Šteiner and I. Ciglar (eds) *Poetoviona in njen ager / Poetovio and its ager (simpozij / conference 18.11.2020)*, Archaeologia Poetovionensis 4: 53–68. Ptuj: Pokrajinski muzej Ptuj – Ormož.

Kušan Špalj, D. 2023. *Aquae Iasae* - novi spomenici posvećeni nimfama iz rimskog svetišta- II dio / *Aquae Iasae* - new Monuments dedicated to nymphs from the Roman Sanctuary – part II, *Vjesnik Arheološkog muzeja u Zagrebu* 56: 153–211.

Kušan Špalj, D. 2024. Recent discoveries in the sanctuary area of the Roman settlement *Aquae Iasae*

(Varaždinske Toplice), *in J. Horvat, S. Groh, K. Strobel, M. Belak (eds) Roman urban landscape: towns and minor settlements from Aquileia to the Danube, Opera Instituti Archaeologici Sloveniae* 47: 447– 470.

Kušan Špalj, D. and D. Nemeth-Ehrlich 2012. *Aquae Iasae*-Varaždinske Toplice, arheološka istraživanja rimskog izvorišnog bazena i okolnog prostora, in J. Balen, M. and Šimek (eds) *Arheologija varaždinskog kraja i srednjeg Podravlja.* Izdanja Hrvatskog arheološkog društva 28: 107–129. Zagreb: Hrvatsko arheološko društvo.

Kušan Špalj, D., N. Perok, T. Bilić, M. Nađ, S. Habus and J. Balen 2014. Katalog razstavljenih predmetov/ Catalogue of exibited items, in N. Pirnat Spahić (ed.) *Aquae Iasae - Najnovejše rimske najdbe na območju Varaždinskih Toplic/ Aquae Iasae - Recent Discoveries of Roman Remains in the Region of Varaždinske Toplice:* 131–188. Ljubljana: Cankarjev dom.

Kušan Špalj, D., N. Perok, T. Bilić, M. Nađ, S. Habus and J. Balen 2015. Katalog izloženih predmeta / Catalogue of exibited items, in N. Pirnat Spahić (ed.) *Aquae Iasae- Nova otkrića iz rimskog razdoblja na području Varaždinskih Toplica/ Aquae Iasae- Recent Discoveries of Roman Remains in the Region of Varaždinske Toplice:* Zagreb: 131–188. Arheološki muzej u Zagrebu.

Kušan Špalj, D., N. Perok and T. Karavidović 2019. Construction and Building Technology in Sanctuary of Roman Settlement *Aquae Iasae* with the Review of Conservation Works on the Site, in R. Aguilar, D. Torrealva, S. Moreira, M. Pando and L.F. Ramos (eds) *Structural Analysis of Historical Constructions:an interdisciplinary approach,* Rilem bookseries 18: 96–104. Springer.

Lučić, L. 2013. Rimski natpisi iz Varaždinskih Toplica / The Roman inscriptions from Varaždinske Toplice. *Vjesnik Arheološkog muzeja u Zagrebu* 46: 185–255.

Ljubić, Š. 1879. *Aquae Iasae* (Toplice Varaždinske). *Viestnik hrvatskoga arheologičkoga družtva* 2: 33–34.

Malez, M. 1979. Nalazišta paleolitskog i mezolitskog doba u Hrvatskoj, in A. Benac (ed.) *Praistorija jugoslavenskih zemalja I:* 227–276. Sarajevo: Akademija nauka i umjetnosti Bosne i Hercegovine.

Marković, T., S. Borović and O. Larva 2015. Geochemical characteristics of thermalwaters of Hrvatsko zagorje. *Geologica Croatica* 68/1: 67–77.

Marković, T., Ž. Sladović, O. Larva and Ž. Brkić 2020. Delineacija i karakterizacija tijela geotermalnih podzemnih voda u Republici Hrvatskoj. Unpublished Report, Croatian geological survey (viewed 10 August 2023) https://voda.hr/sites/default/files/dokumenti/prateca-dokumentacija/delineacija_i_karakterizacija_tijela_geotermalnih_podzemnih_voda_u_rh.pdf

Migotti, B., M. Šašel Kos and I. Radman-Livaja 2018. *Roman Funerary Monuments of South-Western Pannonia in their Material, Social, and Religious Context.* Roman Archaeology 45. Oxford: Archaeopress.

Mócsy, A. 1968. Municipium Iasorum, *RE Suppl.* XI: 1003–1004.

Mrav. Z. 2000. Der Besuch Caracallas und der Deus Invictus Serapis-Kult in Pannonien, *Comunicationes Archaeologicae Hungariae* 20: 67–97.

Nemeth-Ehrich, D. and D. Kušan Špalj 2011. The results of the latest excavations at the Roman forum in *Aquae Iasae*- Varaždinske Toplice, in I. Lazar (ed.) *Religion in public and private sphere,* Acta of the 4th International Colloquium, Annales Mediterranei: 211–232, Koper: Univerza na Primorskem.

Nemeth-Ehrich, D. and D. Kušan Špalj 2014. Rimska naselbina *Aquae Iasae* –izsledki arheoloških raziskav mestnega parka v Varaždinskih Toplicah / The Roman Settlement *Aquae Iasae* – Findings of Archaeological Excavations in the Area of the Varaždinske Toplice Municipal Park, in N. Pirnat Spahić (ed.) *Aquae Iasae - Najnovejše rimske najdbe na območju Varaždinskih Toplic/ Aquae Iasae - Recent Discoveries of Roman Remains in the Region of Varaždinske Toplice*: 21–35, 36–49. Ljubljana: Cankarjev dom.

Nemeth-Ehrlich, D. and D. Kušan Špalj 2015. Rimsko naselje *Aquae Iasae* - rezultati arheoloških istraživanja na prostoru gradskog parka u Varaždinskim Toplicama / The Roman Settlement *Aquae Iasae* –Findings of Archaeological Excavations in the Area of the Varaždinske Toplice Municipal Park, in N. Pirnat Spahić (ed.) *Aquae Iasae- Nova otkrića iz rimskog razdoblja na području Varaždinskih Toplica/ Aquae Iasae- Recent Discoveries of Roman Remains in the Region of Varaždinske Toplice:* Zagreb: 21–35, 36–49. Arheološki muzej u Zagrebu.

Ragolić, A. 2014. The territory of Poetovio and the boundary between Noricum and Pannonia / Upravno območje Petovione in meja med Norikom in Panonijo. *Arheološki vestnik* 65: 323–351.

Rendić-Miočević, D. 1992. O akvejasejskoj epigrafskoj baštini i o posebnostima njenih kultnih dedikacija. *Vjesnik Arheološkog muzeja u Zagrebu* 24-25: 67–76.

Rendić-Miočević, A. and M. Šegvić 1998. Religions and cults in south Pannonian regions, in J. Fitz (ed.) *Religions and cults in Pannonia*: 7–16. Székesfehérvár: Fejér Megyei Múzeumok Igazgatósága.

Schejbal, B. 2003. Nova razmatranja o Aquae Balissae i narodu Jaza: Pejzaž – Vode – Etimologija – Kultovi – Mitologija, pitanje atribucije i kontinuiteta. *Opuscula archaeologica* 27: 393–416.

Schejbal, B. 2004. Municipium Iasorum (Aquae Balissae), in M. Šašel Kos and P. Scherrer (eds) *The Autonomous Towns of Noricum and Pannonia, Pannonia II (Situla 42)*: 99–129. Ljubljana: Narodni muzej Slovenije.

Selem, P., 1997. *Izidin trag, egipatski kultni spomenici u rimskom Iliriku.* Split: Književni krug.

Solter, A. 2016, *Arheološki muzej u Zagrebu : život od 19. do 21. stoljeća.* Zagreb: Arheološki muzej u Zagrebu.

Šašel Kos, M. and P. Scherrer (eds) 2004. *The Autonomous Towns of Noricum and Pannonia, Pannonia II (Situla 42).* Ljubljana: Narodni muzej Slovenije.

Šimunić, A. 1998. Geološko-tektonska osnova termomineralnih vrela u Varaždinskim Toplicama. *Radovi Zavoda za znanstveni rad Varaždin* 2: 9–29.

Tkalčić, I. K., 1869. *Toplice kod Varaždina u Hrvatskoj (Varaždinske Toplice)*. Zagreb: Pismeni Karla Albrechta.

Vikić-Belančić, B. 1972. Prilog istraživanju antičkog naseobinskog kompleksa u Varaždinskim Toplicama. *Vjesnik Arheološkog muzeja u Zagrebu* 6 - 7: 75–127.

Vikić-Belančić, B. 1975. Keramika grublje fakture u Južnoj Panoniji s osobitim obzirom na urne i lonce. *Arheološki Vestnik 26*: 25–53.

Vikić-Belančić, B. 1996. Rezultati arheoloških istraživanja lokaliteta u Varaždinskim Toplicama. *Radovi Zavoda za znanstveni rad HAZU Varaždin* 8-9: 11–34.

Vikić-Belančić, B. and M. Gorenc 1958. Arheološka istraživanja antiknog kupališta u Varaždinskim Toplicama od 1953-1955. g. *Vjesnik Arheološkog muzeja u Zagrebu* 3 (1): 75–127.

Vikić-Belančić, B. and M. Gorenc 1961. Istraživanja antiknog kupališta u Varaždinskim Toplicama od 1956. godine do 1959. godine. *Vjesnik arheološkog muzeja u Zagrebu* 2: 181–223.

Vikić-Belančić, B. and M. Gorenc 1970. Završna istraživanja antičkog kupališnog kompleksa u Varaždinskim Toplicama. *Vjesnik Arheološkog muzeja u Zagrebu* 4: 121–157.

Vlahović, S. 2020. Nekoliko crtica o otkrivenim kasnoantičkim fragmentima fresaka i arheološkim nalazima iz ulice braće Radić u Varaždinskim Toplicama. *Radovi zavoda za znanstveni rad HAZU Varaždin* 31: 9–29.

Abbreviations

AE L'Année Epigraphique

AIJ Hoffiler, V. and Saria B. (eds) 1938. Antike IInschriften aus Jugoslavien, Heft 1: Noricum und Pannonia Superior. Zagreb: F. Pelikan - St. Kugli.

CIL *Corpus inscriptionum Latinarum*

HD *Epigraphische Datenbank Heidelberg*

ILJug Šašel, A. and Šašel J. *Inscriptiones Latinae quae in Iugoslavia inter annos MCMLXII et MCMXL repertae et editae sunt*, Situla 25, 1986.

lupa F. und O. Harl, http://lupa.at (Bilddatenbank zu antiken Steindenkmälern)

Healing Spas in the Arverni Territory (France, Auvergne Rhône Alpes)

Lise AUGUSTIN-ROLLAND
Université Clermont Auvergne (UAR 3550; ArAr, UMR 5138) /
Ingénieure d'études, 4 rue Ledru, 63000 Clermont-Ferrand, France.
lise.augustin@uca.fr

Élise NECTOUX
French Ministery ofCuture (ArAr, UMR 5138; ArScAn, UMR 7041) /
Conservatrice du patrimoine, Service régional de l'archéologie d'Auvergne-Rhône-Alpes,
4 rue Pascal, 63000 Clermont-Ferrand, France.
elise.nectoux@culture.gouv.fr

Hélène DARTEVELLE
French Ministery ofCuture (ArAr, UMR 5138; ArScAn, UMR 7041) /
Ingénieure d'études, Service régional de l'archéologie d'Auvergne-Rhône-Alpes, 4 rue Pascal, 63000 Clermont-Ferrand, France.
helene.dartevelle@culture.gouv.fr

Bertrand DOUSTEYSSIER
Université Clermont Auvergne (UAR 3550) / Ingénieur de recherche, 4 rue Ledru, 63000 Clermont-Ferrand, France.
bertrand.dousteyssier@uca.fr

Élise FOVET
CNRS, Université Clermont Auvergne (UAR 3550) /
Ingénieure de recherche, 4 rue Ledru, 63000 Clermont-Ferrand, France.
elise.fovet@uca.fr

Gabriel ROCQUE
Service d'archéologie préventive du département de l'Allier (Citeres, UMR 7324) /
Operation manager, 1 avenue Victor Hugo BP 1669, 03000 Moulins. France.
rocque.g@allier.fr

Abstract: The Arvernian territory is located in the heart of the Massif Central (central France), a highland region largely shaped by ancient volcanism and teeming with thermal waters, hot or cold, salty or not, exploited at least since the Roman period and very widely used in the 19th century.

Curative bathing is attested to since the beginning of the Roman Empire, in different forms: from simple springs equipped to receive ex-votos to thermal facilities, some situated near important urban centres (Vichy-Cusset, Royat-Chamalières), and others remotely located in mountains (small urban centre of Le Mont-Dore). This territory is strewn with thermal baths and healing springs where practices are diverse but always under gods patronage.

This article aims to present an overview of the current research in this region, carried out by various teams. After a general presentation of the Arvernian territory (mineral water resources and the spatial organisation during Roman period), we will show the current state of archaeological knowledge on Roman thermalism in this area, mainly focused on Vichy-Cusset and Le Mont-Dore.

Keywords: Healing spas, territory, pilgrimage, sanctuaries, Gallo-Roman thermalism.

Introduction

The Arverni territory is located in the heart of the Massif Central, a medium-altitude region largely shaped by ancient volcanism. Due to its geological formation, this territory has a substantial hydrothermal potential, with mineral sources of widely varying temperature and salinity (Figure 1).[1] Throughout Antiquity, hot springs[2] were used extensively for their healing properties in various ways (Figure 2). The use of cold mineral springs in curative spas is now well established in Vichy-Cusset, in the same manner as in neighbouring areas. Addressing curative balneology on the scale

[1] We focus on sites that used mineral waters at least partially. Indeed, it is accepted that healing spas did not only rely on mineral waters (Aupert 1991: 188; Aupert 2012: 308), and that some facilities were clearly bipartite, with only one part being supplied by mineral water, as at *Aquæ Cæsaris*, in Tébessa, Algeria (Thébert 2003: 371).

[2] BRGM (French Bureau of Geological and Mining Research) states that a spring is considered to be hot when the temperature at its emergence reaches 30°C or above.

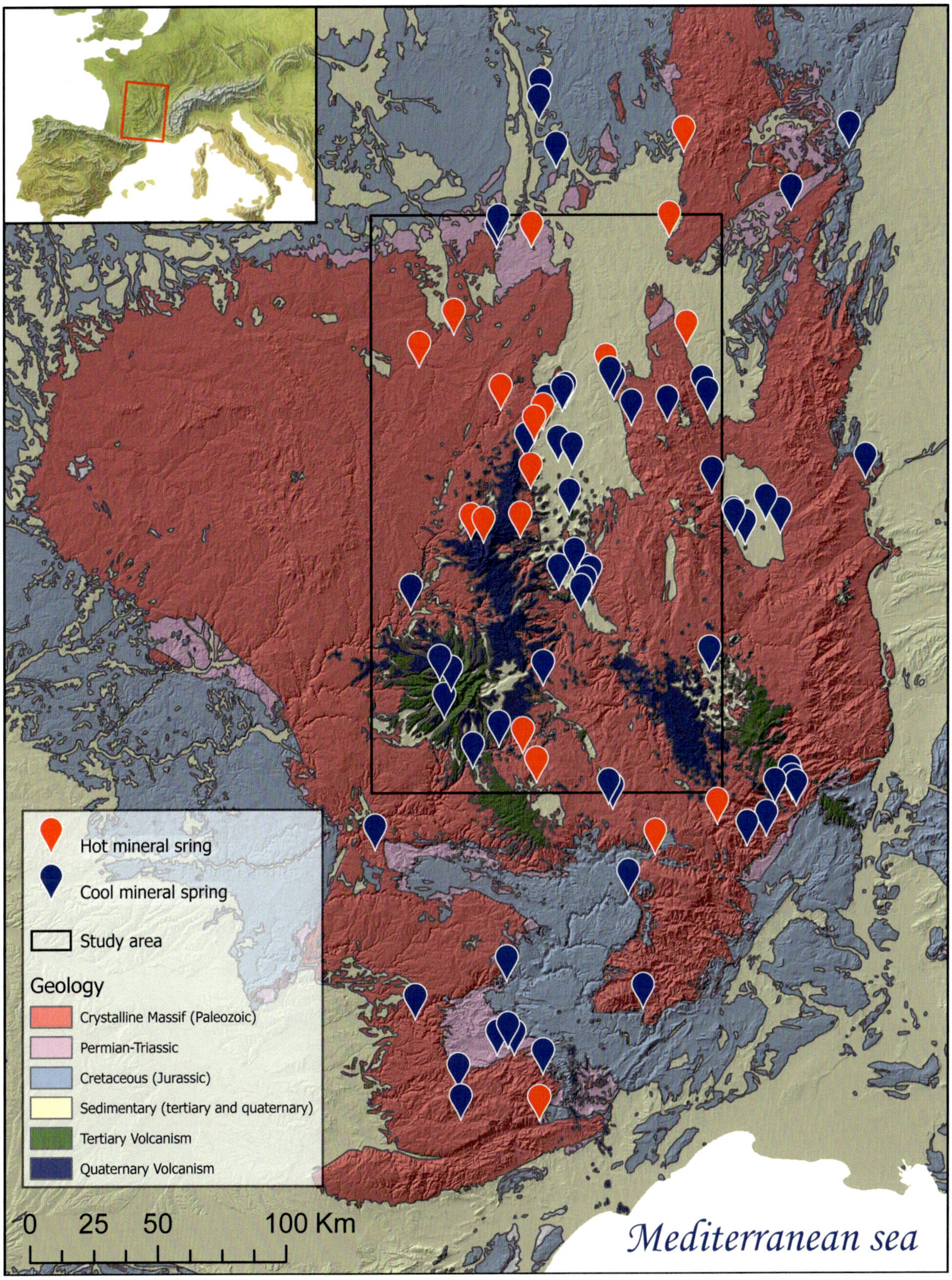

Figure 1. Mineral springs of the Massif Central. Author: É. Fovet (after Boineau, Maisonneuve 1971; Risler 1974).

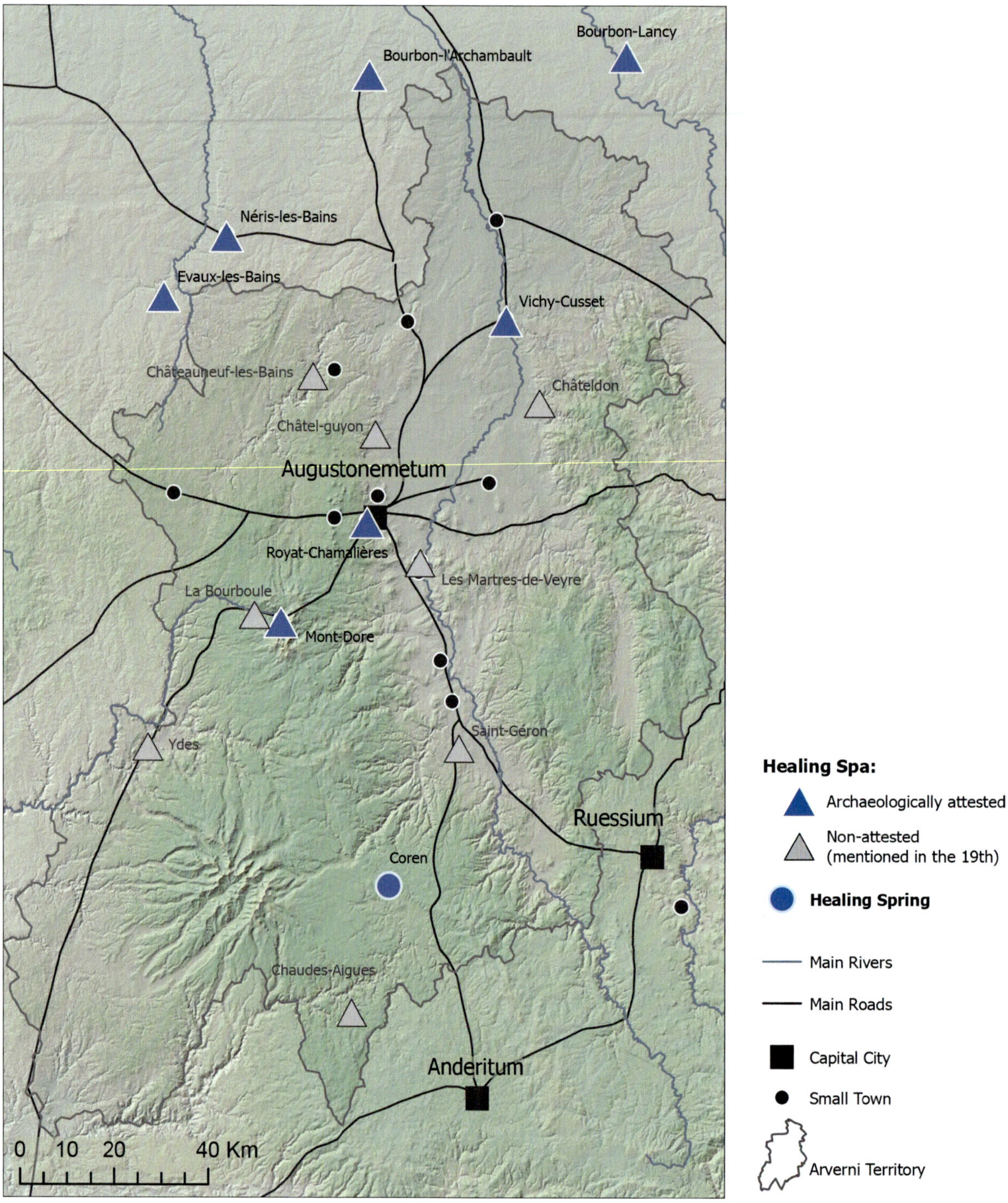

Figure 2. Roman healing spas in the Arverni territory. Authors: É. Fovet, M. Dacko, É. Nectoux, B. Dousteyssier. Base map: after IGN.

of an ancient *cite*, or tribal territory, entails asking questions about the natural potential of the region, the attested sites[3] and their distribution, as well as regional customs.[4] On the scale of a particular site, accessibility, the types of installations and the remains of specific furnishings need to be examined.

In the 19th century, regional balneology was flourishing. It took many different forms, from modest rural facilities to elegant upper-class resorts. There was a genuine

[3] The definition of healing balneology is difficult to apply to remains that are only partially preserved or that were excavated in the past. As such, J. Scheid (1991: 209) warns: 'It is difficult, for all these reasons, to assign healing properties to spas found near sacred sites, as well as to consider as hydrotherapeutic every sanctuary equipped with spas, or even nymphaea or labra'.

[4] As studied by S. González Soutelo (2012).

commercial interest in evoking the roots of the practice in Antiquity, which drove source operators and owners to base their reputations almost systematically on the age of their springs. This enthusiasm led to the discovery of a large number of archaeological remains, as well as the identification of prominent sites within the Arverni territory. But the downside is that the historiographical weight of these ancient discoveries, sometimes badly described or misinterpreted, has caused some sites to be dismissed (such as Châteauneuf-les-Bains, Châtel-Guyon, Châteldon, La Bourboule[5], Saint-Nectaire), while others are still considered potential sites which should be studied more thoroughly (Les Martres-de-Veyre, Chaudes-Aigues). Some authors have tried to identify the cities named on the Peutinger Table, with the term '*Aquis/Aquæ...*', without basing their hypotheses on concrete remains.

This research history has contributed to a biased vision of ancient thermal baths, which now needs to be rectified. The archaeological documentation is incomplete (outdated excavations), and the remains have often been destroyed, are inaccessible or heavily altered, and yet a reassessment of the data is still possible. Within this context, several teams are working on the three symbolic sites of the late Arverni territory (the Royat-Chamalières and Vichy-Cusset complexes, and the Mont-Dore site). We will not focus here on saline springs, since we lack evidence of their use for healing purposes in Roman times. This renewed archaeological approach, based on a critical re-examination of the data, demonstrates the complexity and the plurality of archaeological truths. This presentation is an opportunity to bring these findings together through a territorial approach, a milestone in the domain of regional research.

AUGUSTONEMETUM (H. Dartevelle)

Augustonemetum ('the sanctuary of Augustus'), the centre of the Arverni territory on which the present-day city of Clermont-Ferrand was built, was created at the dawn of our era on the Via Agrippa, a major route linking Lyon (capital of the Gauls) and Saintes (Aquitaine's capital). It was established at the foot of the Chaîne des Puys and the fault escarpment opening onto the Limagne plain, in a small protected sedimentary basin. Located well away from the Allier River but dominated by numerous volcanic mounds and particularly rich in thermo-mineral sources, this place was an ideal setting for the city. Several satellites, among them a sanctuary, thermal baths, a theatre, usually associated with settlements, were indeed built on the outskirts of the city, organized around the exceptional Temple of Mercury at the summit of the Puy de Dôme, one of the largest mountain sanctuaries of the Western Roman territory (Dartevelle 2022a; Dartevelle 2022b). The Royat spas are discussed here in their territorial context, inherently connected to the city of *Augustonemetum*.

The Royat spas

The so-called 'Royat spas', mainly located in the municipality of Chamalières, are situated in the downstream section of the Royat valley, carved out by the Tiretaine River, between a lava flow and an arkose bank, 3km west of the urban centre of Clermont-Ferrand. Five springs are currently tapped on the thermal site: Eugénie, César, Saint-Mart, Saint-Victor and Auraline (the latter was recently bored). When they emerge, these waters are generally rich in bicarbonate, chloride and sodium, and highly gaseous, with temperatures between 27° and 34°C. There, one can find treatments for arthrosis, arteritis, and Raynaud syndrome.

Most of these sources were tapped during Antiquity, yet their chronology remains uncertain, like that of the bathing complex. Were they at the origin – at the beginning of our era – of the development of an urban area and a burial site on the Via Agrippa, in the vicinity of *Augustonemetum*? The exploitation of the arkose quarry at Puy de Chateix for the first public buildings (*Augustonemetum*, or even the early version of the Temple of Mercury) might have contributed to this development. Undoubtedly, the Royat spas were a milestone in the pilgrimage to the Temple of Mercury, only 7km away. Their connection to the theatre near Montaudou was considered, as was the case in Moingt or Salt-en-Donzy in the Loire region, where there was a place of worship combining spas, a theatre and a sanctuary. This idea was finally ruled out since the Montaudou theatre is facing another direction, toward the rising sun, and is associated with a different sanctuary and urban area, 1.5km southwest of the ancient city.

The first mention of this thermal complex dates back to the 16th century. It is known primarily from ancient and poorly documented discoveries, made when the thermal springs were first exploited in the 18th century. One of the pools, still visible today, was restored and designated as a Historic Monument (Figure 3). Ancient records mention pipes, canals and underground masonry, enigmatic vaulted cellars, clogged pipes, water catchments, hypocausts, marbles and mosaics, entablatures, column capitals and mouldings, etc. As regards the catchments, several discovery reports mention wells made of concrete or pine timbers. One particular and explicit example, a report written by A. Petit in 1876 near the Saint-Victor source states:

[5] P. Aupert (2012: 308) mentions the presence of Borvo, water deity, in La Bourboule, but the archaeological files are particularly incomplete.

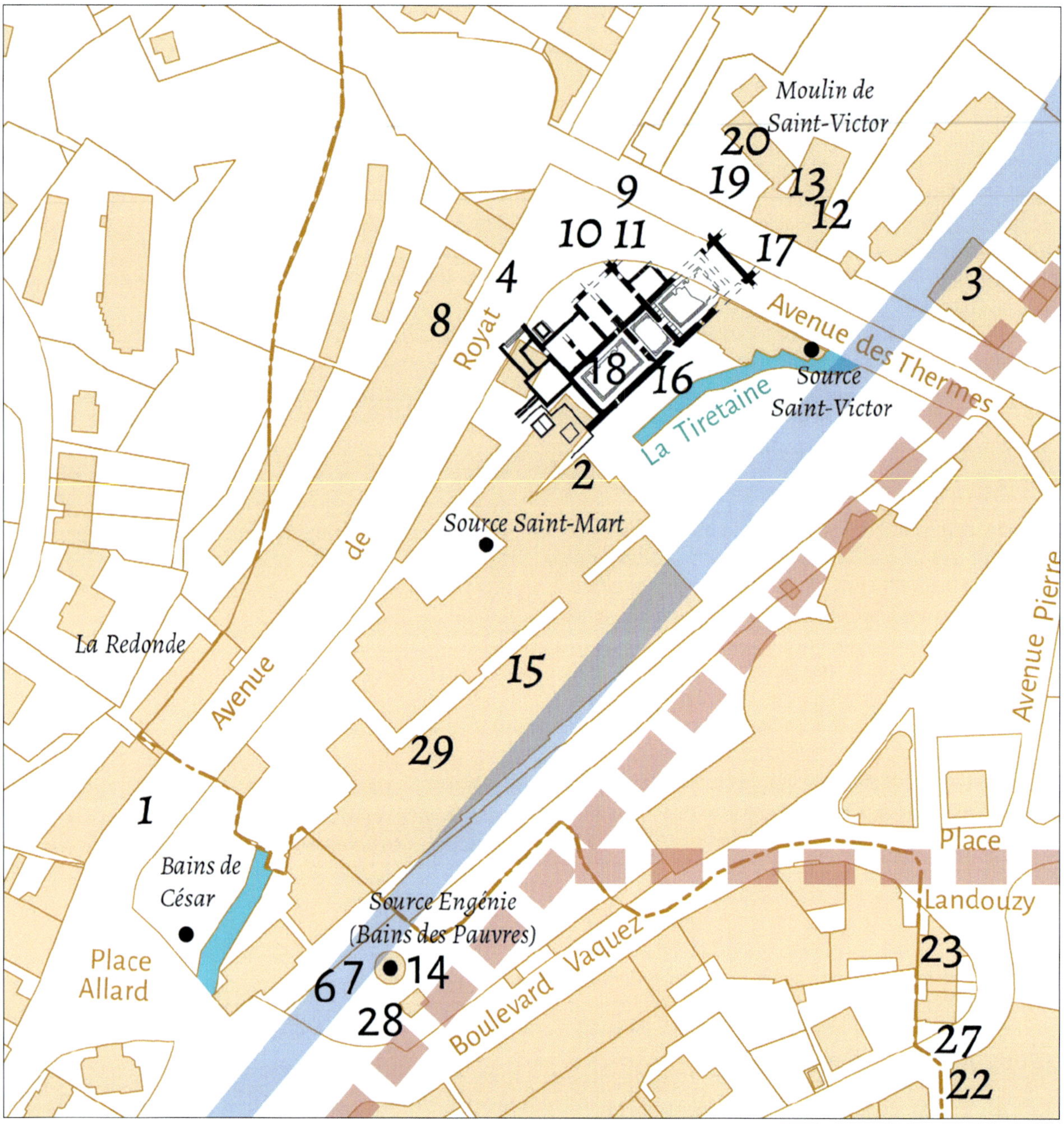

Figure 3. Royat-Chamalières, localisation of the discoveries on a cadastral plan. Extracted from: Dartevelle 2022a, t.2: 162. The numbers refer to remains discovered near the thermal baths.

'a square well, made of fir timbers, 1.20m long. On each side, overlapping timbers were interlocked with alternating rods and grooves; the edges equipped with tenons and mortises ensured the immobility of the framework... Beneath this structure, 6m deep, we unearthed a thick lead pipe, with a diameter of 0.15m...' (Petit 1884: 5). The map of the remains made by Petit is incomplete (2800m^2) and thus does not allow us to reconstruct any routes. At least three pools in the same alignment, yet different in size, each had two rows of seats, confirming the immersion practice (cf. Figure 3). To the northwest, hypocaust-heated rooms adjoined the pools. More pools were discovered downstream in 1946 (Desforges *et al.* 1970: 375-376; Vallat and Le Barrier 2022: note 20).

Hot springs bubbling up at a temperature of 35°C were reported at a depth of two metres near the pools (Petit 1884). However, it is difficult to correlate the sources with the filling of the pools without taking another thorough look at the available documentation. A. Petit noticed the absence of concretions inside one of the pools and hypothesised that it was filled with freshwater. It is likely that the Tiretaine fulfilled this role too, at least for the cold pools, cooling the hot water, flushing latrines and greywaters. The presence of at least one polygonal arkose basin, described as close to the Sainte-Eugénie source, suggests that the water was drunk. A water fountain was also located near the Saint-Victor source 'with a taste of wine, yet very unpleasant to drink' (Belleforest 1575).

Did the construction of the spa complex happen at the same time or after the springs were tapped? Given the current state of academic research, the question of the site's genesis and evolution remains unanswered. We have to imagine *Augustonemetum* in the 1st century AD as a city under constant construction. The public buildings were likely built once the roads and the first residential areas were finished, over the course of the 1st century. They were made of arkose, while trachyte is associated with the middle of the 2nd century, a time when the city was being embellished. Despite the absence of tangible dating evidence, the construction of a spa complex in Royat, an idea which seems at first rather extravagant, would be more coherent with the mid-2nd century, when the city's appearance was embellished with new buildings on the pilgrimage road to the Temple of Mercury.

The Source des Roches in Chamalières

Formerly called the 'Source de Beaurepaire', the Source des Roches emerged at the bottom of the Montjoly hillside. It flowed at temperatures between 19.5° and 20°C, directly from the chalky and marly soil of the Limagne borders, at the end of the Royat lava flow that originated from the Petit Puy de Dôme. Its water is chloro-bicarbonaceous, ferruginous, salty, rich in sodium and magnesium, as well as in carbon dioxide, and was supposed to cure several diseases, including rheumatism. Until 1843, it flowed freely within the city gardens.

Protected by an oak forest, the Source des Roches appeared in Antiquity, first isolated from the city and yet located in its immediate outskirts. The sanctuary was frequented for a long time, at least until the Late Roman Empire, on a regular basis with the donation of anatomically-shaped pieces of wood (3000), between the end of the 1st century BC and *c.* AD 70. Its use began the day after the conquest, through a coin-throwing ritual (VERCA, *c.* 50-30 BC [Gruel 2022]), thus before the actual construction of the city, which dates back to the first decades of the 1st century AD. These elements demonstrate that the Gauls already knew about the source. No remains of buildings or improvements have been found on the site and its surroundings. The variety of the organs and limbs represented by the ex-votos does not indicate any particular pathology, but rather suggests a healing practice. In addition, a lead curse tablet (a judicial curse about a private litigation) invokes the deity of the Maponos spring (Clémençon 2022: 122). Many cups and pitchers were discovered, indicating that the water was consumed (Figure 4). Just like the ex-votos, the ceramics were probably mass-produced and sold on site. The study of these objects is the subject of a collective research project examining the entire site from a new perspective, initiated by A. Wittmann (Inrap[6]).

The outskirts of the ancient city

Nowadays, this sanctuary seems exceptional from an archaeological perspective, given the extraordinary preservation of the remains due to the damp environment. Yet its prominence at the time may have been relative, in the midst of other sanctuaries springing up in this favourable geological context. Such sanctuaries may have been destroyed or are still to be unearthed. *Augustonemetum* was built on a volcanic formation (the Clermont-Ferrand mound), at an altitude of approximately 20m amid the basin. Its outskirts, long considered as a swampy area of little interest, actually offer a wealth of potential in terms of mineral resources that were exploited during Antiquity.

To the northwest, in the Fontgiève neighbourhood corresponding to the suburbs of the ancient city and currently known for its petrifying sources (hard water springs), the catchment of a source was collected in a monolithic arkose tank, completed by a rim made of marble and limestone slabs (Martinez 2021: 47-51). It was protected by a 31.5m^2 rectangular building, built during the last third of the 2nd century. Pine kegs were made on the upper floor, with capacities ranging from 0.74 to almost 6 litres. Were they used to transport or even sell mineral water? Did the water have healing properties? Was it a nymphaeum? On the western border of *Augustonemetum*, where the toponyms are highly evocative (Les Salins [derived from 'salt'], Puits Artésien ['Artesian well']), several sources, associated with Gallo-Roman ceramic deposits, were recently unearthed (D. Tourgon and Evéha, 2022 excavation of the Hôtel-Dieu 3, study ongoing). In the context of ongoing preventive archaeology, recent discoveries of especially well preserved remains, found deep and in a damp environment, have contributed greatly to reorienting urban archaeological issues in these previously neglected areas.

AQUIS CALIDIS (L. Augustin-Rolland and G. Rocque)

The municipalities of Vichy and Cusset are located in the southeast of the current Allier department, which was the northern part of the Arverni territory, at approximately 46km from the main city. They lie to the east of the Grande Limagne, on the western border of the Montagne Bourbonnaise, in the alluvial plain of the Allier River, near its confluence with the Sichon River

[6] French National Institute for Preventive Archaeological Research.

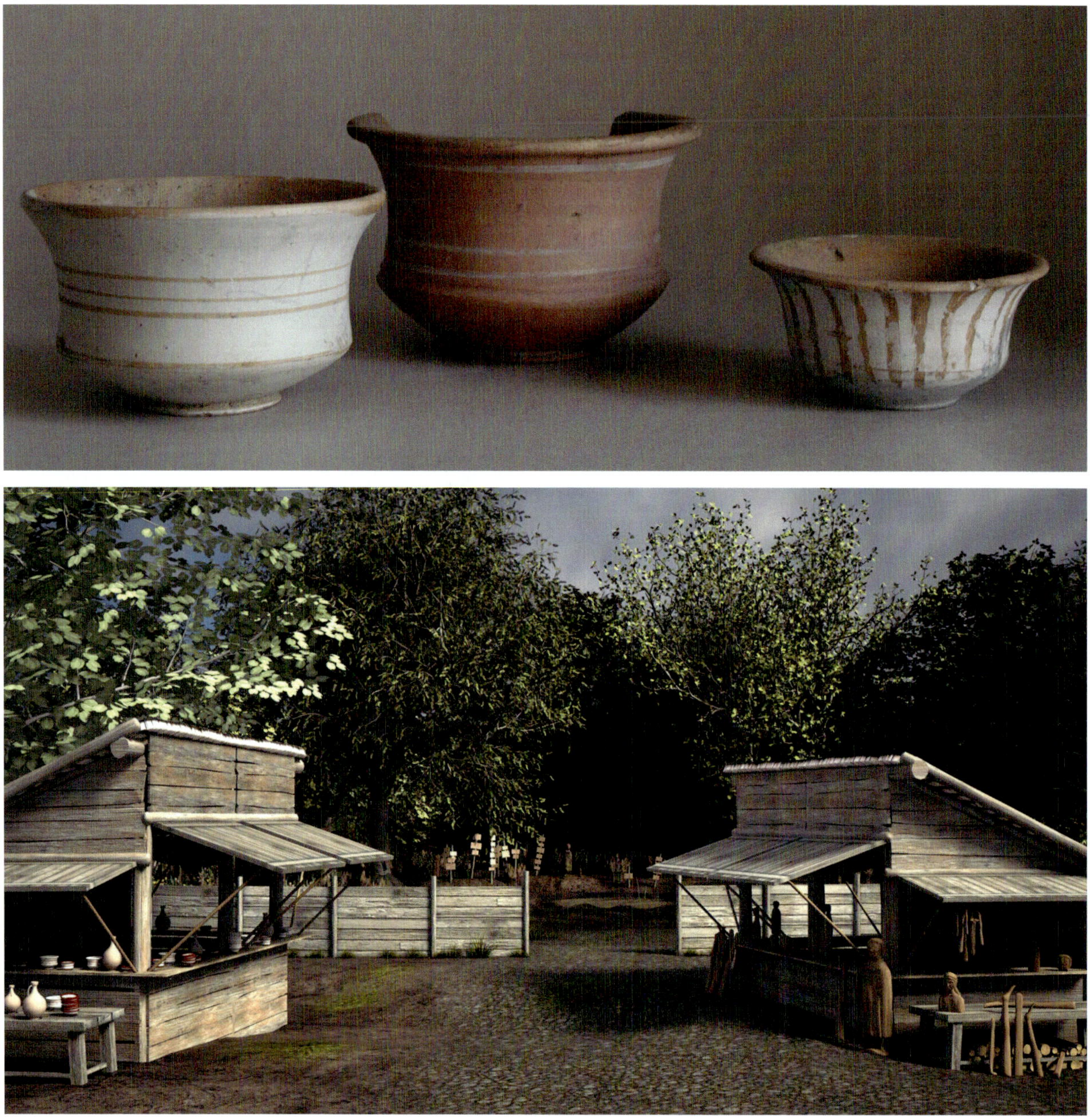

Figure 4. The Source des Roches, outdoor sanctuary excavated in 1970-71.
a: Painted cups discovered in 1968 in the Source des Roches. Photo: M. Veschambre.
b: Cups and ex-votos were probably made by craftsmen and sold in a shop near the sanctuary. 3D reproduction: Court-Jus Production. http://www.augustonemetum.fr.

which flows through Cusset from east to west, at an altitude of between 240 and 480m.

Vichy

At the dawn of the 1st century AD, the Roman city of Vichy was strategically established at the crossroads of land and fluvial transportation routes: notably, the confluence of major public roads connecting the northern part of the Arverni territory to those of neighbouring tribes – Segusiavi, Aedui, and Bituriges (Dacko 2016). This site is located on the right bank of the Allier River – called 'Elaver' by ancient writers – at a crossing of this waterway which was probably a prominent communication route to the Loire region and the Aedui and Bituriges territories. It is now quite evident that the origins of the town of Vichy can be traced back to the Roman era, given the large amount of ancient remains unearthed since the middle of the 19th century. Development began during Tiberius's reign (Figure 5), reaching an estimated maximum surface area of around fifty hectares (Corrocher 1981: 100). It was laid out around a main traffic route, going from east to west, with an area dedicated to housing

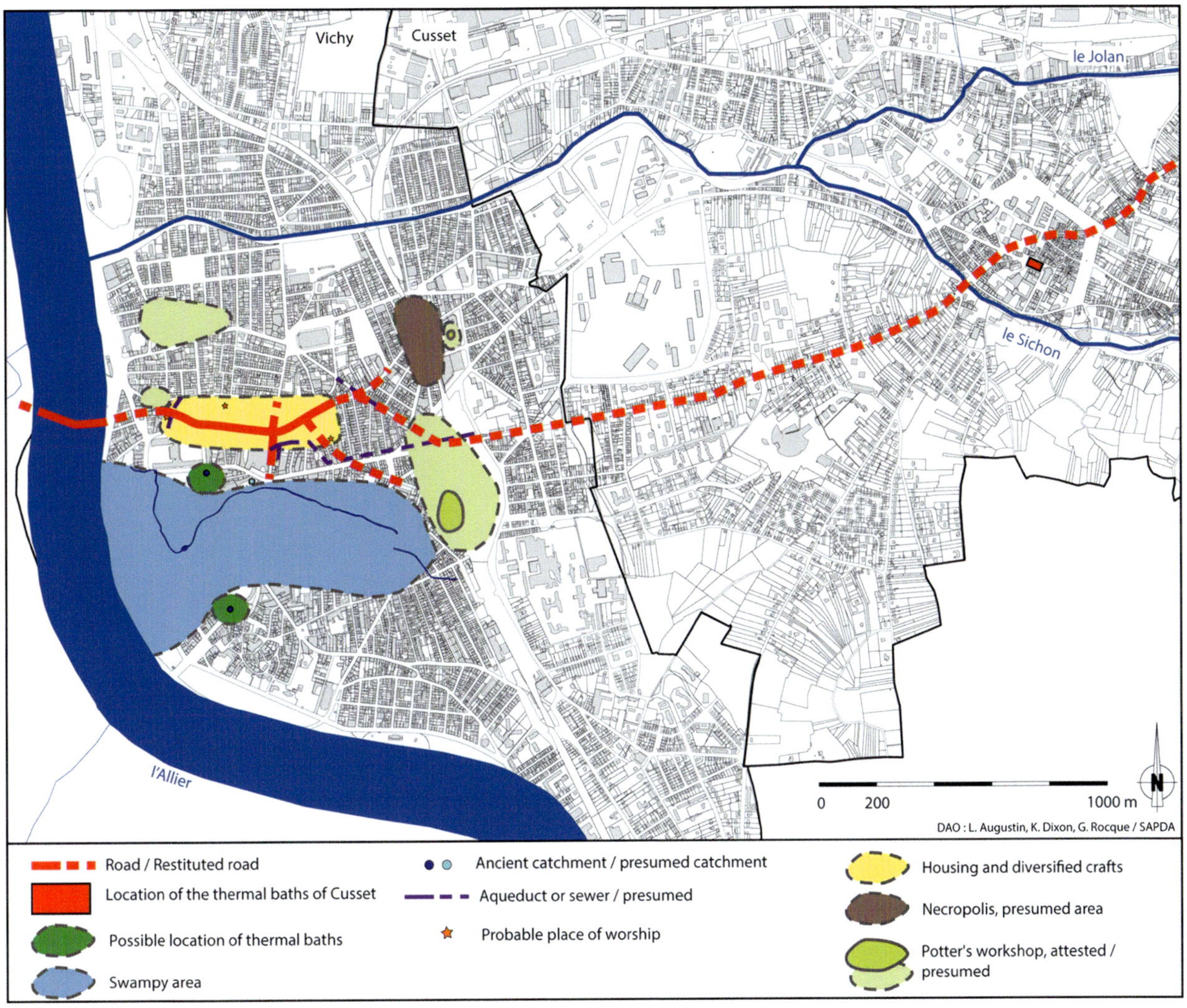

Figure 5. Connections between Vichy and Cusset. Authors: L. Augustin, K. Dixon, G. Rocque / SAPDA.

and diverse crafts on either side. There is little documentation about temples and public buildings. The presence of objects of worship and of a few elements of monumental architectural suggests their existence, but their importance and locations remain unknown. Outside the urban area, spaces devoted to the production of ceramics or to the cremation of corpses have been found.

It has also been confirmed that this particular site corresponds to one of the stops on the Peutinger Table: called '*Aquis Calidis*' ('the hot waters'), and it is represented by a vignette depicting a rectangular building with eight openings surrounding a roofless central space, suggesting the presence of a thermal area. In the heart of the town at least two natural springs have been tapped and developed during the Roman era: the Chomel (42°C) and Hôpital sources (32°C), located respectively north and south of the current Parc des Sources. These bi-carbonated, saline, carbo-gaseous waters originate from the Chaîne des Puys and head to Vichy, traveling about 50km across the Limagne plain. Vichy became known as the 'queen of spa towns', under Napoleon III and its sources are still being used today as a drinking cure for digestive and metabolic disorders.

The ancient catchments of both sources were identified at the beginning of the 1940s, during cleaning and refurbishment work, and they are still in use (Figure 6, a-b). The Chomel Gallo-Roman catchment well is made of an octagonal lining of wooden planks, held in place at the corners by stakes. The Hôpital catchment is a circular masonry well of ashlar topped with an octagonal stone base. Solid tile-concrete blocking and waterproofing were deployed around the periphery of these structures (Augustin *et al.* 2020: 132-133). Similar catchment wells have been discovered in Mont-Dore, as well as in Néris-les Bains and Bourbon-l'Archambault, in the neighbouring Bituriges territory. Inside these three resorts, the water spouted into catchment wells that were built inside the large basins before being transported to the monumental baths.

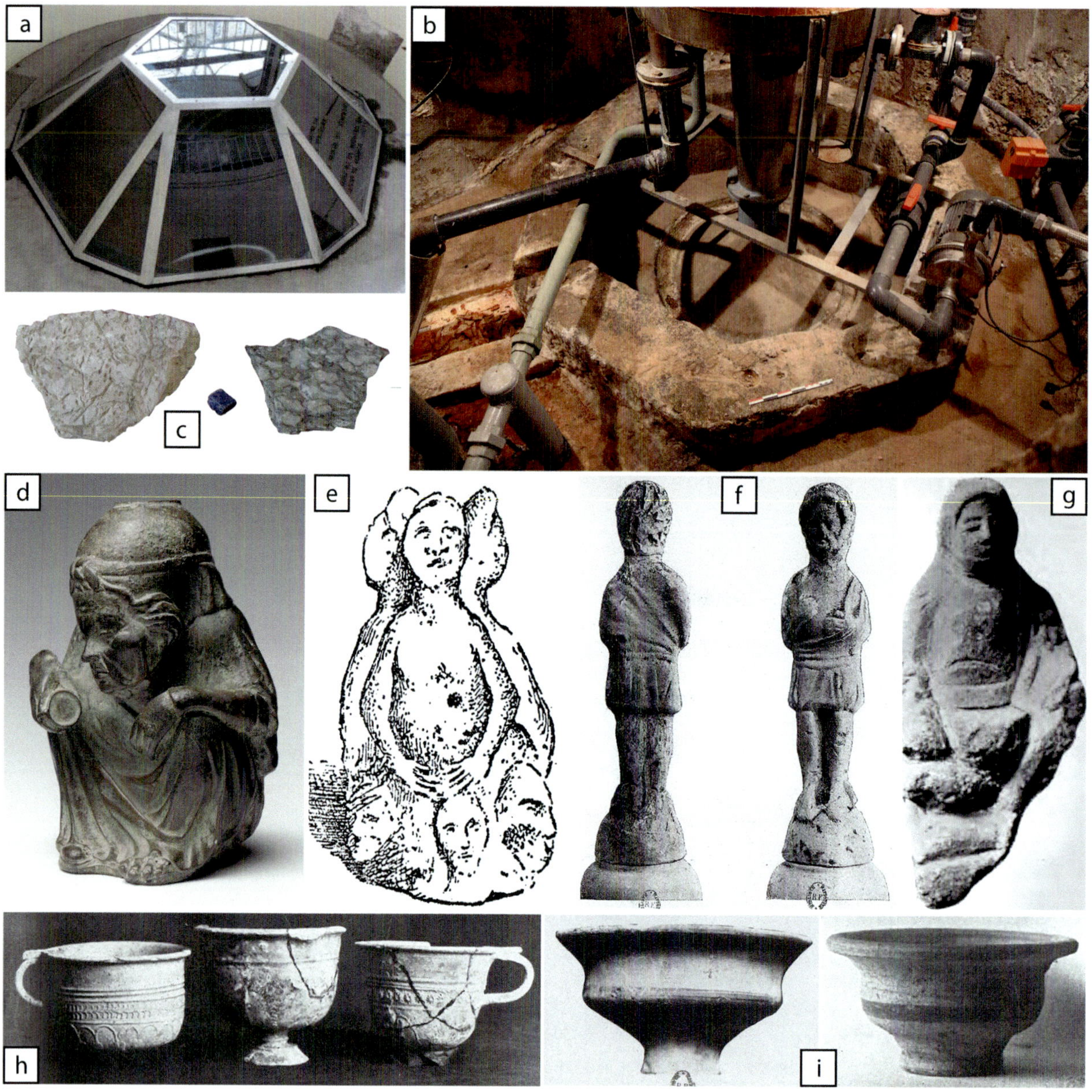

Figure 6. Vichy: remains attesting to a curative practice.
a and b: Current views of the (a) Chomel and (b) Hôpital ancient water catchments. Photos: L. Augustin, 2019.
c: Marble fragments and mosaic tesserae unearthed in 2021 near the Chomel source. Photos: S. Baraton, 2021.
d: Ex-voto, small bronze vase of the 'old rheumatic', depicting an old woman, hunched and obviously sick, dressed with a tunic and holding a cup (Musée du Louvre, Département des Antiquités grecques, étrusques et romaines, BR2936). Photo: © RMN-Grand Palais (musée du Louvre) / Hervé Lewandowski.
e: Ex-voto, drawing of a stone bas-relief depicting a woman giving birth to twins. Extracted from: Corrocher 1982: 137.
f: Ex-voto, white terra cotta figurine depicting a man with his arm in a sling. Extracted from: Mallat, Cornillon 1906: 38.
g: Ex-voto, draft of a stone statue depicting a man sitting on one leg. Extracted from: Espérandieu 1928, n° 1626.
h: Offerings, local lead-glazed cups unearthed in 1878 near the Chomel source. Extracted from: Morlet 1957: 49.
i: Offerings, small ceramic cups with carinated walls, in white slip and decorated with an ochre band discovered *c.* 1834-35 near the sources. Extracted from: Mallat, Cornillon 1906: 34; Morlet 1957: 107.

In Vichy, recent research has failed to unearth similar pools, and the way thermal waters were exploited during Antiquity remains largely unknown. However, the quest for a grand thermal complex has been the focus of research since the mid-19th century. Local scholars have repeatedly interpreted vestiges and remains as being part of public baths (elements of monumental architecture, remains of basins, marble shards...) and have put forward various hypotheses about their location, but the site of the Gallo-Roman thermal facility is still uncertain (Augustin *et al.* 2020: 61-65). Given the current state of research, two possible

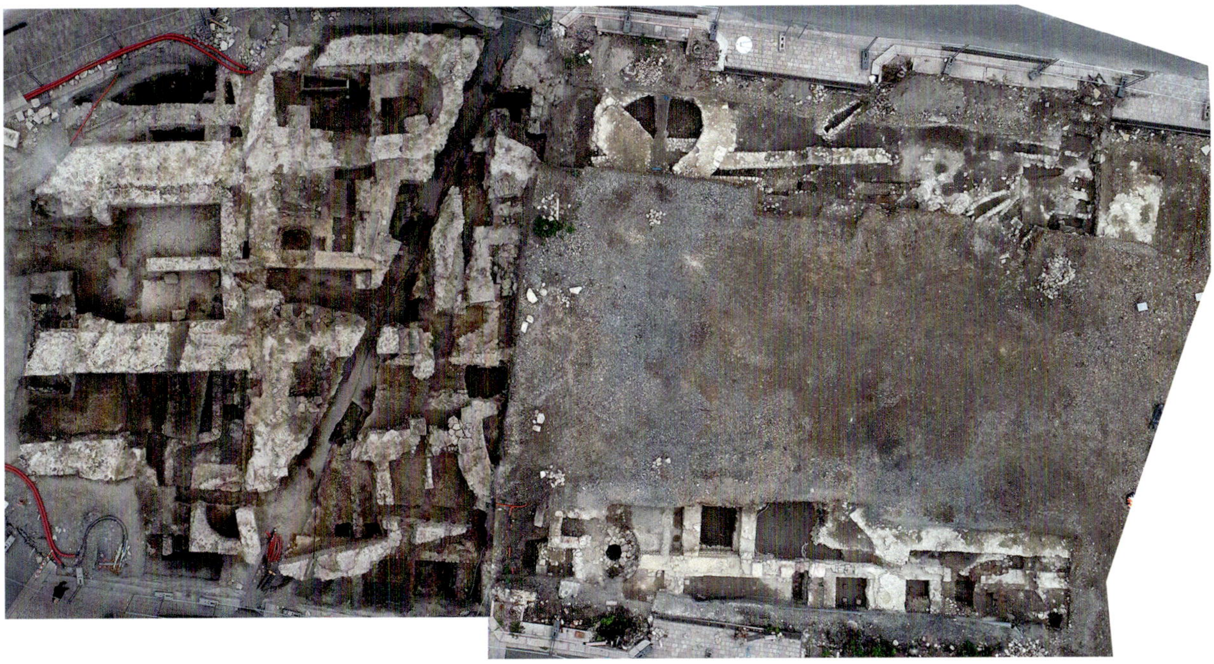

Figure 7. Cusset, aerial view of the 2018 excavation. Photo: T. Eyraud, G. Rocque / SAPDA.

sites merit further study: south of the Parc des Sources by the Hôpital source (B. Michaudel, Inrap, study in progress), and/or north of the park, near the Chomel source where basins lined with hydraulic plaster, shards of marble slabs, a tesserae of glass-paste mosaic and carbonate concretions have recently been unearthed – all associated with ancient demolition elements – (Baraton *et al.* 2021: 321) which suggests the presence of a Gallo-Roman building with a thermal or cult-related function (Figure 6, c).

The therapeutic properties of Vichy's thermal waters were clearly known during the Roman period, as suggested by the ex-votos unearthed during previous excavations (a white terracotta figurine depicting a man with his arm in a sling; a draft of a stone statue depicting a man sitting on one leg; a small bronze vase depicting an old woman, hunched and obviously sick, wearing a tunic and holding a cup; a stone bas-relief depicting a woman giving birth to twins) (Figure 6, d-g). Discoveries of drinking utensils near the sources also indicate that the waters were consumed for their curative qualities. Locally produced lead-glazed ceramic cups (form Déch. 59) were unearthed in 1878 near the Chomel spring. Dating back to the 1st century AD and encrusted with hydrothermal deposits, the cups were probably used to drink water from the source before being given as offerings. A cleaning of the sources conducted *c.* 1834-35 led to the recovery of several small ceramic cups with carinated walls, in white slip and decorated with an ochre band. Dating from the 1st and early 2nd centuries, they were probably locally made. Ancient writers agreed that these small vessels were likely used to drink thermal water before being thrown into the source as offerings (Figure 6, h-i). A significant number of similar examples were discovered near the Source des Roches in Chamalières (Romeuf and Dumontet 2000: 49-52).

Cusset

Less than 3km east of the heart of the Roman city of Vichy, the ancient settlement of Cusset remains largely unknown. Important remains were discovered in the city centre during construction works in 1992-93 (Corrocher 1999), and also in 2018 during a preventive excavation which enabled researchers to assess the size and importance of the area (Chaléat *et al.* 2021), but the remains seemed relatively isolated and no evidence of a dense habitation was found nearby (Figure 7). The 2018 excavation conducted on the Place Victor Hugo uncovered a large ancient thermal complex, with a surface of at least 730m^2, and probably extending over 2280m^2, thus 57m long and 40m wide (Figure 8). Our knowledge of the building is still too limited to fully understand how it functioned and how the bathers moved around. Five rooms at least were heated by a hypocaust system (three to the southeast and two to the northwest). One of them has a very particular layout: it has an elongated shape and its surface is at least 40m^2, and to the south it features a large exedra and could be interpreted as a caldarium, like those unearthed in Aigues-Vives (in the Gard region) and Eyguières (Bouches-du-Rhône) (Bouet 2003: 5-6, 93-94). Several cold rooms and courtyards were uncovered but remain difficult to interpret. At least one cold pool

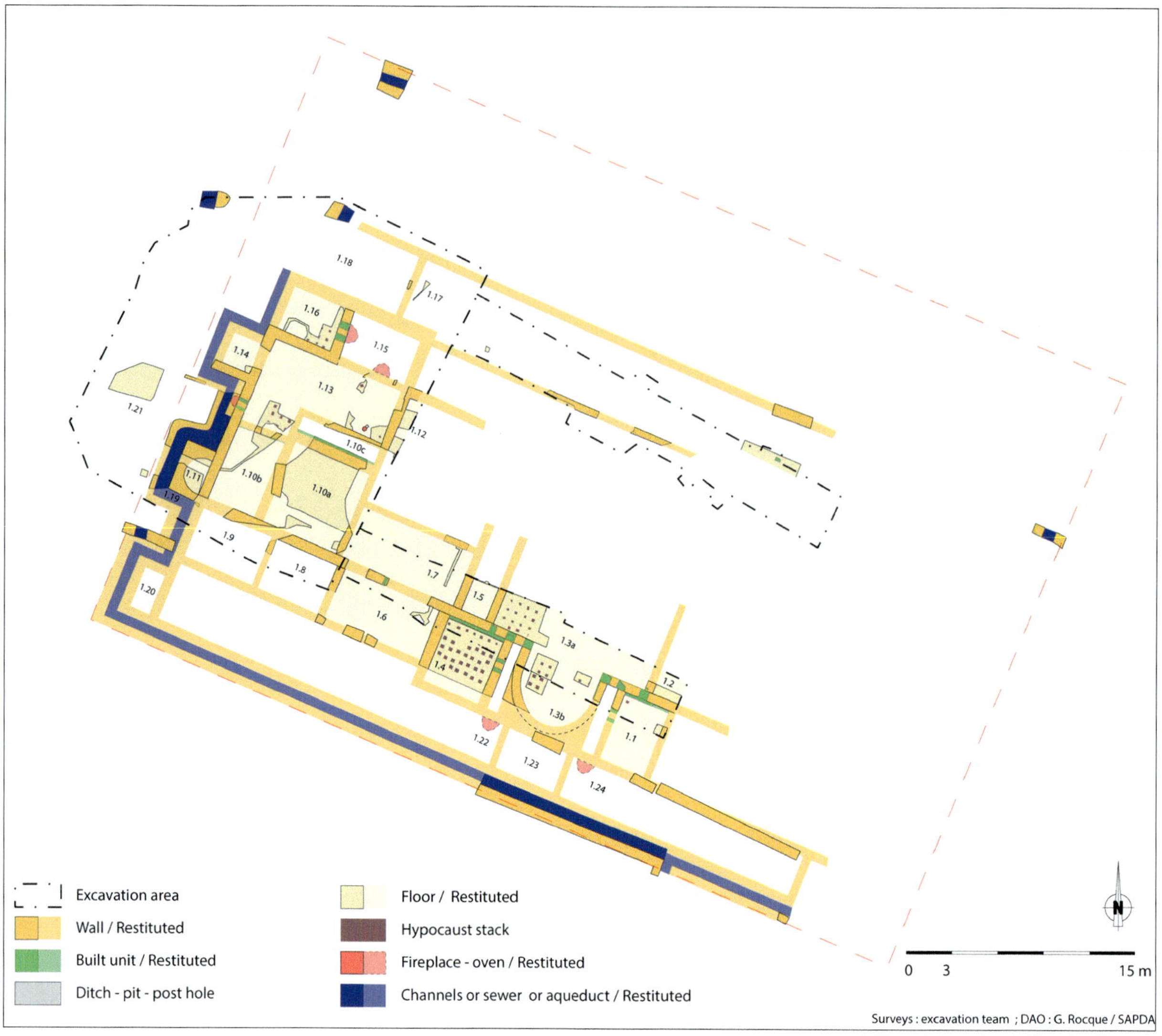

Figure 8. Cusset, general map of the building. Author: G. Rocque / SAPDA.

was adjacent to the west façade of the spas. Two other basins can be identified on the same façade, but it is not known whether they contained hot or cold water. A gutter, or a sewer, runs alongside the building's façade and permitted wastewater drainage, as well as the sanitation of the facility by collecting rainwater and water infiltrations. The origin of the waters used in this facility is still unknown,[7] but a catchment of the Vichy hot springs has already been ruled out, due to the higher topography of the spas. Besides, while numerous mineral sources are known to exist in Cusset, none seem to be really hot (they do not exceed 13.5°C) and all of them were bored in the 19th century.[8] This building was most likely a public bath, considering its size and the importance of its hot rooms. It was probably built between the Flavian dynasty and the beginning of the 2nd century – a period during which large numbers of monuments were built in Gaul – and it remained in use until the 4th-5th centuries. At the very beginning of the Early Middle-Ages, the building underwent several transformations: some hypocausts were filled in, the ancient floors of the rooms were destroyed and rebuilt, and the heating pipes were sealed. It is impossible to determine the role of this new building, which did not seem to retain its function as a spa.

Conclusion

The ancient settlements of Vichy and Cusset were connected by a road leading to Roanne (*Rodunna*), which has never been the subject of archaeological excavations, and yet its route can be reconstructed from ancient references (Fanaud 2005: 193-194) (cf. Figure 5). According to current research, an important secondary

[7] The analysis of the concrete and plaster samples collected in the pools revealed both carbonate deposits and matrix dissolution areas that can be attributed to either hydrothermal waters or waters from source rocks (Augustin *et al.* 2020: 134).

[8] Except for the Chambon source which might have naturally flowed on the banks of the Sichon River in 1818 (Surmely 2004: 315).

city emerged at Vichy in the ancient period, but no evidence of a spa has been found. In Cusset, it was quite the opposite, as a vast spa complex, probably public, seemed to be relatively isolated. Consequently, several theories can be put forward about the organisation and connection between these two entities. The spa town of *Aquis Calidis*, mentioned on the Peutinger Table may have developed around two main centres. Domestic and artisanal activities surrounding a place of worship could be organized around the thermo-mineral sources. This healing custom – connected to the quality of the water, which is still recognised today – would have been based on the drinking ritual. The public spas were probably located in Cusset, on one of the main access routes to the city. Moreover, these baths could have been used to purify travellers before they entered the place of worship. The existence of several thermal buildings can be suggested: the first in Vichy, located on the hot springs, probably had a curative function, while the second, in Cusset, would have served a more traditional, hygienic function. Finally, the idea that there were several healing spas must be kept in mind: one in Vichy, located on hot springs, and one in Cusset, connected to the cold mineral springs. Indeed, the use of cold mineral waters in healing spas was confirmed in Moingt, near the Segusiavi territory, called '*Aquæ Segetæ*' ('the water of the goddess Segeta') on the Peutinger Table.

MONT-DORE (Élise Nectoux, Bertrand Dousteyssier, Élise Fovet)

A geographical and historical overview of the site

The Mont-Dore thermal baths are located on the northern face of the Sancy massif, in the upper Dordogne valley, at an altitude of 1040m, and 30km south of Clermont-Ferrand as the crow flies. The hot springs emerge from natural cavities within the lava flow, at temperatures between 32° and 44°C. Two of the eight sources known today at the spa have been tapped since Antiquity. The healing properties of the waters – administered as baths – were attested to in the earliest written sources from the Late Middle Ages and in the Early Modern period.

The ancient monumental complex was discovered at the beginning of the 19th century, when it was destroyed to make way for the modern spas. It combines so-called 'side by side' spas – equipped with three large pools – with a temple, and both monuments are connected by a courtyard with porticos (Figure 9). Two hot spring catchments were built, and a third source probably directly supplied a hot pool.[9] Part of the architectural decoration can be traced back to the second half of the 2nd century (Dousteyssier and Nectoux 2016: 716); a detailed study is currently being conducted by a multidisciplinary team.

The ancient village that accompanied the spas is known only from the fragile remains mentioned rather anecdotally in the 19th (Bertrand 1819: 16)[10] and 20th centuries. Archaeological excavations are sorely lacking on this particular site, which is estimated to cover just a few hectares (Dousteyssier and Nectoux 2016: 718). Often mistaken (Bertrand 1823: 74-80) for the *Aquis Calidis* represented on the Peutinger Table or the *Calentes Baiæ* mentioned by Sidoine Appolinaire in his *Correspondences* (*Epist.*, V, 14), Mont-Dore cannot lay claim to these designations that must be reserved for other sites. Its ancient name is unknown, yet it should be mentioned that the village was called *Belneis* in 1315, which became 'Bains' during the Early Modern Period.

Curative uses of the waters since Antiquity

The waters are bi-carbonated, saline, carbo-gaseous and highly siliceous. These natural properties stimulate the immune system, have antiseptic and cleansing benefits for respiratory tissues, and can act as a softener for the skin and mucous membranes, as well as a vasodilator and muscular relaxant. These properties have been recognised since Antiquity. Were lung diseases and rheumatisms treated in Mont-Dore, as in the famous Baiae in the Gulf of Naples?[11] The natural phenomena associated with these springs may have also contributed to conferring virtues on the waters. In the 19th century, Dr Bertrand (1823: 106-107) noticed cycles – lasting between one and two hours – during which the waters would rapidly trigger tingling sensations, excessive sweating and faster heartbeat, forcing the clients to shorten their baths. Bertrand noticed that the phenomenon would suddenly stop when it rained, and that the flow of water produced intense gurgling as a storm approached. The presence of carbon dioxide was mentioned and considered as dangerous for the bathers who would settle inside the 'ancient-shaped' building overlooking the Bain de César source (Bertrand 1819: 10).

The thermal complex was connected to a temple through a courtyard with porticos, indicating – by its organisation – a strong link to the sacred (Aupert 1991: 186). Yet the temple was not built on a source and thus cannot be considered a water sanctuary. Moreover,

[9] It must be mentioned that Dr Bertrand (1819), who thoroughly described the remains, did not mention it.

[10] 'The new promenade lies opposite the baths, between the village and the right bank of the Dordogne River. Within the surface it occupies, we found the remains of walls, as well as a large amount of bricks. Between 0.70 or 0.80m deep, the ground was filled with shards of ancient pottery, ornamented with bas-reliefs. It should be noted that in our mountains, similar fragments are found nowhere else.' (Bertrand 1819: 16).

[11] The fashionable curative thermal treatments were condensed over a three-week period in Baiae (Oribase X 3,2).

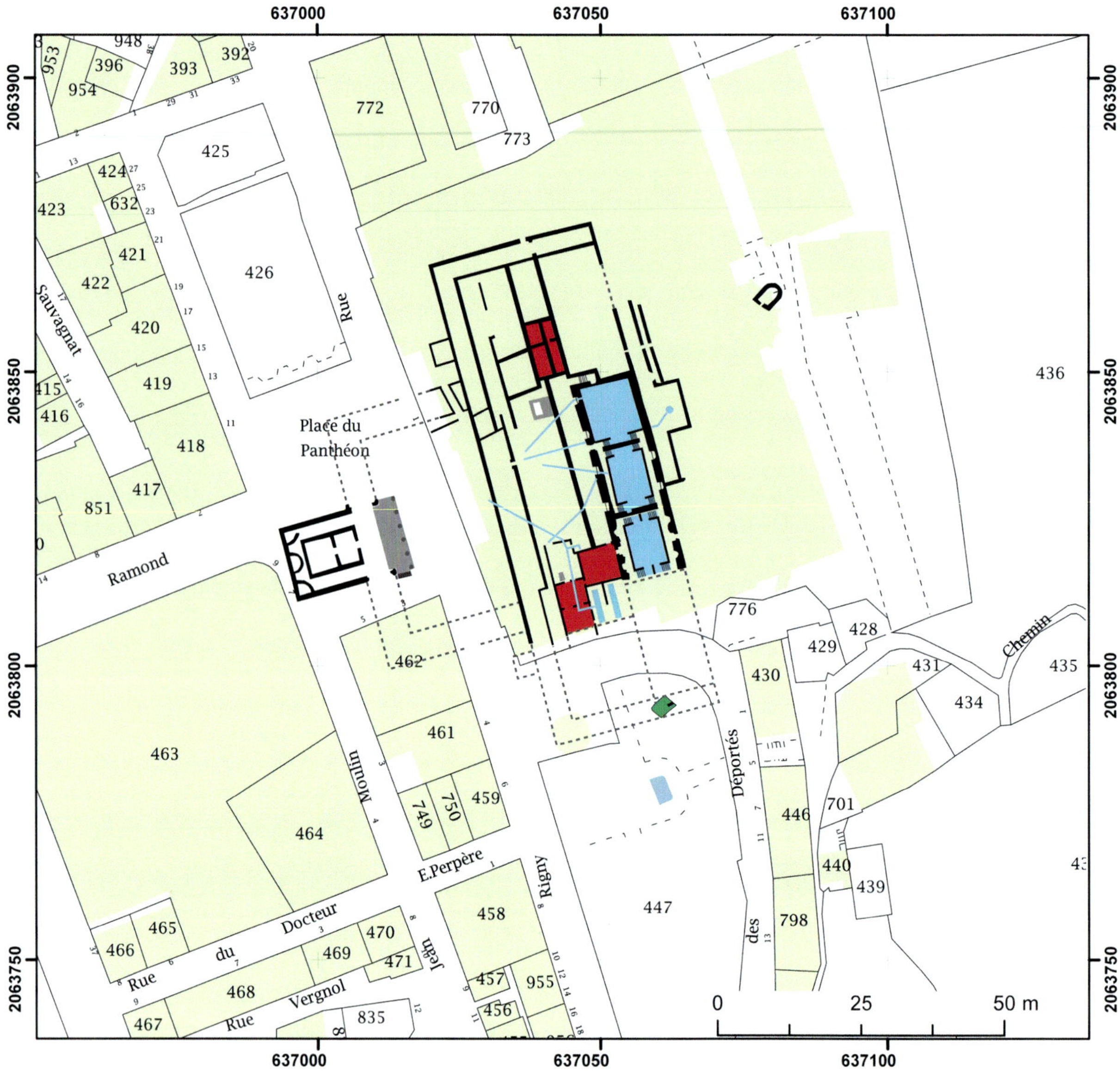

Figure 9. Mont-Dore, general map of the site. Author: B. Dousteyssier.

no ex-voto could be clearly identified on site. So, the theory formulated by Professor Landouzy, and quoted by L. Bonnard (Bonnard and Percepied 1908: 295-296), that the bust known as the 'Old Roman' was a depiction of a man suffering from an emphysematous bronchial syndrome, must be dismissed (Nectoux, Dousteyssier 2021: 344-345). However, the goddess Sianna – to whom a private individual (Iulia Severa) offered an altar – was a helpful deity, undoubtedly linked to the springs (Rémy, Provost 1997: *ILA Arvernes* 43). The excavation of the temple unearthed a group of statue fragments evoking Jupiter: an eagle and a bust that can be readily associated with a horse leg, thus depicting an anguiped rider, a widespread representation in the Arverni territory (Blanchard 2015). Jupiter – often represented in spas (Bonnard and Percepied 1908: 170-171) – was also named on silver votive plaques discovered in Vichy (he was locally nicknamed Sabasius [Rémy and Provost 1997: *ILA Arvernes* 82-83; Augustin 2021]).

The waters were used for immersion, as confirmed by the presence of baths (Duran-Lefebvre's map, 1926) and above all by the structure of the pools: two steps were placed along the bottom of the long sides of the northern oriented hot pools (Bertrand 1819: 19).[12] Here, we agree with H. Broise (2015: 55), who suggests the steps had a curative function, to accommodate seated sessions. There is no evidence to date concerning the ingestion of these waters.[13] We are fully aware that this is an *argumentum a silentio*, but no cups have been unearthed at Mont-Dore, while hundreds of them were

[12] 'Two stone benches, arranged in tiers, lined both of the largest sides' (Bertrand 1819: 19).

[13] Drinking is mentioned in the Early Modern Period.

found at the Source des Roches site in Chamalières (Romeuf and Dumontet 2000: 49-52).[14]

Conclusion

The monumental complex at Mont-Dore is located in what appears to be a very isolated site with a small urban area. It seems that the spas gave birth to the town, not the opposite. Isolated in the mountains and absent from the Peutinger Table – maybe because of its distance from major communication arteries – the site is equipped nonetheless with extensive roadworks[15] (work in progress, É. Fovet), which indicates its importance in the Arverni territory. Given the mountain[16] climate and the isolation of the site, it is possible that the spas were used on a seasonal basis, serving the dual purposes of therapy[17] and pilgrimage. It must not be forgotten that the seasonality of the thermal cures is well documented in the sources by Herodotus and Oribasius (Guérin-Beauvois 2015: 81).

GENERAL OVERVIEW

The three cases presented here cover the same historiographical reality (three 19th century thermal spas of ancient origin, subject to partial and brief excavations), but highlight diverse archaeological realities, regarding both how mineral waters were used and how they were exploited. Some sources had little infrastructure but were highly frequented (such as the Source des Roches in Chamalières), others were tapped for a function that is difficult to identify (in Vichy for example), and others still were developed into thermal buildings (Royat, Mont-Dore, and perhaps Cusset). Thus, the practice of curative balneology, in its strict definition (using hot mineral waters and dedicated facilities) – so essential from the perspective of 19th-century archaeologists – is not invariable indeed, considering the natural potential of the area.

If we exclude from our analysis the healing sanctuaries (such as the Source de Font-de-vie in Cohen, Cantal), where ex-votos were discovered near the water catchments, curative balneology can be described according to three forms:

- prolonged immersion in hot water, in thermal pools equipped with rows of seats (Broise 2015: 55), as at Mont-Dore and the Royat spas;[18]
- the practice of drinking mineral waters, suggested[19] by the presence of drinking cups (small bowls and cups, anthropomorphic bronze cups) near the sources, as was the case in Vichy-Cusset and at the Source des Roches in Chamalières.
- the offering of ex-votos, as at the Source des Roches and in Vichy.

Comparing these three cases, chosen for their monumental facilities, enables us to think about the form of the urban developments, triggered by the presence of springs in this territory. Two of the thermal facilities studied were built near a large urban area (a capital or a 'lesser' city). Thus, the only site mentioned on the Peutinger Table with an evocative name, *Aquis Calidis* (Vichy-Cusset), corresponds to a complex site, comprising both an urban centre with thermo-mineral water catchments (for a curative use) and monumental public baths, far from the centre of the city, the function of which is still to be deciphered. This site benefits from a geographical situation favourable to urban development, located between the Limagne plain and the Montagne Bourbonnaise, with crossroads and a bridge to cross the Allier River. In addition, numerous activities have been documented there, particularly connected to artisanal crafts. *Augustonemetum* featured a healing thermal centre with baths and a curative source sanctuary – built earlier – surrounded by sacred woods (Prat and Cabanis 2006-07). The remains unearthed nearby suggest the presence of a settlement connected to the spas and built very close to the city centre, an unusual urban feature. Similar outlying spa complexes, close to a town, were discovered in nearby territories, for example in Moingt (Loire) and in Évaux-les-Bains (Creuse). However, the third site studied, Mont-Dore, corresponds to an isolated healing spa, connected to the city by a route which was probably built to serve this site located at the end of a deep valley.[20] The isolation, mountainous climate, as well as the relatively small size of the settlement surrounding the facility suggest that it operated on a seasonal basis (pilgrimage[21] / curative therapy? [22]).

[14] This curative source was abundantly used but it did not lead to the construction of a thermal building.

[15] The importance of the site was studied in the Early Modern Era. One of the precursors of the Auvergnat balneology, the last *intendant* C. de Chazerat (1728-1824), wanted to establish a thermal facility in Mont-Dore. He started by 'opening' a convenient route.

[16] In the 17th century, J. Banc (1605) was indeed surprised to find Roman buildings in 'such a harsh, unpleasant and vexing country'.

[17] P. Aupert (1991: 186) identified the whole Mont-Dore infrastructure as healing spas.

[18] The same apparatus was also present in other recently studied thermal facilities, for example in Chassenon (Doulan *et al.* 2015: 374-376).

[19] Vitruvius and Pliny mentioned this healing practice, as well as immersion in hot springs (Pliny, *Histoire Naturelle*, 31, 9; Vitruvius, 8, 3, 4).

[20] The results of a research program currently underway will provide more detailed information on this subject.

[21] A pilgrimage is strongly indicated between *Augustonemetum* and the Temple of Mercury (at the summit of the Puy de Dôme). Is there a similar phenomenon at the Mont-Dore site?

[22] P. Leveau (2007: 284) discusses the urban forms of curative spas.

The significance of mineral waters in the organisation of the territory can be addressed through the prism of architectural finery. The architectural complexes were part of the monumentalising of the Gallic territories, which demonstrates the importance of mineral waters to the Arverni elite.[23] The chronology of the sites' usage is still to be clarified, especially the phases of abandonment (which is still under study). The evolution of practices can subsequently be approached with greater certainty.

In this way, the study of Arverni balneology – so prominent within the regional historiography – is being re-examined. The exchange of perspectives in this initial collective overview will provide food for thought and open up new avenues of research in the years to come.

Bibliography

Augustin, L., G. Torrent, C. Merciecca, F. Donnadieu, P. Labazuy and B. Carton 2020. Parc des Sources, square de l'Hôpital et square Général-Leclerc. Recherches sur les structures thermales antiques et leur environnement géologique (Vichy, Allier, Auvergne-Rhône-Alpes). Unpublished report, Service régional de l'archéologie d'Auvergne-Rhône-Alpes.

Augustin, L. 2021. Les lamelles votives: un temple de Jupiter Sabasios à Vichy?, in P. Bet and B. Dousteyssier (eds) Éclats arvernes. Fragments archéologiques (*Ier-Ve s. apr. J.-C.). Tome 2*: 226-233. Clermont-Ferrand: Presses universitaires Blaise-Pascal.

Aupert, P. 1991. Les thermes comme lieux de cultes, in *Les thermes romains. Actes de la table ronde organisée par l'École française de Rome, 11-12 novembre 1988* (EFR 142): 185-192. Rome: École Française de Rome.

Aupert, P. 2012. Eau et religion, in J.P. Bost (ed.) *L'eau: usages, risques et représentations dans le Sud-Ouest de la Gaule et le Nord de la péninsule Ibérique, de la fin de l'âge du Fer à l'Antiquité tardive (IIe s. a.C.-VIe s. p.C.)* (*Aquitania*, suppl. 21): 293-321. Bordeaux: Fédération Aquitania.

Banc, J. 1605. *La mémoire renouvelée des merveilles des eaux naturelles en faveur de nos nymphes françaises et des malades qui ont recours à leur emploi salutaire.* Paris: Sevestre.

Baraton, S., L. Augustin, M. Bandiera, M. Duriez, L. Fleury, R. Guillon, M. Labalme, C. Roger and G. Torrent 2021. Vichy, Parc des Sources (03.310, Allier, Auvergne). Des occupations romaines aux thermes du XXe s., un diagnostic au cœur de l'histoire thermale vichyssoise. Unpublished report, Service régional de l'archéologie d'Auvergne-Rhône-Alpes.

Belleforest, F. 1575. *La cosmographie universelle de tout le monde.* Paris: chez N. Chesneau/chez M. Sonnius.

Bertrand, M. 1819. *Mémoire sur l'établissement thermal du Mont-D'Or et les antiquités que l'on vient d'y découvrir.* Clermont-Ferrand: Landriot.

Bertrand, M. 1823. *Recherches sur les propriétés physiques, chimiques et médicinales des eaux du Mont D'Or.* Clermont-Ferrand: impr. Thibaud-Landriot.

Blanchard, F. 2015. *Jupiter dans les Gaules et les Germanies: du Capitole au cavalier à l'anguipède.* Rennes: Presses universitaires de Rennes.

Bonnard, L. and É. Percepied 1908. *La Gaule thermale. Sources et stations thermales et minérales de la Gaule à l'époque romaine.* Paris: Plon.

Bouet, A. 2003. *Les thermes privés et publics en Gaule Narbonnaise. Volume II Catalogue.* Rome: École Française de Rome.

Broise, H. 2015. Thermes « classiques » et thermes « curatifs ». Réflexion sur l'architecture et l'organisation interne des thermes utilisant l'eau des sources thermales chaudes durant l'Antiquité, in J. Scheid, M. Nicoud, D. Boisseuil and J. Coste (eds) *Le thermalisme. Approches historiques et archéologiques d'un phénomène culturel et médical*: 45-63. Paris: CNRS éditions.

Chaléat, F., C. Favart and G. Rocque 2021. Cusset, place Victor Hugo. Évolution d'une place de centre-ville des périodes antiques à contemporaine. *Revue Archéologique de l'Allier* 2: 127-153.

Clémençon, B. 2022. Témoignage de la vie religieuse, in H. Dartevelle (ed.) *Augustonemetum, Atlas topographique de Clermont-Ferrand*: 115-126. Gollion: Infolio.

Corrocher, J. 1981. *Vichy antique.* Clermont-Ferrand: Institut d'Études du Massif central.

Corrocher, J. 1982. Les eaux thermales de Vichy dans l'Antiquité. *Revue archéologique du Centre de la France* 21, 2: 131-144.

Corrocher, J. 1999. *La place Victor-Hugo à Cusset: haut lieu de mémoire (Ier-XIXe s.).* Charroux-en-Bourbonnais: ECB éd./Les Amis du Vieux Cusset.

Dacko, M. 2016. Circuler dans le Massif central à l'époque romaine. Réseaux, infrastructures et équipements routiers. Le cas des cités arverne et vellave. Unpublished PhD dissertation, University of Clermont-Ferrand.

Dartevelle, H. 2022a. *Augustonemetum, Atlas topographique de Clermont-Ferrand.* Gollion: Infolio.

Dartevelle, H. 2022b. *Augustonemetum*, genèse et évolution d'une capitale, in H. Dartevelle (ed.) *Augustonemetum, Atlas topographique de Clermont-Ferrand*: 466-493. Gollion: Infolio.

Desforges, É., G. Fournier, P.F. Fournier, J.J. Hatt and F. Imberdis 1970. *Nouvelles recherches sur les origines de Clermont-Ferrand.* Clermont-Ferrand: Institut d'Études du Massif central.

Doulan, C., D. Hourcade, L. Laüt and G. Rocque 2015. Du sanctuaire rural à l'agglomération, relecture des vestiges de Cassinomagus (Chassenon, Charente), in T. Dechezleprêtre, K. Gruel and M. Joly (eds)

[23] The Arverni epigraphic record does not provide any information about evergetism.

Agglomérations et sanctuaires. Réflexions à partir de l'exemple de Grand. Actes du colloque de Grand, 20 au 23 octobre 2011 (Grand, Archéologie et territoire 2): 365-386. Epinal: CG Vosges.

Dousteyssier, B. and É. Nectoux 2016. Bâtiments publics monumentaux gallo-romains au fond d'une vallée « perdue » de l'Auvergne: Le Mont-Dore (Puy-de-Dôme), in A. Bouet (ed.) *Monumental! La monumentalisation des villes d'Aquitaine et de l'Hispanie septentrionale durant le Haut-Empire. Actes du colloque de Villeneuve-sur-Lot, 10 au 12 septembre 2015* (*Aquitania*, suppl. 37): 693-721. Bordeaux: Fédération Aquitania.

Espérandieu, É. 1928. *Recueil général des bas-reliefs de la Gaule romaine, II Aquitaine*. Paris: Imprimerie nationale.

Fanaud, L. 2005. *Voies romaines et vieux chemins en Bourbonnais*. Moulins: Les Imprimeries réunies.

González Soutelo, S. 2012. Los establecimientos de aguas mineromedicinales en el mundo romano. Un modelo de estudio aplicado al NW de la Península Ibérica, in J.P. Bost (ed.) *L'eau: usages, risques et représentations dans le Sud-Ouest de la Gaule et le Nord de la péninsule Ibérique, de la fin de l'âge du Fer à l'Antiquité tardive (IIe s. a.C.-VIe s. p.C.)* (*Aquitania*, suppl. 21): 321-332. Bordeaux: Fédération Aquitania.

Gruel, C. 2022. Les monnaies des fouilles de la Source des Roches à Chamalières, in H. Dartevelle (ed.) *Augustonemetum, Atlas topographique de Clermont-Ferrand*: 150-151. Gollion: Infolio.

Guérin-Beauvois, M. 2015. *Le thermalisme romain en Italie. Aspects sociaux et culturels aux deux premiers siècles de l'Empire*. Rome: École Française de Rome.

Leveau, P. 2007. Aix-les-Bains et son tombeau-temple: « ruralité » et « urbanité » d'un *vicus* allobroge. *Gallia* 64: 279-287.

Mallat, A. and J. Cornillon 1906. *Histoire des eaux minérales de Vichy*, I, 1-2. Paris: Steinheil.

Martinez, D. 2021. *Un quartier de frange urbaine en milieu humide (IIe-XVe s): les fouilles de la rue Fontgiève à Clermont-Ferrand (Puy-de-Dôme)*. Lyon: Alpara/DARA.

Morlet, A. 1957. *Vichy gallo-romain*. Mâcon: Buguet-Comptour.

Nectoux, É. and B. Dousteyssier 2021. À propos d'un buste antique découvert au XIXe s. au Mont-Dore, in P. Bet and B. Dousteyssier (eds) Éclats arvernes. Fragments archéologiques (*Ier-Ve s. apr. J.-C.). Tome 2*: 344-345. Clermont-Ferrand: Presses universitaires Blaise-Pascal.

Petit, A. 1884. *Recherches sur la découverte à Royat des substructions d'un établissement thermal gallo-romain*. Clermont-Ferrand: impr. Thibaud.

Prat, B. and M. Cabanis 2006-07. Apports de l'archéobotanique à la compréhension de la Source des Roches, Chamalières (Puy-de-Dôme). *Revue archéologique du Centre de la France* 45-46, put online on 8 April 2008, viewed 25 August 2023, < http://journals.openedition.org/racf/663>.

Rémy, B. and M. Provost 1997. *Inscriptions Latines d'Aquitaine (ILA), Arvernes*. Bordeaux: Ausonius Éditions.

Romeuf, A.M. and M. Dumontet 2000. *Les ex-votos gallo-romains de Chamalières (Puy-de-Dôme). Bois sculptés de la source des Roches*. Paris: Maison des Sciences de l'Homme (DAF, 82).

Scheid, J. 1991. Sanctuaires et thermes sous l'empire, in *Les thermes romains. Actes de la table ronde organisée par l'École française de Rome, 11-12 novembre 1988* (EFR 142): 205-216. Rome: École Française de Rome.

Surmely, F. 2004. *Les sources minérales oubliées du Massif central*. Olliergues: Éd. de La Montmarie.

Thébert, Y. 2003. *Thermes romains d'Afrique du Nord et leur contexte méditerranéen. Études d'histoire et d'archéologie*. Rome: École Française de Rome.

Vallat, P. and C. Le Barrier 2022. Feuille 39, Thermes de Royat-Chamalières, in H. Dartevelle (ed.) *Augustonemetum, Atlas topographique de Clermont-Ferrand*: 161-173. Gollion: Infolio.

Website

Augustonemetum. L'agglomération de Clermont-Ferrand et la ville antique, 2009-2023, H. Dartevelle (ed.), ministère de la Culture, viewed 25 August 2023, <http://www.augustonemetum.fr>.

Nunc Baias petamus: A Visit to the Roman Elite Spa Town from an Archaeological Perspective

Matthias NIEBERLE
Universität zu Köln, Archäologisches Institut, Albertus-Magnus-Platz 1, 50931 Köln.
nieberlematthias@gmail.com

Abstract: In this article the famous and well-known spa and health resort of Baiae is examined in light of the archaeological evidence. The numerous advantages of the coastal strip, which contributed to Baiae's outstanding position in comparison with other spa and health resorts, are revealed. Particularly striking are the enormous infrastructural measures established in the Augustan period, which are also critically questioned for the first time. Thanks to these measures, Baiae had an optimal infrastructure, which ensured the reputation and importance of the place in the long term.

Keywords: *Baiae*, Bathing, Roman elite, Otium, Infrastructures.

Introduction

Ancient Baiae was recognised in a coastal strip located about 17km west of Naples in the Phlegraean Fields (Figure 1). This region was already aptly named "the burning fields" in antiquity because of the numerous volcanic craters, such as the still active Solfatara volcano to the west of Pozzuoli, which characterise the landscape. Indeed, the bay of Baiae was formed from a volcano that erupted around 7000 BC. During this eruption, a large part of the eastern half of the volcano was blasted off. Over time, a lake, *Baianus lacus,* formed in the former crater centre (Döring 2012: 28 and 112).

The region's volcanism created not only a scenically spectacular and fertile region with numerous natural bays that could be used as landing sites, but also produced thermal springs and natural hot vapours, known as fumaroles. In addition, the volcanic tuff makes an excellent building material. The rock is easy to quarry, but also load-bearing, making tunnel constructions easily feasible.[1]

Today, the bay of ancient Baiae is framed by the Epitaffio hill in the north and the mighty Castello Aragonese in the south.[2] In the centre is the tranquil village of Baiae with a shipyard and a small fishing and yacht harbour (Figure 2). Here, between the 1940s and the 1960s, a complex landscape of buildings was uncovered, bearing witness to the remarkable Roman past and the once dense settlement of the bay (Borriello and D'Ambrosio 1979: 35-98). The area of about four hectares was opened to the public as the *Parco archeologico delle Terme di Baia* immediately after the end of the excavation work in the 1960s.[3] In addition, thanks to underwater archaeological surveys and excavations, a rich archaeological heritage has been documented underwater, including villas, *tabernae*, bath buildings and other structures.[4] Furthermore, there are numerous other sites distributed over the area investigated by the author, which also impressively reflect the former importance of the coastal strip in Roman times (figure 3).[5]

The bay of Baiae was situated in an area of Greek influence. The city of Kyme, founded by Greek settlers around 750 BC, was only about four kilometres north of the coastal strip. To the east of the bay was Puteoli, the former Dikaiarcheia. Again, further east followed Parthenope and the new foundation of Neapolis, today's Naples (Döring 2012: 14, 17, 67-72). Apart from that, however, the coastal strip was insignificant and there is no evidence of a relevant pre-Roman settlement.

This situation only changed during the conflict between Rome and Carthage. The Gulf of Naples and the Gulf of Puteoli became the focus of Rome's attention because

[1] This is demonstrated by the numerous Roman tunnel constructions in the Phlegraean Fields; cf. Döring 2012: 55-60 (Crypta Neapolitana), 64 (Grotta di Seiano), 96-100 (Grotta della Sibilla, Galleria Scalandrone and Grotta Cocceio), 104-108 (Crypta Romana, Antro della Sibilla), 109 (Tunnel of Baiae).

[2] The Castello Aragonese today houses the Museum of the Antiquities of the Phlegraean Fields, which is well worth seeing. Cf. Miniero 2006: 45-65.

[3] The terrain formed the focus of the author's dissertation work, entitled "Baiae. Genesis, use and function of a Roman spa and health resort" and completed at the end of 2022. Various findings from this doctoral research have already been published: Nieberle 2016; Nieberle *et al.* 2016; Nieberle *et al.* 2017; Nieberle and Oprée 2018; Nieberle 2020; Nieberle 2023 (forthcoming).

[4] Due to the volcanic bradyseism (the generally slow acyclic raising and lowering of the coast) the Roman ground level is about 6-14 m below the present ground level Since 2002, most of the submerged areas of ancient Baiae have been protected as an underwater archaeological park, cf. e.g. Di Fraia 2019: 74f.

[5] The area studied by the author extended from the *Fondi di Baia* to Lake Avernus and also included the northern slope of Lucrine Lake. In total, the study area covered about 4.6 km2 and 125 sites.

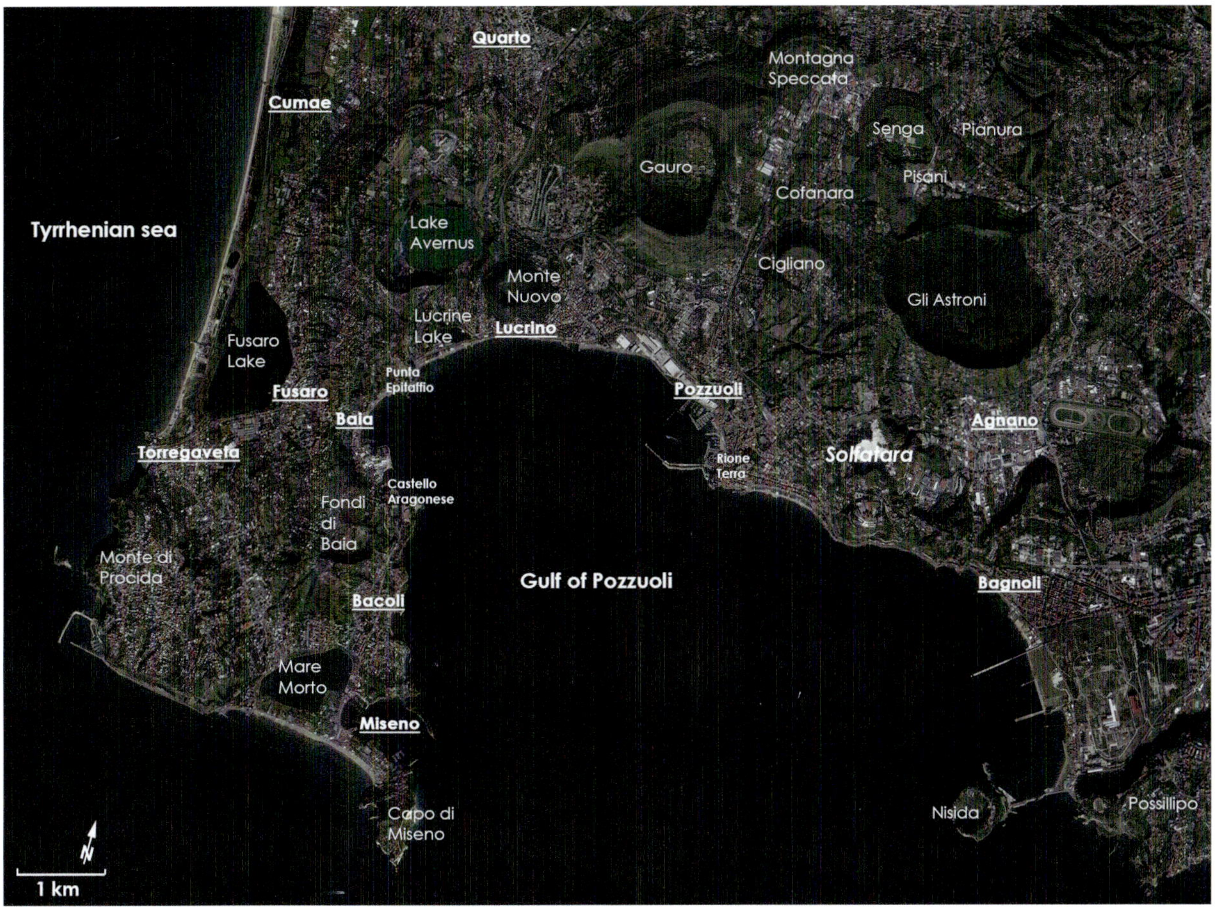

Figure 1. Google satellite image of the Phlegraean Fields with the main towns and volcanoes (Google Earth, November 2015, edited by author).

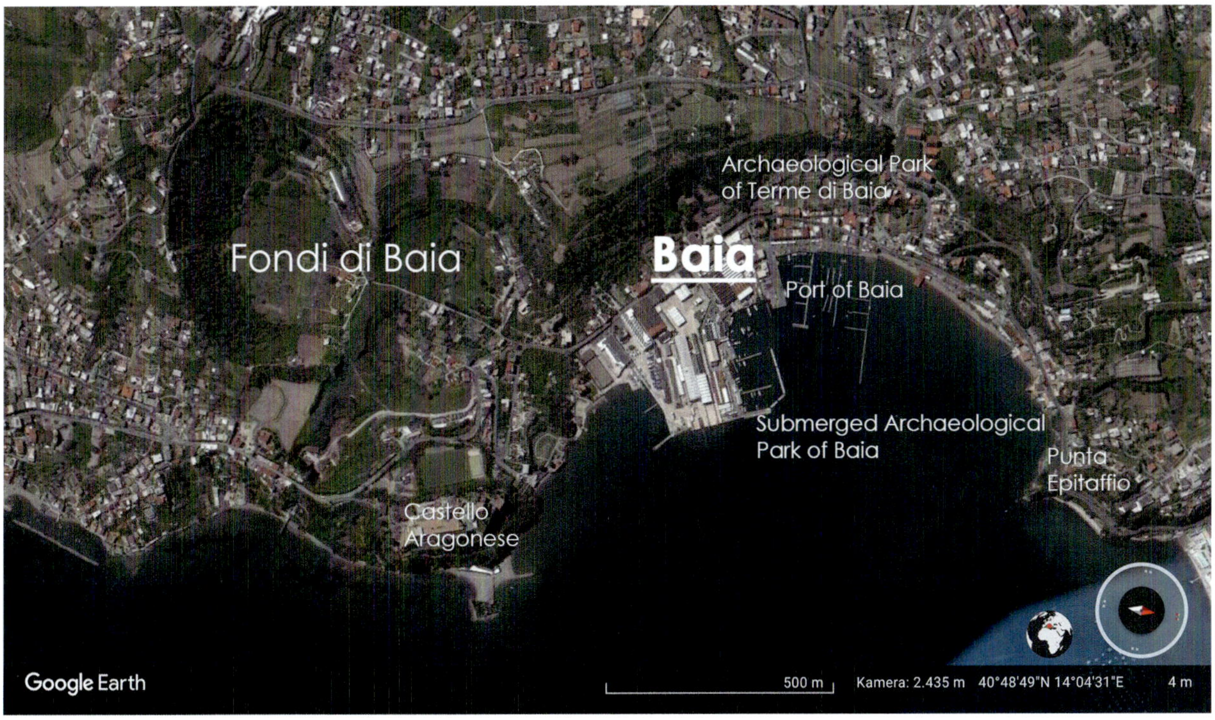

Figure 2. Google Earth image of the bay of Baiae (Google Earth, November 2022, edited by author).

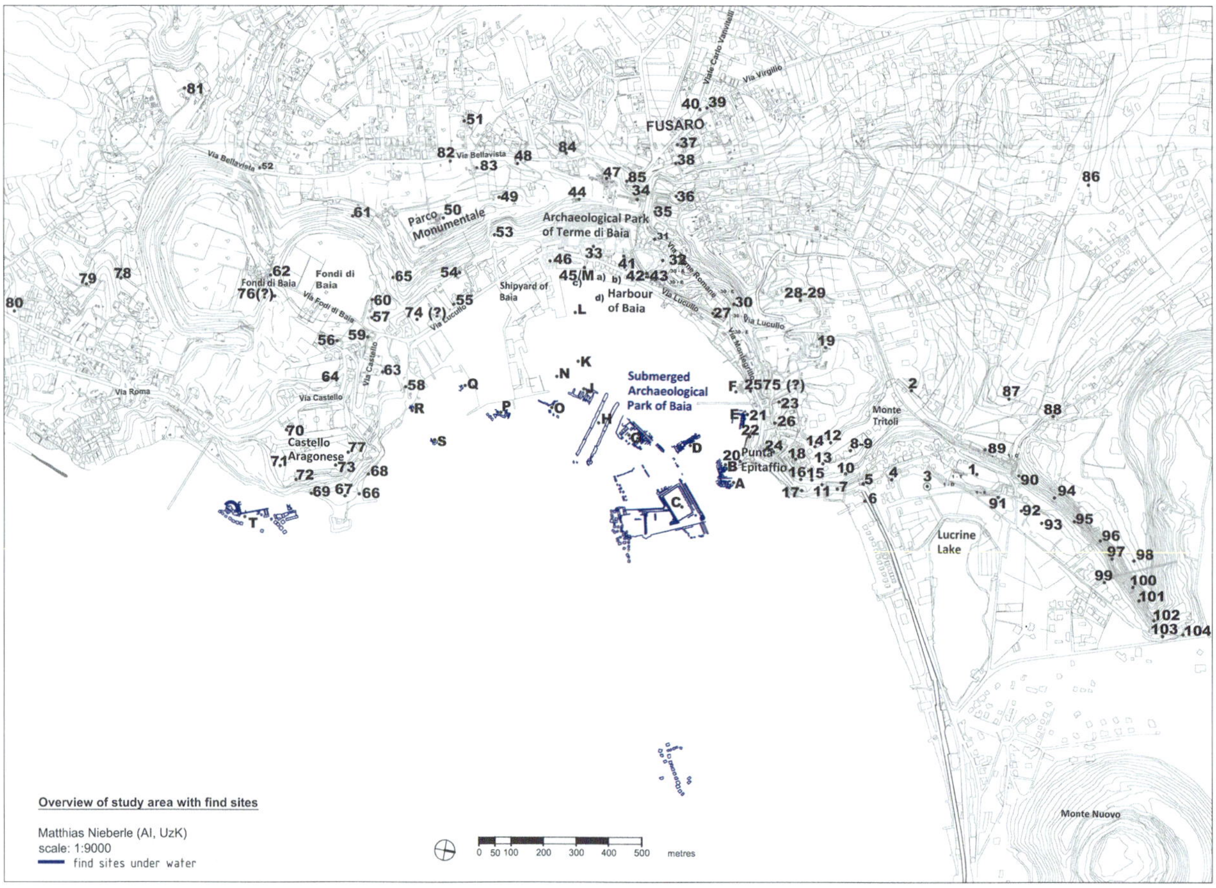

Figure 3. Localization of archaeological features in the study area (author)

of their strategic location and economic importance. In order to secure the Gulf region, the port city of Puteoli was founded in 194 BC. Due to various favourable factors and tax advantages, this new foundation became Rome's main supply port as early as the 1st century BC (Jaschke 2010: 12-15, 263). As a result, the Roman nobility was looking for suitable locations for *otium* villas in the vicinity of this new overseas port and economic centre. Plots of useable land were divided up on the slopes of the Lucrine Lake, near Misenum and directly in the bay of Baiae, cf. Figure 1. The local volcanic rock, which was ideally suited for this purpose, was used in the construction of the villas.

The initial development of the bay

The earliest wall features in Baiae are dated to around the middle of the 2nd century BC and are interpreted as the remains of these villa complexes.[6] Based on the distribution of the features, the first building development of Baiae seems to have been limited to the crater rim and the outside of the crater. There were sufficient usable areas surrounding the villas here for agricultural production (Figure 4). Because of the distribution of the wall features and the postulated usable areas, it is assumed that strategic considerations and agricultural production still played a role with regard to the location and spread of the villas. Despite the suggested rustic areas, it is assumed that the villas were already *villae expolitae*, i.e. very luxurious villas. This is based not so much on the archaeological evidence (only a few indicators of this type of luxury can be found in the archaeological evidence, such as elaborate floors Miniero 2010: 303-308), a megalography (Miniero and Capaldi 2010) and an early bathing facility heated with volcanic gases[7]) but rather on contemporary criticism of the overly carefree and luxurious life in the villas of Baiae (Varro *rust.* 3.17).

The early villa complexes are likely to have been connected to the larger roads via simple pathways. A larger infrastructure concept did not exist at this time. The roads themselves very probably did not correspond to the Roman standard. Only the Via Herculanea led

[6] Miniero *et al.* 2017: 795-797. The lack of features and finds also speaks against a noteworthy pre-Roman settlement of the bay of Baiae; cf. Nieberle 2023, forthcoming; Di Fraia 2019: 37f.

[7] This is the only room in the Piccole Terme built in *opus quadratum* technique (sector J, room07), cf. room 9 in Medri *et al.* 1999: 208 and 211, fig. 4.

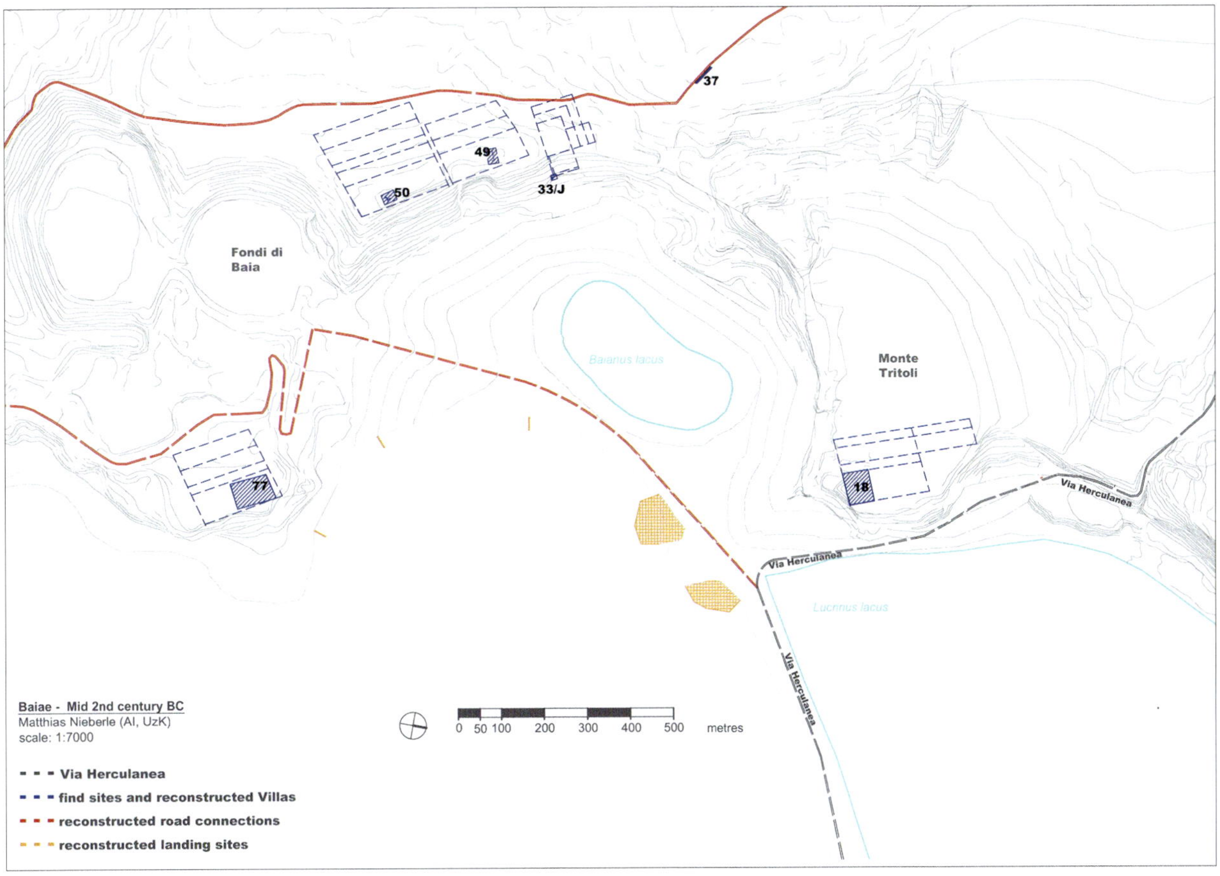

Figure 4. The bay of Baiae in the late 2nd century BC (author)

from Puteoli along Lucrine Lake—here the road ran over a natural dam—to Cumae. On the beach of Baiae, there may have been simple landing stages to moor ships in the bay of Baiae and to load and unload ships.

The hot vapours and thermal water springs

Initially, the bay of Baiae was merely one of several locations for the eccentric villa complexes of the aristocratic upper class. A villa near Misenum even appeared to be more in demand in this early phase (D'Arms 2003: 22f). The thermal water springs in the bay also do not seem to have been in great demand at first. It is true that a passage in Livy is often referred to as the earliest reference to the use of the thermal springs in Baiae (Miniero 2006: 7-10; Maiuri 1958: 72). Livy reports that the former consul Gnaeus Cornelius wanted to visit the *Aquae Cumanae* in 176 BC to cure himself of a partial paralysis resulting from a fall, but he died before reaching the healing baths.[8] It is certain that the *Aquae Cumanae* were healing springs located within the city of Cumae.[9] However, the territory of ancient Cumae is not precisely known and it is therefore unclear where the *Aquae Cumanae* are to be located.[10] Furthermore, thermal springs appeared and still appear at various places within the Phlegraean Fields.[11] Livy explicitly does not speak of Baiae in his account, although the coastal strip was already known at the time of the writing of the *Ab urbe condita*. For this reason, the *Aquae Cumanae* is not the bay of Baiae, but a bath in the territory of Cumae that cannot be localised. In addition, a corresponding spring sanctuary in Baiae, which would prove a long cult tradition, is neither

[8] Liv. 41.16.3-4. The fall was probably the result of a stroke.

[9] It must be mentioned that Baiae belonged to the urban area of Cumae until the 3rd century AD. An inscription, CIL 10, 3698, which can be dated to 289 AD, still names the magistrates of Cumae as priests of the *Mater Deum Baiana*, cf. D'Arms 2003: 52; Medri 1990: 185.

[10] The urban area of *Cumae* also changed. It was truncated as a result of the Roman conquest when, for example, the *lacus Lucrinus* was declared a Roman state territory.

[11] This is reported by Strabo (*Geogr.* 5.4.6): *ἅπαν γὰρ τὸ χωρίον ἐκεῖ μέχρι Βαιῶν καὶ τῆς Κυμαίας θείου πλῆρές ἐστι καὶ πυρὸς καὶ θερμῶν ὑδάτων. Τινὲς δὲ καὶ Φλέγραν διὰ τοῦτο τὴν Κυμαίαν νομίζουσι κληθῆναι, καὶ τῶν πεπτωκότων Γιγάντων τὰ κεραύνια τραύματα ἀναφέρειν τὰς τοιαύτας προχοὰς τοῦ πυρὸς καὶ ὕδατος.* Translation: "since the whole district, as far as Baiae and Cumae, has a foul smell, because it is full of sulphur and fire and hot waters. And some believe that it is for this reason that the Cumaean country was called "Phlegra" and that it is the wounds of the fallen giants, inflicted by the thunderbolts, that pour forth those streams of fire and water". Trans. based on H. L. Jones, LCL 50 (1923). According to this, the Phlegraean Fields would have belonged to the urban area of *Cumae*. Lafon, on the other hand, assumes that they were the thermal springs of Baiae, but that the name Baiae was not yet used for the bay at that time, cf. Lafon 1996. The name Baiae is, however, mentioned in written sources that predate Livy; cf. Lycoph. 694.

known nor reported in the contemporary sources.[12] A central sanctuary and a cult use of the bay would also have prevented or influenced the first development of luxurious villa buildings, because the Roman nobility specifically sought a certain seclusion for the construction of *otium* villas in order to be among their own kind.[13]

This only changed when fumaroles came into focus around 100 BC. This discovery is closely associated with a certain Gaius Sergius Orata.[14] Orata succeeded in harnessing the volcanic hot vapours naturally emitted in the bay of Baiae and the surrounding area for various purposes. First, he used the hot gases to breed oysters and ornamental fish. The breeding of exquisite ornamental fish was a hobby that was particularly popular among the wealthy society of Rome in the 1st century BC (Varro, *Rust.* 3.17.2-9). In a further step, he succeeded in heating entire rooms with the volcanic hot gases, primarily the bathrooms of villas. The skilful speculator bought villas in the area, equipped them with the optimised breeding facilities and the newly heated bathrooms and then sold the facilities at a great profit (Cic. *De Orat.* 1.178).

With regard to the baths of the villas heated with hot steam, Orata also benefited from the almost simultaneous emergence of hydrothermal therapy. The Greek physician Asclepiades of Bithynia, who practised in Rome, advised his patients to take sweating cures, whereby sweating was induced without the patient overexerting themselves. It is a remarkable coincidence that this form of therapy developed just at the moment when the possibility of using the fumaroles in Baiae was recognised and harnessed to a greater extent.[15] In any case, the volcanic vapours in Baiae were ideally suited for Asclepiades' form of therapy. Subsequently, the volcanic resources formed the unique selling point of the bay of Baiae. Because the coastal strip thus stood out positively from other villa locations, the density of villa buildings increased abruptly (Figure 5).

The focus of the newly built villas was now on the volcanic resources, primarily the hot vapours, but also the thermal springs. For this purpose, the inner side of the former volcanic crater was now developed, where corresponding volcanic resources were found. A bathing facility in the villa was a standard elsewhere, but in Baiae the baths were ideally heated with hot steam. This is particularly evident in the bathing facilities of this phase within the Archaeological Park.[16] The baths were partially dug into the mountainside to develop resources and served as an attraction and new leisure activity for the distinguished villa society. Figure 6 shows the bath of the so-called Villa of Sosandra dug into the volcanic slope.

Indispensable for this development was a sufficient supply of thermal springs and hot vapours. The location of the remains and indications of bathing facilities clearly demonstrate that the region of the Gulf of Naples, and in particular the bay of Baiae, was extremely richly blessed with these two volcanic resources. Due to the location of the baths, it is also possible to infer the volcanic resource that was used in each case. The thermal springs emerged at the foot of the slope. The fumaroles, on the other hand, could also be used for the baths at higher altitudes.[17] A high density of baths can be found in the area of the Archaeological Park and on the slopes of Monte Tritoli in the north of the bay, cf. Figure 7.[18]

In favour of the benefits of the volcanic resources, the newly built villas dispensed with agricultural areas. Instead, the inside of the crater was cleverly used for several terrace levels, corresponding to the *caveae* of a natural theatre. The orientation was now towards the east with a view of the *Baianus lacus* (Cf. Figure 5).

Although it cannot be proven, this increase in the number of villas was probably connected with an expansion of the transport infrastructure (Cf. Figure 5). It is assumed that a road was now also laid out on the inner side of the *Baianus lacus* in order to provide access to the villas that were built on the inner side of the volcanic crater. In addition, landing places on the outer *Baianus lacus* were now indispensable in order to supply the villa inhabitants with all the necessities of life. Another advantage was the geographical proximity

[12] In thermal spring sites with a long tradition of use, a corresponding sanctuary is often the central element around which the thermal spa develops. Examples of thermal spring sites with a corresponding sanctuary, which have usually been frequented since prehistoric times, include *Aquae Sulis* or *Aquae Taurine*, cf. Guérin-Beauvois 2015: 323-326; Dvorjetski 2007: 88 and 90; Köhler 2013: 211f.; Künzl 2013. Similarly, pre-Roman cult activity can be demonstrated in *Aquae Aponi* (Montegrotto Terme), *Aquae Sinuessanae* and in Vicarello, cf. Dvorjetski 2007. From this, E. Künzl concludes: "Thermal spas were usually associated with a sanctuary", see Künzl 2013: 120. It is therefore all the more surprising that this is not the case in Baiae, the most famous and important thermal spa. In fact, this discrepancy has not yet been questioned.

[13] Initially, *homines novi*, such as Cicero, apparently also had difficulties acquiring property in Baiae; see Guérin-Beauvois 2015 : 138; Klingenberg 2019 : 216; Lafon 2001: 188f.

[14] Cic. *De Orat.* 1.178; Val. Max. 9.1; Plin. *Nat.* 9.167-169. N. De Haan has already presented a coherent thesis on the development of the hypocaust and the role of the Orata, cf. De Haan 2010: 22-35.

[15] On the person of Asclepiades see DNP 2 (1997) 89-92, s. v. Asclepiades of Bithynia (Vivian Nutton). The astonishing coincidence is not discussed further. It is pointed out, however, that Asclepiades' medical prescriptions were primarily addressed to the wealthy.

[16] Cf. Nieberle 2023 forthcoming, Figure 3.

[17] Maura Medri already noted this observation in 2013; cf. Medri 2013: 134-135.

[18] Because the area of the Archaeological Park is better documented, this assumption is possibly based on a bias. Whether there were other focal points of volcanic resources in the bay will possibly be clarified in the course of further research.

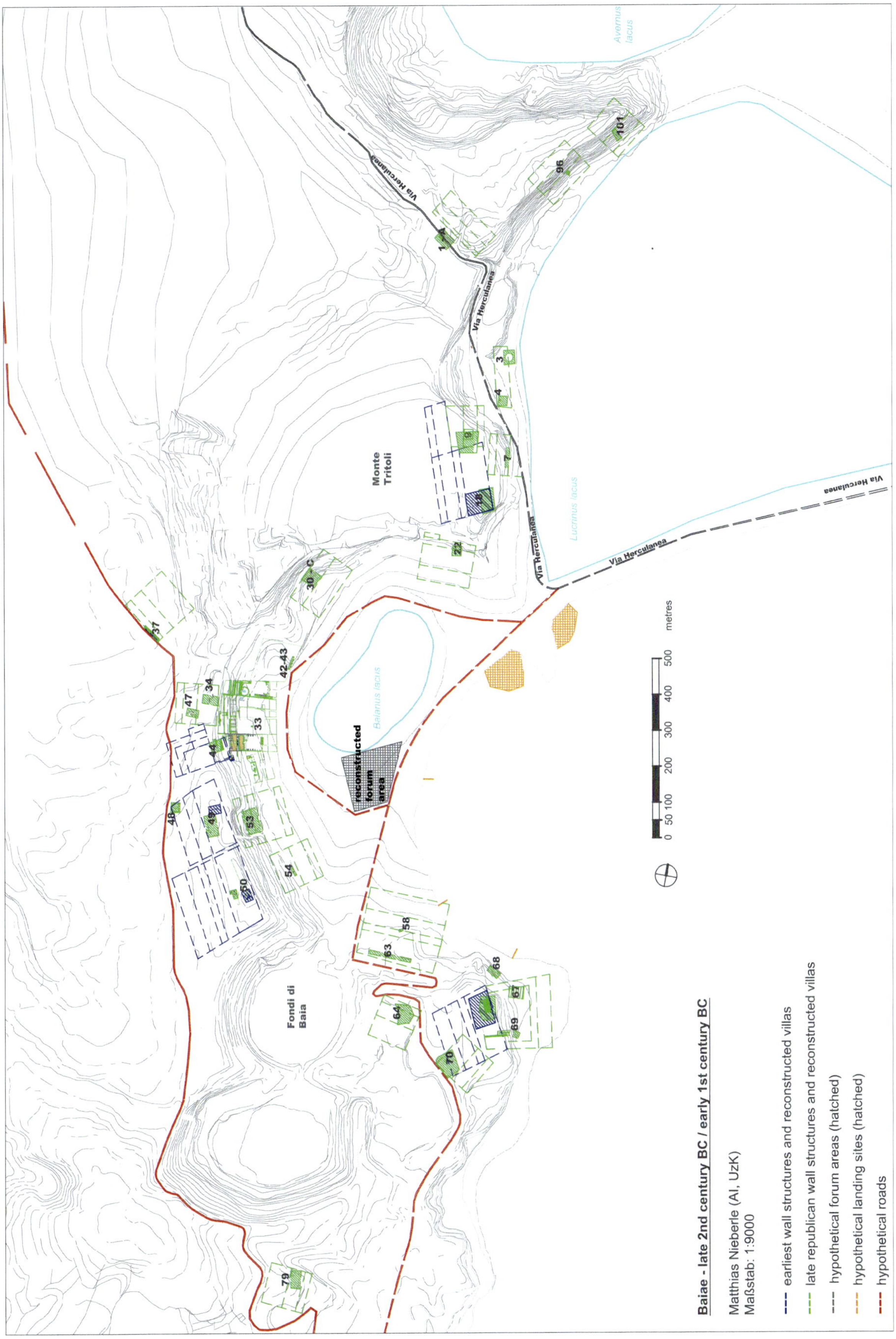

Figure 5. The bay of Baiae in the early 1st century BC (author)

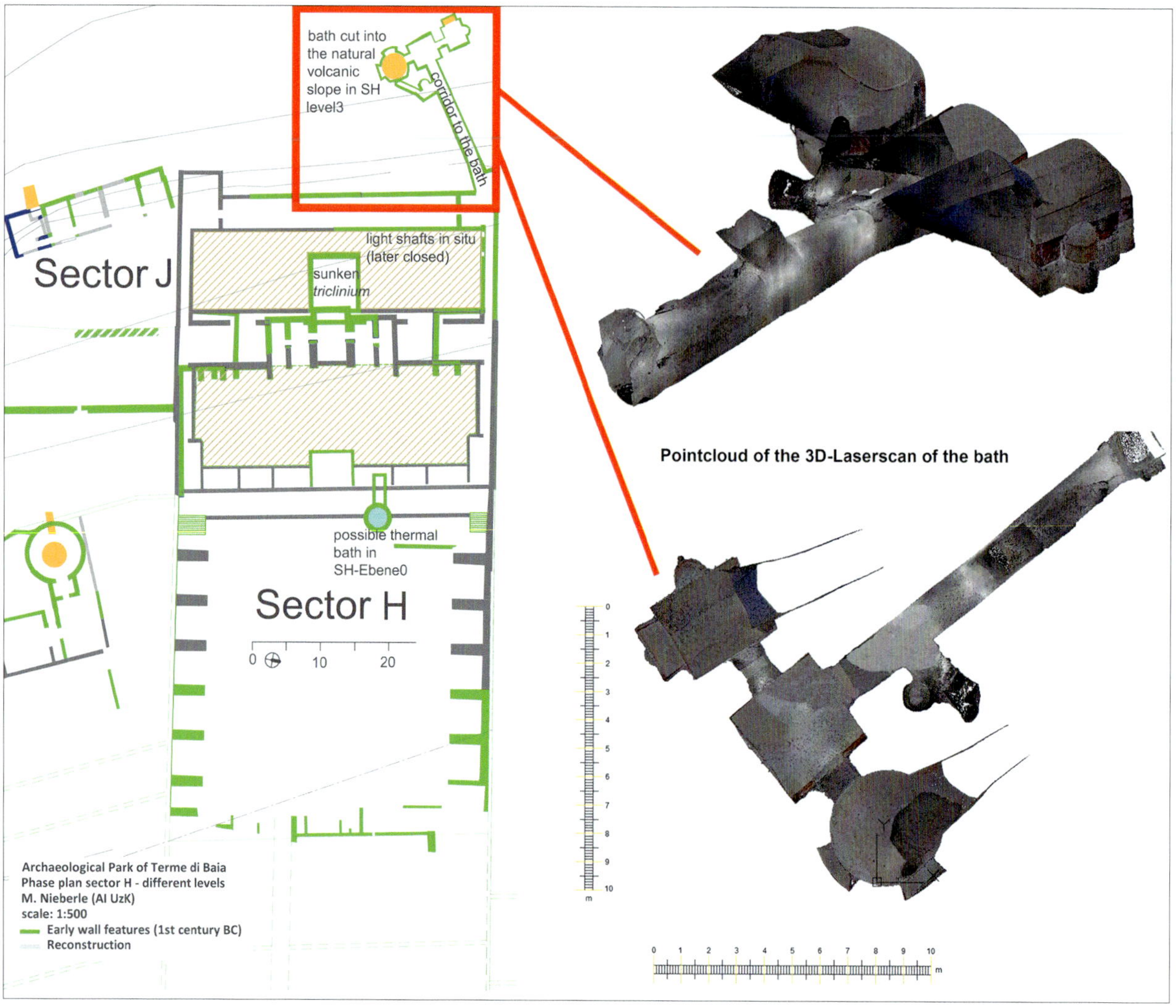

Figure 6. The bath in level 3 of Sector H (the so-called Villa of Sosandra) cut into the volcanic slope (Laserscanning and Pointcloud by S. Geiermann. Scandric 3D SOLUTIONS GmbH / author)

to the overseas port of Puteoli, so that all conceivable luxury goods were available in Baiae.

The establishment of an elite spa resort

After spa bathing had established itself in the bay, the previous villa landscape with a thermal bathing character was transformed into a spa and thermal bathing resort in a luxurious villa setting. The *otium villeggiatura* was further developed into the *otium* bathing experience in Baiae (Nieberle 2020). An essential prerequisite for this genesis was that the nobility, to whom the offer was directed and who could afford this form of leisure, already resided in the villa complexes on site. The bay of Baiae owed its particular fame to this development and was at the forefront of a trend. For a new leisure activity of the wealthy upper class had emerged, anticipating the modern phenomenon of spa and wellness culture. Other thermal spa sites now also became the travel destinations of the wealthy Roman upper class, with visits to the respective thermal spa sites depending on the respective medical or healing therapy fashion of the time.[19]

But how did Baiae manage to maintain its importance, especially since the amenities mentioned were not limited to Baiae?

Optimal infrastructure

An important criterion for Baiae's special position was its optimal infrastructure. In this respect, the bay benefited from the conflicts between Augustus and Sextus Pompeius. In the course of the conflict with

[19] Emperor Augustus was treated thanks to a cold-water cure on the recommendation of his physician Musa. Subsequently, cold-water cures became temporarily fashionable and bathing resorts such as *Clusium* (Chiusi) in Etruria became favoured. These changing fashions were followed by numerous people of the upper class, such as Horace, who complains that the water is too cold for him (Hor. *Epist.* 1.15).

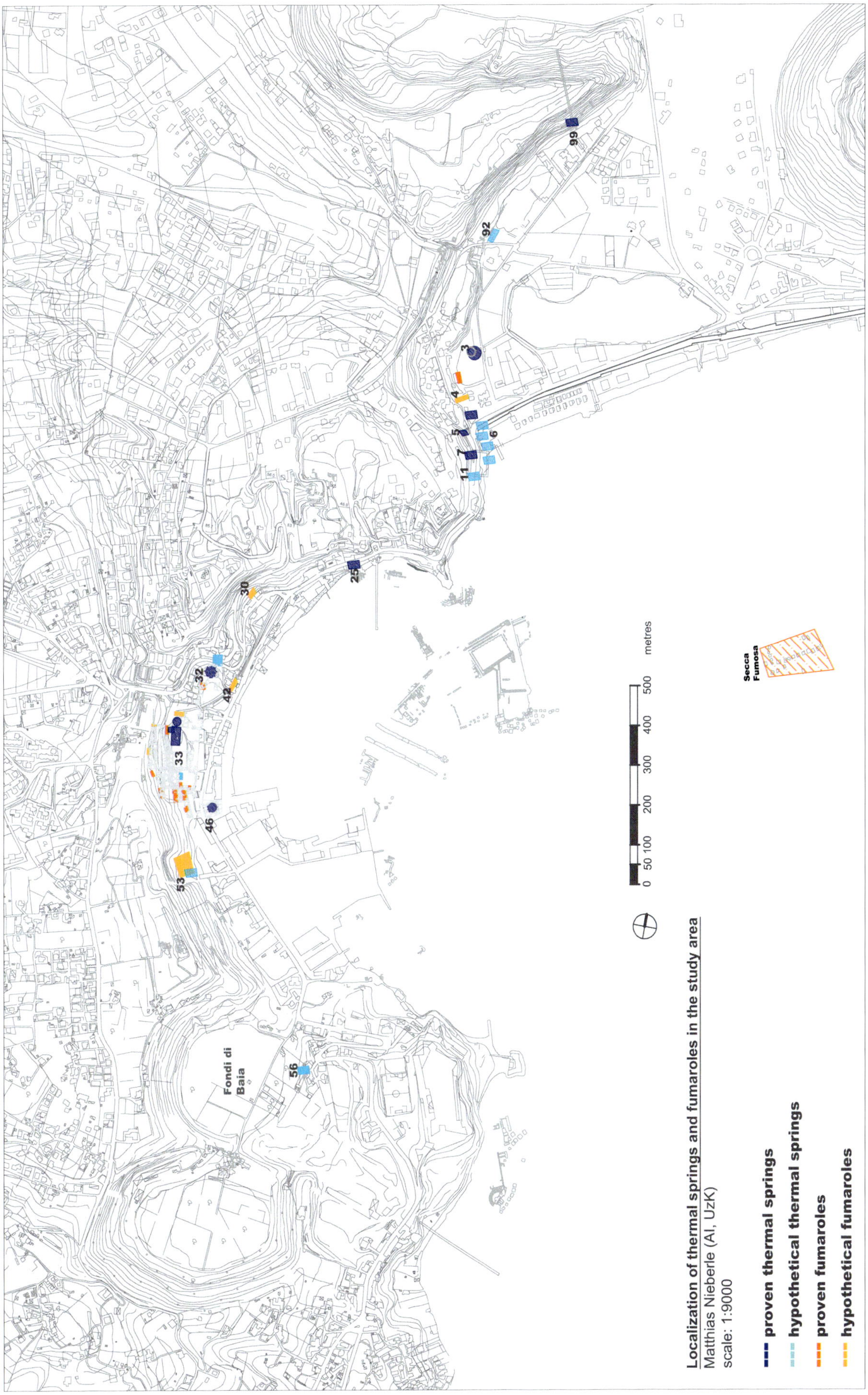

Figure 7. Distribution of volcanic resources in the bay of Baiae (author)

Sextus Pompeius, Augustus and Agrippa chose Lucrine Lake and Lake Avernus as the base for a naval fleet (Cf. Figure 1). The decision to build the new harbour, Portus Julius, at this location was primarily for strategic reasons, since the overseas port of Puteoli was decisive for Augustus in the war.

As a further measure, new transport routes were created. These new routes included numerous tunnel connections, such as the *Crypta Romana*, which runs under the acropolis of Cumae and connects the harbour with the lower town (Döring 2012: 104-106), the *Grotta della Sibilla*, which leads from Lake Avernus to Lucrine Lake (Döring 2012: 96f.), *the Grotta Cocceio,* which leads from Lake Avernus to Cumae (Cf. Döring 2012: 99f.), the Galleria Scalandrone, which leads from Lucrine Lake to Monte Tritoli (Camodeca 1997: 195-199; Amalfitano *et al.* 1990: 178-180), as well as at least one tunnel in the bay of Baiae.[20] The tunnels and traffic routes primarily served to supply the soldiers in the new naval base. At the same time, however, they considerably shortened the travel time within the Gulf of Naples and effectively connected the villas and the elite spa and health resort of Baiae to the existing transport network. Thanks to the volcanic rock, these works could be carried out quickly and with comparatively little effort. In order to establish a secure entrance to the Portus Julius, Agrippa had an artificial access channel built. Another artificial canal connected Lucrine Lake and Lake Avernus so that both lakes could be used as harbour basins. Only a short time before, it had been recognised that *opus caementicium*[21] also hardens under water after the addition of Pozzolana earth (volcanic ash).[22] It was only thanks to this invention that building huge underwater structures was made possible.

It is noteworthy that a canal entrance to the *Baianus lacus* was probably created at the same time as these works (Brandon and Hohlfelder 2014: 81-85; Brandon *et al.* 2008) (Figure 8). In this way, the lake could be used as a civilian harbour (Lucrine Lake and Lake Avernus were reserved for military use at this time) and enabled a quick and direct journey to Baiae, but also the supply of the villa inhabitants via the sea (Döring 2012: 156). The *Baianus lacus* could also be used for small excursion boats. Ancient authors also refer to boat parties and boat trips at night (Weeber 2014: 90-93). In addition to the artificial canal entrance, the Baian coastal causeway was secured with *pilae.* The *pilae* are pillars made of *opus caementicium* that served as breakwaters and thus secured the coast from the surf (Miniero 2006: 20). Thanks to the *pilae,* the areas near the beach could also be developed with buildings and villa complexes.[23] The beach villas, together with the hillside villas, shaped the landscape that was typical of Baiae and which has been transmitted to us through the letters of Pliny the Younger (Plin. *Epist.* 9.7).

Shortly after the battle of Actium in 31 BC, the soldiers were finally relocated to neighbouring Misenum, where a new military port was created. Conversely, the previously fortified areas around Lucrine Lake and Lake Avernus could be returned to civilian use and developed with villas.

Immediately before the relocation of the fleet, an aqueduct was also built, primarily to supply the soldiers of the fleet in Misenum with drinking water. The newly constructed freshwater conduit transported the water from the Apennine Mountains in the southeast over about 106 km to Misenum (Döring 2012: 215-222; Illiano 2022: 64f.; Keenan-Jones 2010). All towns and villas along this route benefited from this new freshwater supply, as they no longer depended solely on precipitation. At the same time, the additional water supply enabled greater water use.[24] A major beneficiary of the aqueduct was Baiae, because up to that time an adequate supply of drinking water had been the crucial shortcoming of the coastal strip and the surrounding area, as there was no sufficient supply.[25] The lack of fresh water and all the benefits associated with drinking water had to be covered by rainwater cisterns before the aqueduct was built. Thanks to the artificial freshwater pipeline, the water supply for the villas in Baiae was assured.[26] In addition, the hot thermal water could be cooled with fresh water. Furthermore, it was possible to cleanse oneself after a thermal bath. The aqueduct formed another essential aspect for the long-term establishment of Baiae as a spa and health resort.

[20] The author postulates another tunnel that led from the Fondi di Baia to Misenum. However, concrete evidence for this tunnel cannot be provided.

[21] Vitr. 2.6.1. on Roman concrete: Lamprecht 1993: 33-45.

[22] The exact date of this discovery and when it became widespread are unclear. Because the villa complexes of the early 1st century BC already used this achievement for their artificial fish breeding facilities (cf. Varro *Rust.* 3.17.9), it can be assumed that the discovery was made in the late 2nd century BC or early 1st century BC. The export of the Pozzolana earth was an important industry; cf. Jaschke 2010: 65.

[23] The best-known example of a beach villa in Baiae is the Villa of the Pisones; cf. Di Fraia *et al.* 1985-86: 262-280.

[24] For general information on this topic, see De Haan 2010. The presence of the aqueduct did not mean that there was an unlimited supply of fresh water. The supply of the fleet soldiers at the end of the conduit had priority. For this reason, and because of the length of the conduit and the numerous connections, access to the water was strictly regulated.

[25] Only one drinking water spring at Lake Avernus has survived, cf. Strab. *Geogr.* 5.4.5. Because of the high outlet temperature of the thermal water springs—in some cases they emerge at more than 50 degrees—and because of their high mineral content, they are not suitable as drinking water springs.

[26] The course of the Augustan aqueduct in the bay of Baiae is shown in Figure 8.

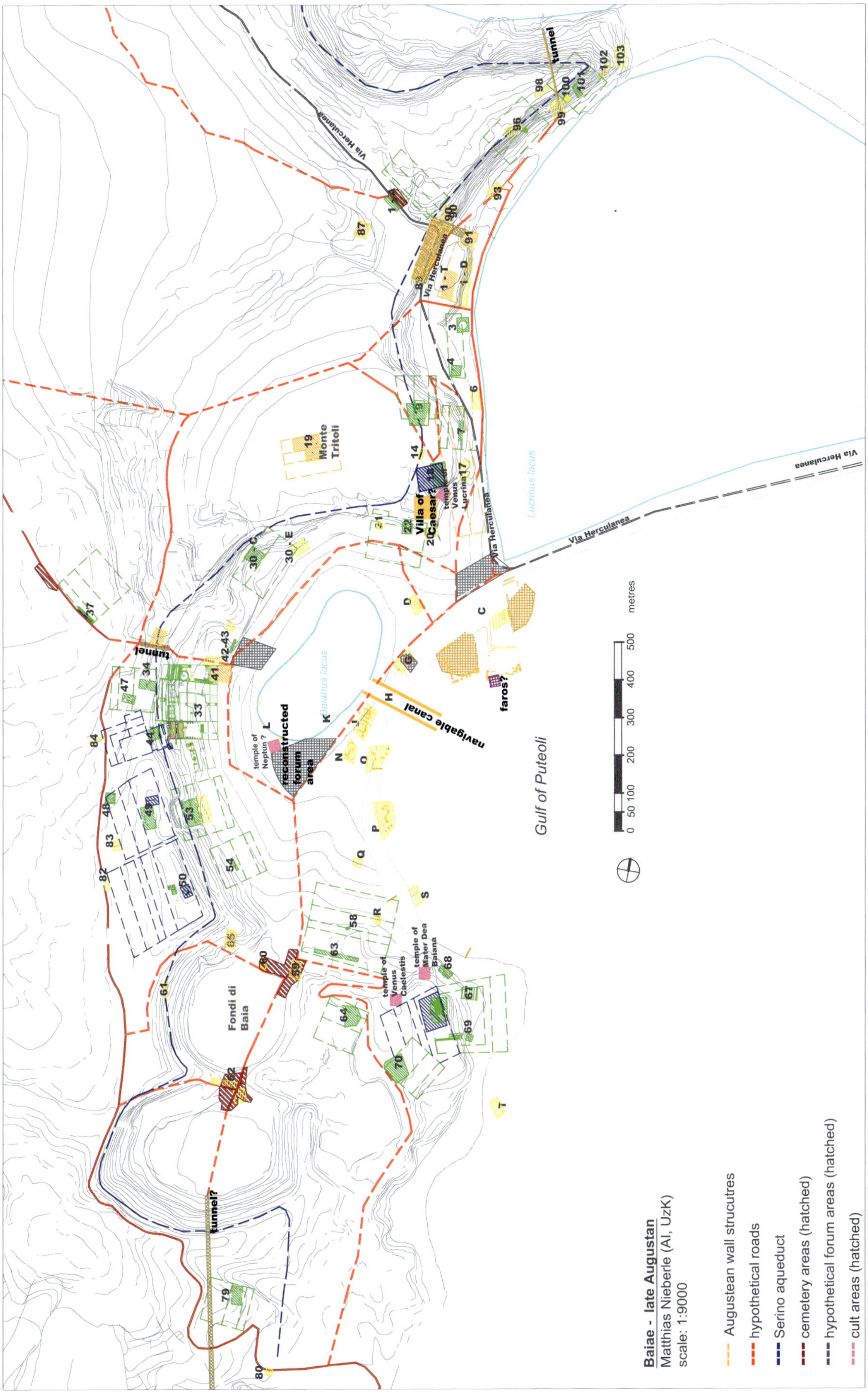

Figure 8. The bay of Baiae in the Augustan period (author)

Infrastructure

The aforementioned infrastructural measures of Augustus are not only impressive in their scope and magnitude but are also interesting because Augustus apparently avoided Baiae.[27] One reason for this conspicuous absence of the first princeps could have been Baiae's dissolute reputation. However, it was precisely against this vice and immorality that Augustus campaigned after the establishment of the Principate, issuing several decrees for stricter adherence to traditional *mores*.[28] Accordingly, he also took consistent action against his only natural daughter, who had too obviously violated these morals by visiting Baiae, among other things.[29]

Accordingly, there must have been another motive for why Baiae and the surrounding area benefited so much from Augustus' measures. In the author's opinion, the main reason was probably the senators residing here and the wealthy clientele on whom the first princeps depended. Augustus secured their favour, possibly also with the help of the military threat of the naval base at Portus Julius, by optimising the infrastructure of the entire Gulf region and especially that of the bay of Baiae (see Figure 8).

In the end, thanks to Augustus, Baiae had good transport connections, its own harbour and an adequate water supply. The excellent infrastructure was another unique feature of the spa town of Baiae and consolidated its exceptional position. Understandably, the density of the villa complexes in the bay increased again in Augustan times (Cf. Figure 8).

The fact that the elite owned villas in Baiae meant that Augustus' successors were also particularly fond of the place. Caesar's villa was extended into an imperial palace, which the following emperors also liked to use as a holiday domicile. Thanks to literary sources, almost all emperors up to the Severan period are attested in Baiae. The continued favour of the elite and especially the emperors is another special feature of Baiae which elevated it over other spa and health resorts. Emperor Nero even began the construction of a navigable canal, the *fossa Neronis*, which was to connect Rome with the Gulf of Naples. Traces of this megalomaniac project can still be found in the landscape today (see Figure 3, no. 86). Baiae would also have benefited enormously from this project. Emperor Nero, who was very attached to Baiae (it is said that he even planned a gigantic basin to enclose all the thermal springs of Baiae there) can be credited with the fact that the *fossa* was also intended to provide quick access to the bathing resort.

Thanks to the wealthy clientele and their willingness to innovate, as well as the intersocial competition among the elite, further specific architectural forms were developed in Baiae in addition to the baths heated with fumaroles and fish farms, which served to showcase the volcanic resources. One example of this special architecture are the enormous domed buildings, which are found with particular frequency in the area under investigation and were probably built here for the first time (Nieberle 2023, forthcoming).

The fact that the importance of Baiae, in contrast to comparable spa and health resorts, did not survive into the present day was also due to volcanism. Due to local bradyseism, the coastal strip slowly sank into the sea, probably from the 2nd century AD onwards. This sinking of the coast led to the drying up of numerous thermal water springs and hot vapours. Although attempts were made to counteract this subsidence with extensive construction measures and by raising the levels of the waterways near the coast,[30] the collapse could not be stopped. As a result, the emperors turned to other holiday destinations.[31] Although Baiae was still important as a villa location in the 4th century AD,[32] it had lost its unique selling points as both a fashionable spa and health resort and an imperial holiday residence. Due to various internal and external political developments, the coastal strip eventually lost all relevancy and disappeared into insignificance from the 6th century AD onwards, a circumstance that has continued to this day.[33]

Conclusion

In view of the infrastructural measures described above, the bay of Baiae was probably the best-developed and best-connected spa and health resort of antiquity from the Augustan period onwards. Its easy accessibility contributed to the fact that the place became known far beyond the borders of Italy. Despite its good connections, however, it was unaffordable for most people to rest and recover in Baiae. This was because

[27] Augustus was reported to have stayed in the Gulf of Naples, but not in the bay of Baiae; cf. Yegül 1996: 157.

[28] It is a remarkable coincidence that Augustus was cured of a terrible illness by a cold-water cure (!); see Suet. Aug. 81. Thanks to the cure prescribed to the princeps by his personal physician Antonius Musa, Augustus did not even have to visit Baiae for health reasons.

[29] On Julia and here corresponding, see Suet. *Aug.* 53-55.

[30] The Severan building measures are particularly impressive. During this period, a general raising of the levels of coastal sites can be observed throughout the Gulf of Pozzuoli; see Maniscalco 1997: 95-107 and 128-134; for the Macellum in Pozzuoli in particular, see Scherillo 1977: 105f.

[31] Alexander Severus is the last emperor who, according to tradition, erected buildings in Baiae, SHA *Alex.* 26.

[32] The frequentation of Baiae until the late 4th century AD was last recorded by G. Di Luca (Di Luca 2020: 2). This view is also shared by Maniscalco; cf. Maniscalco 1997: 67.

[33] Despite various reactivation measures, such as in the 13th century under Frederick II (for which see Di Bonito and Giamminelli 1992: 6; also Pontieri 1977: 388-395), the area's former importance as a health resort and thermal spa was never regained.

the elite had settled in Baiae even before its emergence as a spa and health resort. In fact, the Roman nobility, with its lavish tastes and the prevailing competition within this social class, first conditioned the formation of extravagances including spa bathing. At the same time, the Roman aristocracy was concerned that Baiae remain an elite location. Conversely, this also meant that whoever wanted to belong to this elite also had to be present on site. This applied to the first princeps as well as to his successors. The positive reports from this select environment in turn ensured lasting interest and propaganda that put the spa in an even better light than the actual circumstances and the optimised infrastructure already did. With this knowledge, Horace's statement: *Nullus in orbe sinus Baiis praelucet amoenis*[34] is quite understandable.

Bibliography

Amalfitano, P., G. Camodeca and M. Medri (eds) 1990. *I Campi Flegrei. Un itinerario archeologico.* Venezia: Marsilio.

Borriello, M.R. and A. D'Ambrosio 1979. *Baiae-Misenum (Forma Italiae I, 14).* Florence: Olschki.

Brandon, C.J., J.P. Oleson and R.L. Hohlfelder 2008. The concrete construction of the Roman harbours of Baiae and Portus Iulius, Italy: The ROMACONS 2006 field season. *International Journal of Nautical Archaeology* 37(2): 374 – 379.

Brandon C.J. and R.L. Hohlfelder 2014. Narrative of the ROMACONS fieldwork, in C.J. Brandon, R.L. Hohlfelder, M.D. Jackson, J.P. Oleson and L. Bottalico (eds) *Building for eternity. The history and technology of Roman concrete engineering in the sea*: 55–102. Oxford: Oxbow Books.

Camodeca, G. 1997. Una ignorata galleria d'età augustea fra Lucrinum e Baiae e la più antica iscrizione di un curator aquae Augustae, 10 d.C, *Annali di archeologia e storia antica* 4: 191-199.

D'Arms, J.H. 2003. Romans on the Bay of Naples. A social and cultural study of the Villas and their owners from 150 B.C. to A.D. 400, in J.H. D'Arms and F. Zevi (eds) *Romans on the Bay of Naples and other essays on Roman Campania*: 1–226. Bari: Edipuglia.

De Haan, N. 2010. *Römische Privatbäder. Entwicklung, Verbreitung, Struktur und sozialer Status.* Frankfurt am Main: Peter Lang.

Di Bonito, R. and R. Giamminelli 1992. *Le terme dei Campi Flegrei. Topografia storica.* Milano, Roma: Jandi Sapi.

Di Fraia, G. 2019. Baia: un quarantennio di studi e ricerche, in M. Erto (ed) *Bacoli. 1919-2019: cento anni di storia: volume commemorativo del centenario dell'autonomia amministrativa del comune di Bacoli* (Flegrea 1): 37-94. Nocera Superiore: D'Amico Editore.

Di Fraia, G., N. Lombardo and E. Scognamiglio 1985-86. Contributi alla topografia di Baia sommersa, *Puteoli - Studi di Storia Antica*, 9-10: 211-299. Pozzuoli: Azienda autonoma di soggiorno, cura e turismo.

Di Luca, G. 2020. Il paesaggio del *Sinus baianus* tra abbandono e riutilizzo, in A. Cristilli, A. Gonfloni and F. Stok (eds) *Experiencing the landscape in antiquity. I Convegno Internazionale di Antichità -Università degli Studi di Roma 'Tor Vergata'*: 1-8. Oxford: BAR Publishing.

Döring, M. 2012. *In der wundersamsten Gegend der Welt. Die Phlegraeischen Felder am Golf von Neapel.* Adenstedt: Parmenios.

Dvorjetski, E. 2007. *Leisure, pleasure and healing. Spa culture and medicine in ancient Eastern Mediterranean.* Supplements to the journal for the study of Judaism 116. Leiden: Brill.

Guérin-Beauvois, M. 2015. *Le thermalisme romain en Italie. Aspects sociaux et culturels aux deux premiers siècles de l'Empire*, Bibliothèque des Écoles françaises d'Athènes et de Rome 364. Rome : École Française de Rome.

Illiano, G. 2022. Lo studio del water management per la ricostruzione delle trame insediative tra Baiae e Misenum: Nuovi dati e prospettive di ricerca, in: E. Tamburrino (ed) *Aquam ducere IV* (Proceedings of the international conference "Water and the Roman cities and settlements". Feltre, 3rd-4th november 2017): 63-73. Seren del Grappa (BL): Edizioni DBS.

Jaschke, K. 2010. *Die Wirtschafts- und Sozialgeschichte des antiken Puteoli.* Pharos (Studien zur griechisch-römischen Antike 26). Rahden: Verlag Marie Leidorf.

Keenan-Jones, D. 2010. The Aqua Augusta and Control of Water Resources in the Bay of Naples, in N. O'Sullivan (ed) *Proceedings of The Australian Society for Classical Studies 31*, viewed 20 February 2023, http://ascs.org.au/news/ascs31/.

A. Klingenberg 2019. Zwischen republikanischer Tradition und kaiserzeitlicher Realität. Der soziale Abstieg von Senatoren und die senatorischen Rollenbilder im frühen Prinzipat, in K.-J. Hölkeskamp and H. Beck (eds) *Verlierer und Aussteiger in der "Konkurrenz unter Anwesenden". Agonalität in der politischen Kultur des antiken Rom*: 207–224. Stuttgart: Franz Steiner Verlag.

Köhler, J. 2013. Aachen und die römischen Thermalbäder, in R. v. Haehling and A. Schaub (eds) *Römisches Aachen. Archäologisch-historische Aspekte zu Aachen und der Euregio 1*: 207-260. Regensburg: Schnell und Steiner.

Künzl E. 2013. *Die Thermen der Römer.* Stuttgart: Konrad Theiss.

Lafon, X. 1996. Baies, une nouvelle forme de thermalisme (IIe-Ier siècles avant J.C.), in D. Jarrassé (ed) *2000 ans de thermalisme. Économie, patrimoine, rites et pratiques ; actes du colloque tenu en mars 1994 à Royat (Puy-de-Dôme)* (Publications de l'Institut d'Études du Massif

[34] Hor. *Epist.* 1.1.83. "No bay in the world surpasses the lovely Baiae." Trans. by author.

Central Collection «Thermalisme et civilisation» 4): 11-22. Clermont-Ferrand: Centre d'études sur le thermalisme.

Lafon, X. 2001. *Villa Maritima. Recherches sur les villas littorales de l'Italie romaine : 3. siècle av. J.C.-3. siècle ap. J.C*, Bibliothèque des Écoles françaises d'Athènes et de Rome 307. Roma: École française de Rome.

Lamprecht, H.-O. 1993. *Opus caementitium*. Bautechnik der Römer 4. Düsseldorf: Beton-Verlag.

Maiuri, A. 1958. *Die Altertümer der Phlegräischen Felder. vom Grab des Vergil bis zur Höhle von Cumae*, Führer durch die Museen und Kunstdenkmäler Italiens 32. Rome: Libreria dello Stato.

Maniscalco, F. 1997. *Ninfei ed edifici marittimi severiani dal palatium imperiale di Baia*. Appendici di Aniello Parma e Fara Nasti. Naples: Massa Editore.

Medri, M. 1990. Il quadro storico, in P. Amalfitano, G. Camodeca and M. Medri (eds) *I Campi Flegrei. Un itinerario archeologico*:185–189. Venezia: Marsilio.

Medri, M., G. Soricelli and A. Benini 1999. In Baiano sinu. Le Piccole Terme di Baia, in J. DeLaine, D.E. Johnston (eds). *Roman Baths and Bathing. Proceedings of the First 13 International Conference on Roman Baths held at Bath, England, 30 March - 4 April 1992* (Journal of Roman Archaeology suppl. 37): 207-219. Portsmouth: Journal of Roman Archaeology.

Medri, M. 2013. In baiano sinu. Il vapor le aquae e le piccole terme di Baia, in M. Bassani, M. Bressan and F. Ghedini (eds). *Aquae salutiferae : il termalismo tra anticoe contemporaneo : atti del convegno internazionale, Montegrotto terme, 6-8 settembre 2012* (Antenor quaderni 29): 119-144. Padua: Edizioni Quasar.

Miniero, P. 2006. *Baia. The Castle, Museum and Archaeological Sites.* Naples: Electa Napoli.

Miniero, P. 2010. La villa romana inglobata nel Castello Aragonese di Baia. Campagna di scavo 2003-2004, in S. Adamo Muscettola, C. Gasparri, G. Greco and R. Pierobon Benoit (eds) *Dall'immagine alla storia: studi per ricordare Stefania Adamo Muscettola* (Quaderni del Centro studi Magna Grecia 10): 303-316. Pozzuoli: Naus Editoria.

Miniero, P. and C. Capaldi 2010. Affreschi in II e III stile dalla villa romana di Baia, localita' Tritoli, in I. Bragantini (ed) *Atti del X Congresso internazionale dell'Association internationale pour la peinture murale antique* (Annali dell'Università di Napoli "L'Orientale". Sezione filologico-letteraria Quaderni 18): 387- 394. Naples: L'Orientale Università degli Studi.

Miniero P., M. Di Marco, F. Guardascione 2017. Ville romane in Baiano sinu: recenti rinvenimenti e riflessioni, in G. Greco, B. Ferrara and L. Cicala (eds) *Kithon Lydios : studi di storia e archeologia con Giovanna Greco* (Quaderni del Centro studi Magna Grecia 22): 795–810. Napoli: Naus Editoria.

Nieberle, M. 2016. The Archaeological Park of Baiae. New Hydrological Findings and Considerations, in G. Wiplinger (ed.) *De aquaeductu atque Aqua urbium Lyciae Pamphyliae Pisidiae. The Legacy of Sextus Juius Frontinus, Tagungsband des internationalen Frontinus-Symposiums, Antalya, 31. Oktober - 9. November 2014* (BABESCH Annual Papers on Mediterranean Archaeology suppl. 27): 203-214. Leuven: Peeters Publishers.

Nieberle, M., M. Broisch, S. Geiermann and J.-M. Broser 2016. Neue Forschungen zum antiken Baiae - Teil 1, *Kölner und Bonner Archaeologica 6*: 91-115.

Nieberle, M., P. Vivacqua, M. Di Gerio, S. Geiermann and J.-M. Broser 2017. Neue Forschungen zum antiken Baiae - Teil 2. Vorbericht zur zweiten Kampagne 2017, *Kölner und Bonner Archaeologica 7*: 125-144.

Nieberle, M. and J. Oprée 2018. Neue Forschungen zum antiken Baiae - Teil 3. Ein architektonischer Entwurf zur Anbindung von Sektor A an den archäologischen Park von Baia, *Kölner und Bonner Archaeologica 8*: 177-192.

Nieberle, M. 2020. Das römische Baiae. Ein otium-Badeort par excellence?, in H.W. Hubert, A. Grebe and A. Russo (eds) *Das Bad als Mußeraum* (Otium. Studien zur Theorie und Kulturgeschichte der Muße 13): 25-39. Tübingen: Mohr Siebeck.

Nieberle, M. 2023. Water Display at its Best. *The Example of Baiae*. in G. Wiplinger (ed.) *Forthcoming*.

Pontieri, E. 1977. Baia nel medioevo, in E. Cerulli, F. Castagnoli, S. Mazzarino, P. Mingazzini, P. Romanelli and P. Z. Montuoro (eds) *I Campi Flegrei nell'archeologia e nella storia. Convegno Internazionale (Roma 4-7 maggio 1976)* (Atti dei convegni lincei 33): 377-410. Rome: Accademia Nazionale dei Lincei.

Scherillo, A. 1977. Vulcanismo e bradisismo nei Campi Flegrei, in E. Cerulli, F. Castagnoli, S. Mazzarino, P. Mingazzini, P. Romanelli and P. Z. Montuoro (eds) *I Campi Flegrei nell'archeologia e nella storia. Convegno Internazionale (Roma 4-7 maggio 1976)* (Atti dei convegni lincei 33): 377-410. Rome: Accademia Nazionale dei Lincei.

Weeber, K.-W. 2014, *Baiae - Stadt der hundert Genüsse, Herberge aller Laster*. Mainz: Nünnerich-Asmus Verlag & Media GmbH.

Yegül, F. 1996. The thermo-mineral complex at Baiae and "De balneis Puteolanis", The Art Bulletin 78: 137-161.

Architecture Adapted to Thermal Springs. Some Examples of Roman Engineering Solutions to Thermo-Mineral Water Abstraction in the Western Empire

Matteo MARCATO
Independent researcher
matteo.marcato.87@gmail.com

Silvia GONZÁLEZ SOUTELO
Universidad Autónoma de Madrid (UAM) and Madrid Institute for Advanced Studies (MIAS). Campus Cantoblanco. Faculty of Filosofía y Letras, Dep. Prehistory and Archaeology
silvia.gonzalezs@uam.es

Abstract: When considering the constructive characteristics of bath buildings with thermo-mineral waters in Roman times, one of the essential factors to consider was the need to adapt the bath building(s) to the site of the source of the thermal springs so as to protect and take advantage of the physical-chemical and salutary qualities of these waters.

Because of the problems posed by the collection of these waters, Roman engineers sought different technical solutions for the use of these valuable natural resources. Different examples have been documented that we can analyse and interpret, individually and as a complete typology, based on the brief descriptions presented of these findings. From studies carried out in the western regions of the Roman Empire (González Soutelo 2015; González Soutelo and Ramón Sánchez 2016; Ghedini *et al.* 2018; Marcato 2017; Ramón Sánchez and González Soutelo 2019), we present an analysis of some of the best examples from the provinces of Roman Gaul, including comparative proposals based on selected cases from Iberian and Italian territories.

Thanks to this study, it has been possible to identify a type of construction solution based on slabs of *opus caementicium* used for the capture and isolation of thermal springs. The first step for the engineers was to prepare the ground out of which the thermo-mineral waters gushed, to the level of the bedrock; the flow was then channelled with formwork and conductions according to the design of the establishment and topography; lastly, concrete layers were laid over the sites to ensure, inter alia, firm ground for subsequent constructions, the isolation of thermal and mineral springs from other surface water, and the elevation of constructions to levels that would protect them from local rivers and possible flooding in those areas closest to streams.

With this new study we have been able to recognise some specific characteristics of these water collection methods and their uses, clearly demonstrating their technical complexities and the economic and political implications linked to the construction of this type of thermal establishment.

Keywords: concrete layer, Roman construction, hydraulic systems, thermal water, water catchment.

Introduction

Within the study context of thermal architecture and the construction of thermo-mineral baths in Roman times,[1] analysis of the adaptation of these buildings to the terrain to optimise the use of these springs was one of our main objectives. Clearly, such endeavours demonstrate the levels of construction capacity in Roman times, and the technical skills; the economic costs, testify to the importance that this natural resource already had for the ancient world, in particular from the Roman era.

Based on the examples we have been able to analyse from the Iberian Peninsula (González Soutelo and Matilla Séiquer 2017; González Soutelo 2020), specifically those focusing on water collection systems (González Soutelo 2015; Carneiro 2017; Ramón Sánchez and González Soutelo 2019), e.g. the Roman spa of Lugo (González Soutelo 2015; 2016; González Soutelo and Ramón Sánchez 2016), it is very evident that these types of infrastructures are of great importance to these buildings. Of course, the varied and complex topographies around the upwelling points called for innovation and creativeness in terms of providing optimum facilities.[2]

In our search for the various construction solutions used to control and manage the mineral-medicinal waters at each site (González Soutelo 2019), the territory between Gaul and the neighbouring provinces is undoubtedly one of the most illustrative – although there are many

[1] Research undertaken within the framework of the project 'Healing spas in Antiquity: analysis of Roman thermalism from an architectonical and functional point of view' (MIAS/UAM), coordinated by one of the authors of this paper.

[2] In accordance with previous proposals, this research should be understood in the light of recent works in other areas of the empire (Annibaletto 2014; Ghedini *et al.* 2018) that have sparked interest in studying this type of infrastructure.

other significant examples throughout the empire – both from the point of view of the unique constructions they present, and from the long tradition of relevant studies developed within the French context, which is based on three factors: (1) the growing interest in this subject since the 19th century,[3] including extensive and meticulous compilations and descriptions, as well as detailed graphic representations of these structures;[4] (2) the abundance of hyperthermal springs throughout this territory, mainly in the area of the Central Massif; and (3) the importance of these thermal complexes within the social, political, and organisational configuration of this territory, even before the Roman conquest.

In this article, we will focus on the construction models used in Roman times for the adaptation, collection, distribution, and isolation of thermal springs, including the foundations on which the spa buildings were to be erected later. It became apparent that the preparation of slabs of *opus caementicium* offered construction solutions[5] that were much more common than we initially considered for this type of building (González Soutelo 2014). Its uniqueness and constructive qualities are well represented at various French thermal sites, where it is possible to assess the levels of economic and technical advancement achieved during the Roman era that enabled the effective control and management of these springs.

At Évaux-les-Bains, and, indeed, applicable to the other sites looked at in this study, Georges Janicaud observed: 'Ce très simple procédé de captage s'est révélé si parfait, qu'au bout de plus de 1800 ans, on n'a pas eu à y retoucher pour la création de l'établissement thermal actuel' (Janicaud 1934: 409).

[3] See works that are still current and constantly cited, i.e. Greppo 1846 and Bonnard 1908 – especially the latter, for the study of thermalism in all its facets, starting with correspondence on the discoveries made during the construction of the modern spa, which continues to be a reference in this field – as well as Grenier 1960, and the collected and updated works coordinated by Pelletier 1985 and Chevallier 1992a, 1992b.

[4] The plans and graphic documentation presented in the French accounts of the late 19th and early 20th centuries are remarkable for their quality and meticulousness; they provide valuable documentation for the study of these infrastructures. See, e.g., the description of the plans at Évaux-les-Bains.

[5] The creation of a concrete slab as a foundation for buildings was a common practice in Roman times, mainly in the case of works intended for the construction of larger buildings, as well as structures of significant volume and weight that required a solid platform, fundamentally on land that was not very stable or inconsistent. Other factors that could have been taken into consideration were the need to level the construction surface, search for insulation against possible filtrations in the ground that could affect the stability of the building, and the subsequent maintenance and chronologies (van Deman 1912; Oleson *et al.* 2004; Coutelas 2012).

Case studies

As already mentioned, the techniques that developed to prepare the terrain properly, in the face of multiple difficulties, for the effective capture, use, and distribution this resource, which, with its technical complexities and economic costs, reflect the important role that mineral-medicinal waters played for many populations in many lands. Thus, to the well-known examples of buildings usually cited for their exceptional construction in *opus caementicium*, we can also add numerous examples of Roman spas that used this technique/technology to adapt to the topography and existing water sources.

In addition to examples from the Iberian Peninsula (Ramón Sánchez and González Soutelo 2019), the search for construction parallels has identified many sites employing these infrastructures within the province of *Gallia* (Figure 1), and we will go on to mention some of the better studied examples.[6]

Évaux-les-Bains

In the Roman era, many roads connected Évaux-les-Bains with other centres within the *Aquitania* region, including Clermont-Ferrand (*Augustonemetum*), Ahun (*Acitodunum*), Bourges (*Avaricum*), and Néris-les-Bains.

The thermal waters here range in temperatures between 27°C and 57°C and are mostly high in sodium sulphate, silicates, and ferruginous in content. The springs are located in a narrow valley, *c.* 30m below the current village. In Roman times, a long, covered gallery connected the thermal area with the top of the Évaux hill, where the main Roman settlement was probably located (Lintz 1992: 95-96; Maniquet 2014; Roger 2008: 170-176).[7]

Excavations of the Roman thermal structures were undertaken in different phases between 1833 and 1858, during the construction of the modern spa. These not only revealed a monumental complex, but also the scale of interesting engineering work done to manage the flow of these curative waters.[8]

[6] In the Gallia provinces our sites included: Bagnères-de-Bigorre and Bagnères-de-Luchon, in the Roman province of Aquitaine; as well as Saint-Honoré and Bourbon-Lancy in the Lugdunensis province; Amélie-les-Bains and Balaruc-les-Bains in the *Gallia Narbonensis* province; and Luxeuil-les-Bains, in the *Germania Superior* province.

[7] For an overview of Évaux-les-Bains in the Roman era, see: Dussot 1989: 110-113; Lintz 1992; Maniquet 2014.

[8] New archaeological work has been carried out at the site in 2022 by the Service régional de l'archéologie of the Direction régionale des Affaires culturelles (DRAC) of Nouvelle-Aquitaine. Their results will allow for a better understanding of the different sectors of this thermal complex and its construction characteristics. For an excellent recreation of the site and the work carried out, see https://www.youtube.com/watch?v=M-H18-k65gI (viewed 1 February 2023).

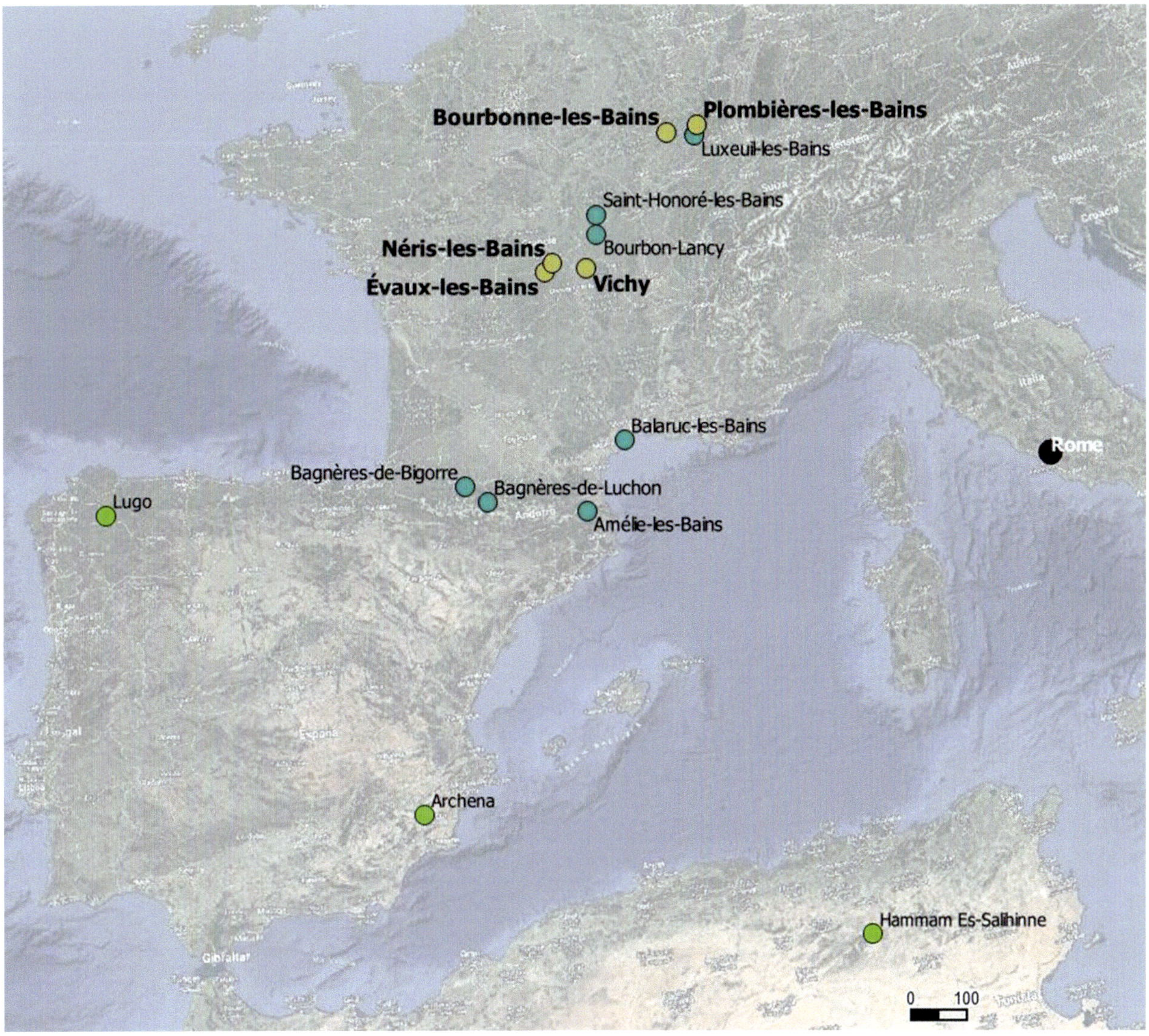

Figure 1. Map with the main thermal towns cited in the text (by authors)

In search of the mineral springs and the best conditions for the use of the thermal waters, the Romans excavated the local rock slope within a square area of *c.* 60m and 10m deep; they discarded the waste downstream to create a platform. Once the upwelling points were reached, cleaned out, and properly collected, a concrete slab, i.e. an artificial platform of *opus caementicium*, was created to cover an area of *c.* 3600m^2. Sand, brick fragments, pozzolana, and lime were the components of the *opus caementicium* layer. Using wooden formwork and masonry constructions, the engineers opened more than 40 wells of various shapes (e.g. square, triangular, circular, oval, rectangular), before covering them with this *opus caementicium* layer, which could reach a thickness of 3.5m over some of these springs. Occasionally the wells were lined with lead sheets. The construction solutions for these wells varied according to the nature of each catchment, but in general terms they reveal the enormous complexity in articulating the hydraulic network of the complex through pipes or channels embedded within the concrete slab. The Romans built the thermal complex on this platform. The modern spa would continue to depend on these Roman catchments (Launay 1895: 616-621; Janicaud 1934: 408-425; Roger 2008: 164-170), being built over the Roman remains (Figure 2). Recent investigations have led to a reconsideration of the function and the hypothesis of a single concrete slab, in favour of localised layers with different functions (Roger 2008: 170), but only continued research and the study of the new data from recent archaeological excavations (2022) will help clarify this.

The first construction phase of the thermal bath dates from the 1st century AD, with a progressive abandonment from the middle of the 3rd century AD, after its destruction by fire (Janicaud 1934: 403-404; Roger 2008: 163, 170).

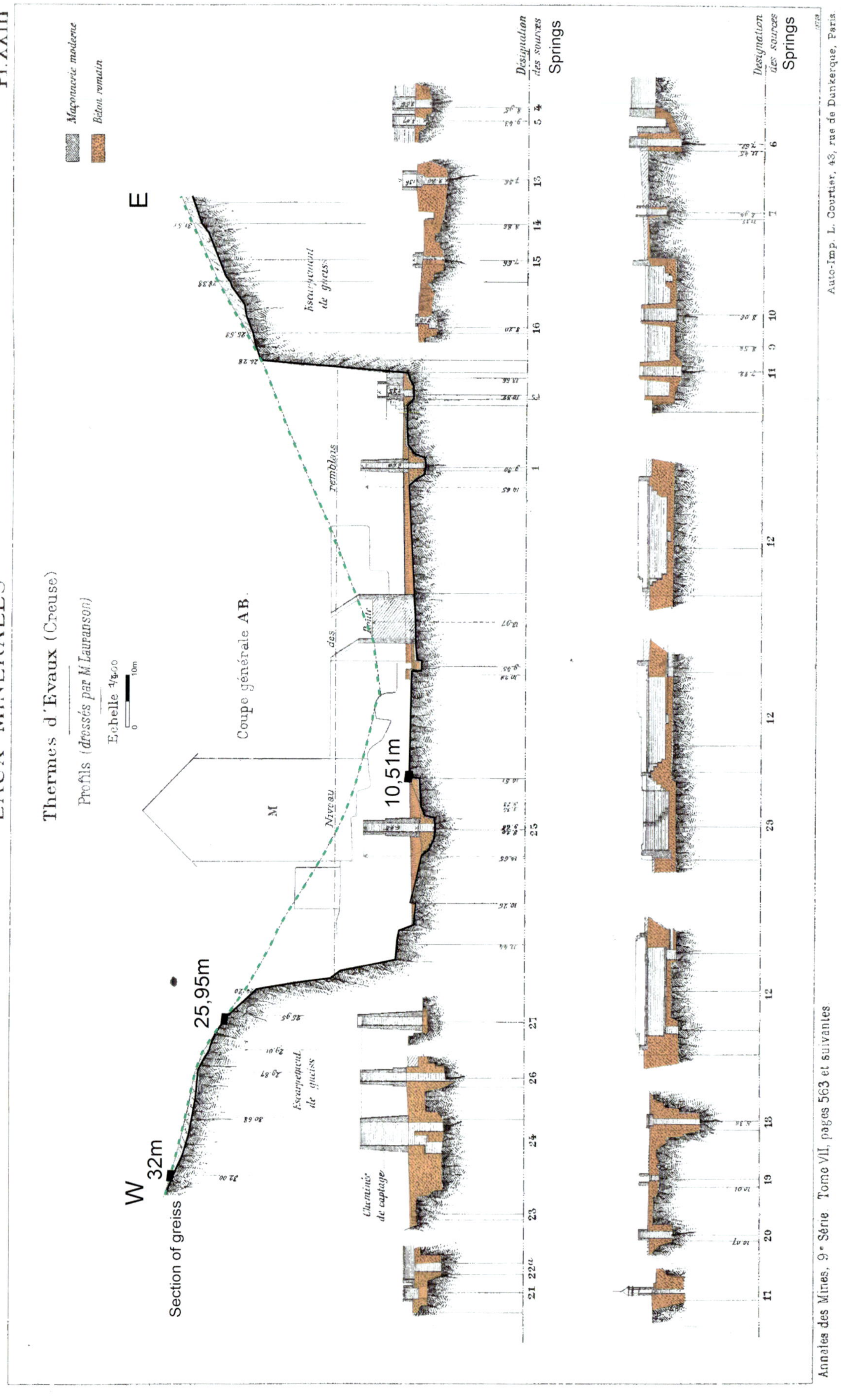

Figure 2. Section of Évaux-les-Bains thermal site, including the Roman cut and preparation of the bedrock to catch thermal springs, as well as the section of the Roman thermal wells, adapted by a slab of *opus caementicium* and *opus signinum* (both of them in orange), after the plan of Launay (1895: Fig. 23)

Néris-les-Bains

Néris-les-Bains (*Neriomagus/Aquae Nerii*) is in an area with numerous routes that connected this centre with Bourges (*Avaricum*), Clermont-Ferrand (*Augustonemetum*), Nevers (*Noviodunum*), Limoges (*Augustoritum*), and Poitiers (*Limonum*), as well as other thermal sites, e.g. Évaux-les-Bains and Bourbon-l'Archambault in the Roman province of Aquitania.

The thermal waters (53°C, radioactive and rich in gases and trace elements) gush from the granite base of a narrow valley, which, over the centuries, has gradually filled in.[9] It is interesting to note that a monumental road at Néris-les-Bains also connected the thermal complex at the bottom of the valley with the inhabited area above (Franceschelli 2017).

In 1832, excavations at the spring uncovered, at a depth of *c.* 5m from the level at the time, the catchment system of the Roman period, consisting of a concrete layer in which five circular wells were dug. It is possible that, as at Évaux-les-Bains, the Roman engineers excavated the rock *in situ* to lower and level the point of the emergence of these thermal waters. The central well (*Puits César*) had a diameter of 1.72m and the surrounding ones of *c.* 1m. A lead sheet, 5mm thick, increased the impermeability of the *Puits César*. There were also two rectangular basins, which are difficult to interpret now, but they seem to have collected the water from all the other wells and then conveyed it towards the thermal complex through two lead pipes, 21.5cm - 24.5cm in diameter. The total extent of the concrete layer is not known with any certainty. The area of the wells, as can be deduced from L. Forichon's drawing, is *c.* 30m^2, but it cannot be excluded that the concrete covered the entire end of the valley. The *opus caementicium* presents fragments of tiles, and a fine mortar of reddish colour appears to have coated the upper surface of the layer (Forichon 1866: 43-53; Launay 1895: 612-614; Desnoyers 1982: 147-148; Charguéron et al. 2003: 19-21) (Figure 3).

As for the chronology of these structures, precise dating is currently unavailable, but preliminary data indicate that the area of the *Thermes sud*, which depends on water from the springs, has been occupied at least since the 1st century AD (Liegard and Fourvel 1999: 113-114), and the first traces of the surrounding settlement date from the Augustan era (Courchay and Champion 2013: 64).

Vichy

Vichy, the ancient *Aquae Calidae* in *Aquitania*,[10] is on the Allier river, an area full of routes that connected the ancient site with *Augustonemetum*, modern Clermont-Ferrand, and the thermal sites of Nèris-les-Bains and Évaux-les-Bains.

The thermal waters are sodium bicarbonates, and the temperature in the wells used by the Romans varies between 27.8°C and 43°C.

The archaeological investigations carried out over the past centuries present an extensive picture of the ancient structures, which are only known in a fragmentary way through summary accounts. We have more precise information, in particular, about the catchment works brought to light at the springs of Chomel and de l'Hôpital.

In 1942, work at the source de l'Hôpital revealed the presence of a Roman well dug within a dark-grey concrete layer more than 2m deep and composed of large brick and tile fragments, sand, and travertine dust. The mouth of the well was enclosed by an octagonal-shaped *puteal*, made of eight stone blocks of 1m length, bonded with mortar. Stone blocks formed the walls of the well (Morlet 1943: 445; Corrocher 1981: 206; 1982: 133-134) (Figure 4).

In 1943/4, repair and cleaning works at the Chomel spring, north of the source de l'Hôpital, revealed the presence of Roman constructions. Roman engineers had gathered the thermal waters by means of an octagonal well (1.60m per side), built using oak planks and reinforced at the angles with beams. The well had a surrounding layer of *opus caementicium* of considerable thickness (Morlet 1945; Fournier 1947: 464-465; Corrocher 1981: 204-206; 1982: 134-135). François observed the layer as early as 1856, commenting: 'Il est difficile de se faire une idée sans avoir vu les lieux, des efforts qui furent faits à l'époque gallo-romaine pour arrêter la déviation de la source vers le sud-est (...); on établit des massifs de béton considérables, formant barrage, dont l'épaisseur s'élève jusqu'à 5 et 6m et qui descendent jusqu'à 7m de profondeur au-dessous du sol actuel' (François in Fournier 1947: 464). It is interesting to note that works to the east of the Chomel source revealed the presence of another layer of *opus caementicum*, suggesting the laying of the concrete over a considerable area. In this case, there were oak beams at the base, 25-30cm thick and 50cm apart, immersed in a concrete layer more than 1m thick. Above there was plank decking (20cm thick) and a concrete layer (50cm

[9] For an overview of Néris-les-Bains in the Roman era, see: (Corrocher et al. 1989: 165-184; Courchay and Champion 2013)

[10] For an overview of Vichy in the Roman times, see: Corrocher 1981; Corrocher *et al.* 1989: 138-163.

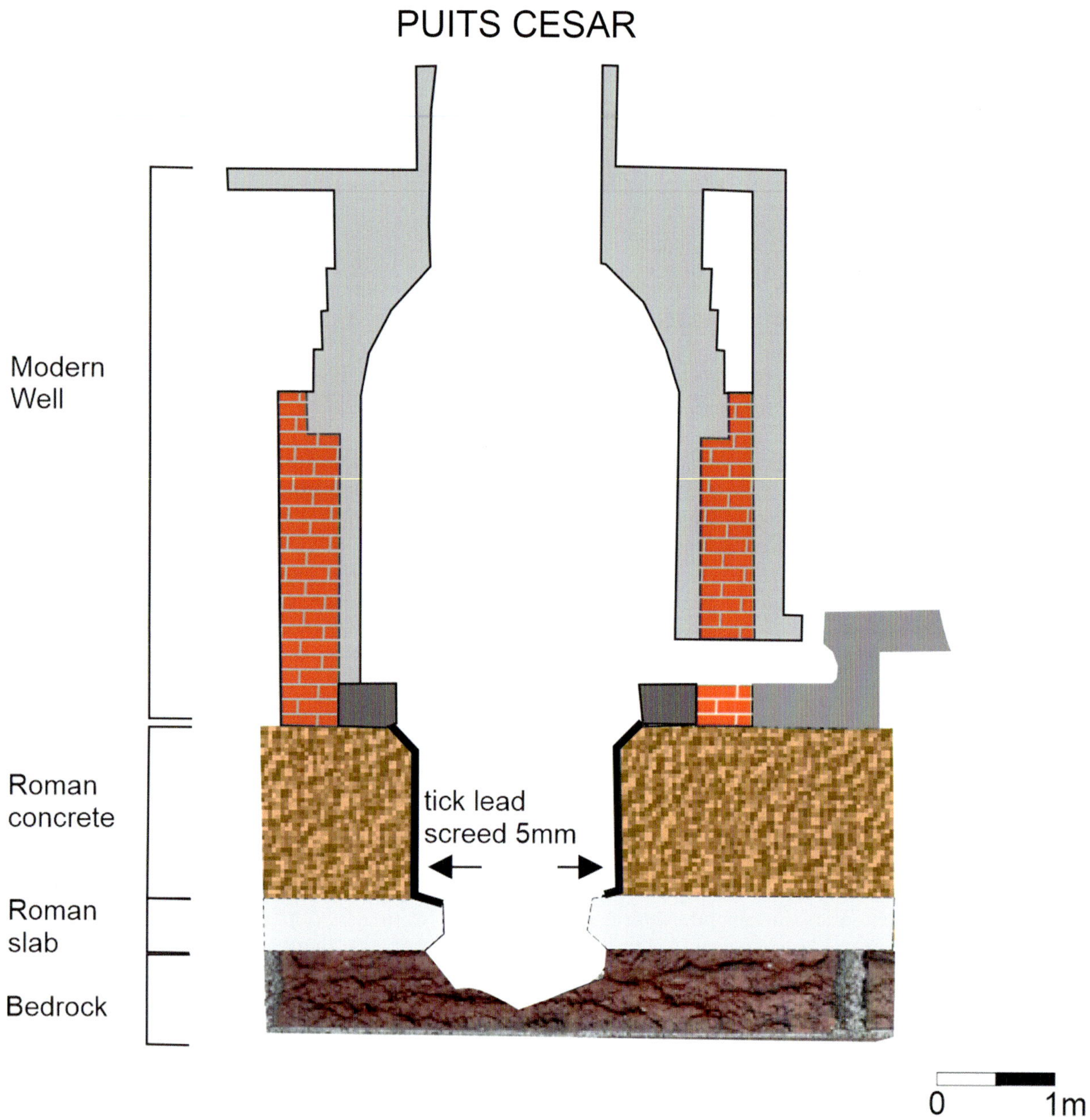

Figure 3. Section of the Cesar well in Néris-les-Bains, including the adaptation of this structure to be used in the modern period (after Chargueron *et al.* 2003: 24)

thick) with fragments of tiles and pebbles (Corrocher 1981: 208; 1982: 136-137).

The Romans also built a catchment system at the Lucas spring, but the information available is scarce, with only a reference to a '*piscine romaine*' and pipes made of trachyte from the Auvergne region (Corrocher 1981: 206; 1982: 132-133).

These sporadic findings make it difficult to understand the overall extent of the *opus caementicium* layers, but their presence undoubtedly testify to the care taken by Romans to control and isolate the waters of Vichy.

At present, a precise chronology of these structures is not available, but they must be framed within the small settlement created in the Roman period, between the 1st and 3rd centuries AD (Corrocher 1982: 143), as is also supported by recent archaeological investigations at the Parc des Sources (Baraton 2022: 3).

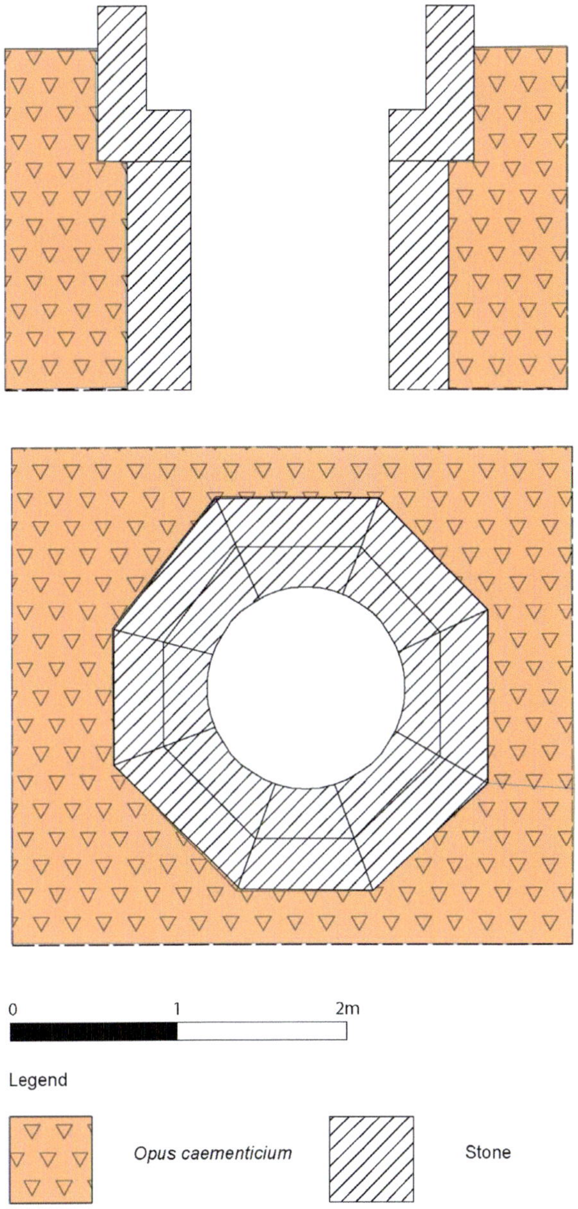

Figure 4. Section and plan of the Hôpital Roman well in Vichy (after Corrocher 1982: 134)

Bourbonne-les-Bains

Bourbonne-les-Bains is just under 40km from Langres, the ancient *Andematunum* – the capital of the *Lingones* in the province of *Germania Superior*. Routes connected the site with Nijon (*Noviomagus*), Besançon (*Vesontio*), and the thermal site of Luxeuil-les-Bains.[11] The waters, high in mineral content (sodium chlorides) and with a temperature of 66°C, gushed into the marshy depths of the valley of the Borne.

The studies and observations conducted by various researchers over the last centuries allow us to hypothesise on the construction phases of the spa complex. At first, Roman engineers carried out excavation works to a depth of 6.5m at the base of the slope, so as to define the spring emergence point, increase its flow rate, and separate the thermal waters from the surface water and that of the Borne stream, which was diverted. The bottom of the excavation was covered with a concrete layer and a masonry wall built around the spring. This structure, later referred to as *Puisard Romain*, is rectangular (2.5m x 3m in its interior) and its base was reinforced by a series of poles. Two walls, built with oolitic limestone blocks from Chalvraines, enclosed the shaft, and fine-grained concrete filled the cavity to ensure maximum watertightness and force the waters to rise high enough, without the need for lifting mechanisms. Around the *Puisard Romain*, various technical solutions were employed to help locate and isolate the mineral medicinal springs, eventually filling the entire area with *opus caementicium*. Over this the engineers went on to erect the spa complex. It is interesting to note that a second group of sources was intercepted by vertical lead pipes in the area of the *Hôpital militaire* (Thévenard 1996: 129-134; Sauer 2005: 5-7) (Figure 5).

As for the chronology of the Bourbonne structures, the study of the architectural elements found in the area led Février and Maligorne to date the first structures between 10 BC and AD 10, with a preference for the earlier date (2009: 42). The same chronological span was confirmed by E. Sauer's study of the coins found inside the *Puisard Romain*, who dates the main phase of the deposition between 9 BC and AD 1 (2005: 89-90), i.e. dating the structures to a slightly earlier period.

Plombières-les-Bains

Our last example is Plombières-les-Bains, a thermal town in the narrow valley created by the Augronne, in a border area between the Roman province of *Germania Superior*, *Gallia Lugdunensis*, and *Belgica*.

The thermal waters spring around the riverbed of the Augronne from a granitic substrate covered by sandstone layers. The thermal complex is characterised by the abundance, variety, and high temperature of its thermo-mineral waters (more than 27 springs). These springs form two groups: to the north of the river, the waters are hyperthermal (up to 74°C) and composed of bicarbonates, sodium, sulphates, and silicates; to the south, the waters are lower in temperature (around 30°C) and have high concentrations of calcium and magnesium.[12]

[11] For an overview of Bourbonne-les-Bains in Roman times, see: Thévenard 1996: 125-138; Sauer 2005.

[12] For an overview of Roman Plombières-les-Bains, see Bouchet and Caumont in Michler 2004: 253-268.

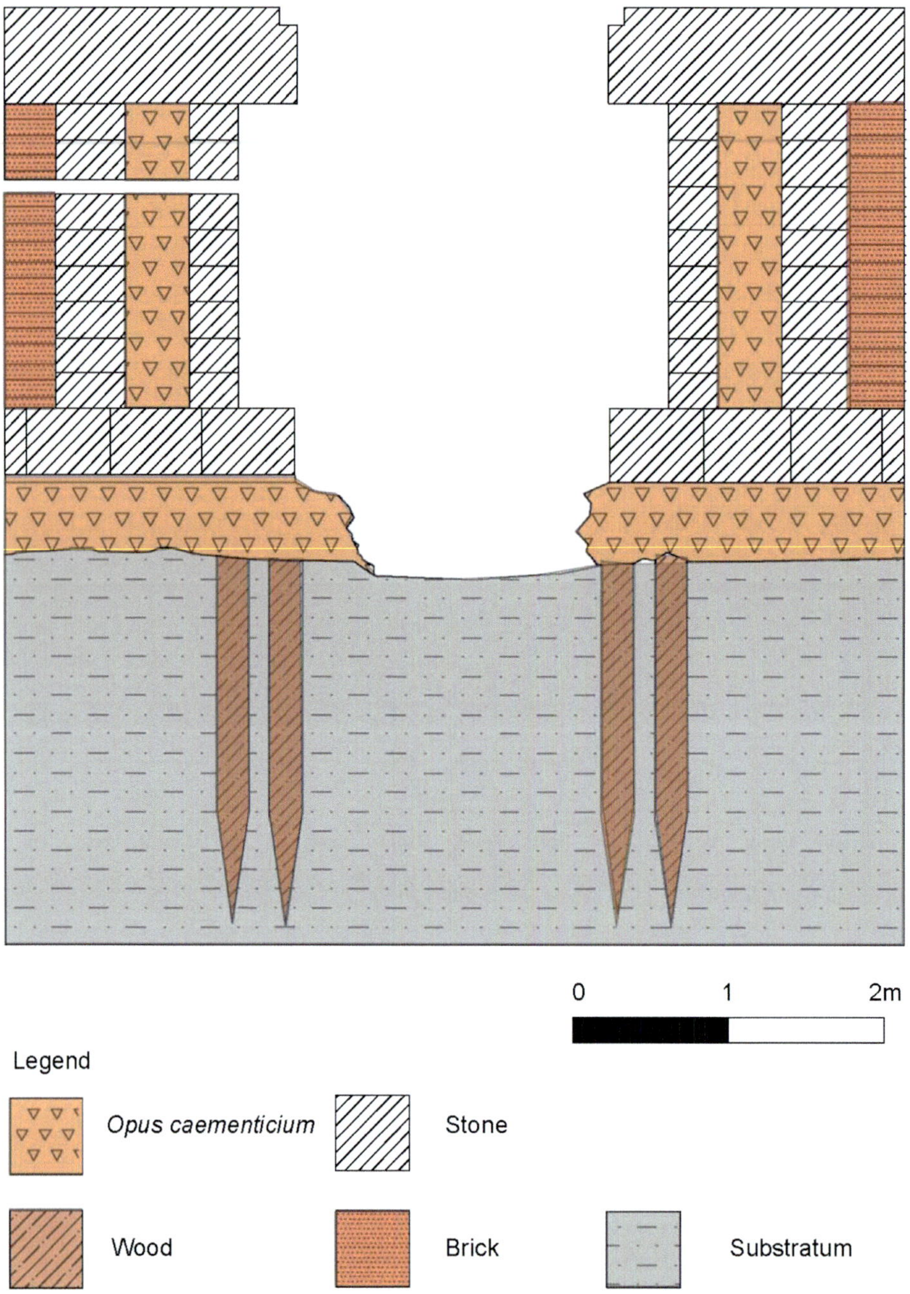

Figure 5. Section of the Roman well in Bourbonne-les-Bains (after G.A. Daubrée 1875, XIII, in Sauer 2005: fig. 2).

To gather and isolate these thermal waters, the Roman engineers diverted the Augronne and covered the exposed valley base with a substantial layer of *opus caementicium* (Figure 6). The stream itself was directed into an artificial canal, 360m long, and the springs were collected through vertical wells (Calmet 1748: 34; Caumont in Michler 2004: 255-256).

The engineering work associated with the *opus caementicium*, already mentioned in detail by Calmet (1748: 33) and subsequently revised by Bonnard (1908: 467), has mainly been studied by K. Bouchet (in Michler 2004: 256-258). The layer extends over a length of 139 m, from at least the *Bain National* in the west to the Étuve Romaine in the east, and for *c.* 20m in a north-south direction. The total area is *c.* 2780m^2, not taking into account the southern area of the canal. The thickness of this concrete layer, which is still visible today in the *Galerie Jutier*, is *c.* 6 m, corresponding to the *Bain National*, and 5m corresponding to the *Salle des Manoeuvres*, but it may be greater at lower points in the valley. To make this *opus caementicium*, the Romans used small pieces of local sandstone and brick and tile fragments, all bound in lime mortar that had hydraulic properties. Two types of catchment systems were created in the concrete layer: horizontal drains connected to a manhole for the

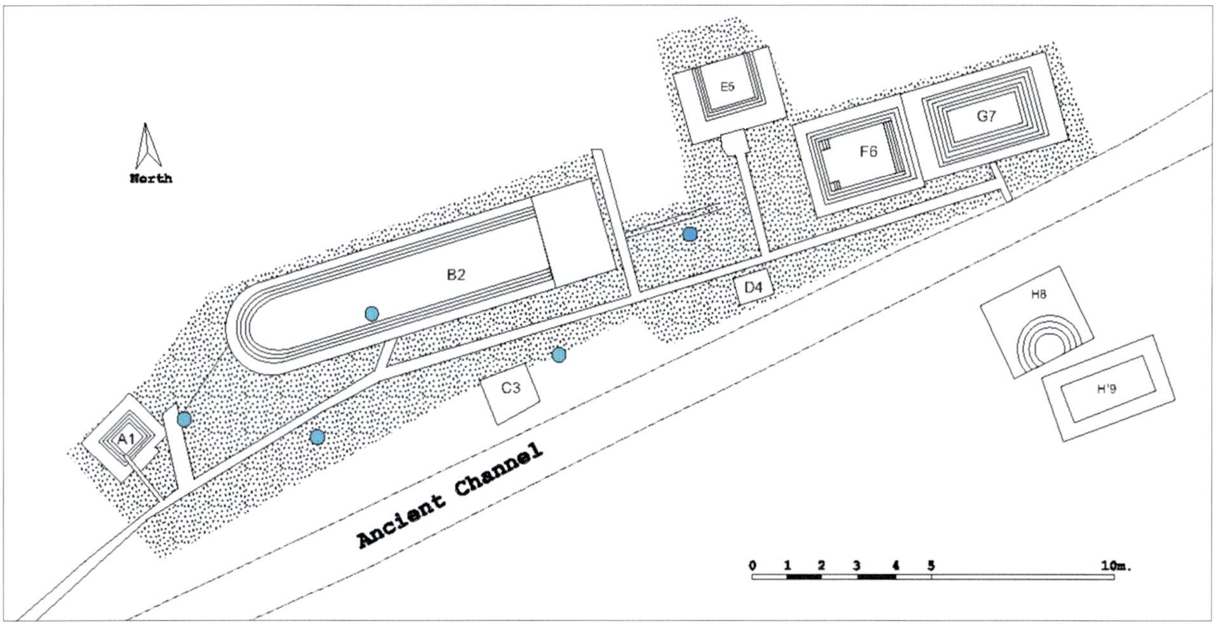

Figure 6a. Plan of the Plombières-les-Bains Roman thermal area, including the pools and the thermal springs exploited in the Roman time, as well as the *opus caementicium* slab discovered in this area. A1: Bain des Capucins; B2: Bain romain; C3: salle des Manoeuvres; D4: Hipocauste?; D5: Bain du crucifix; F6: piscine Jutier; G7: étuve romaine; H8: Bain des Dames; I9: hypocauste du bain des dames (after K. Bouchet in Michler 2004, fig. 268).

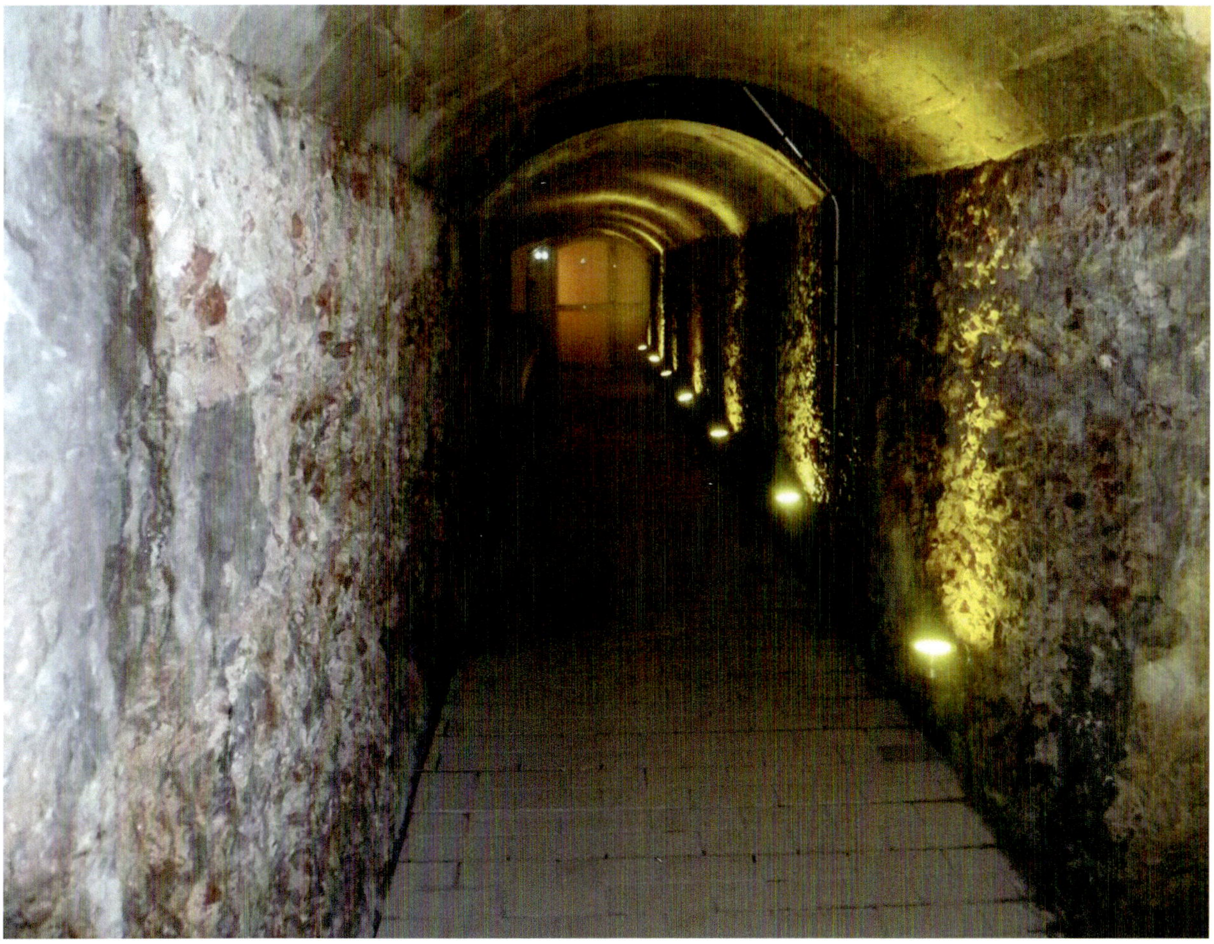

Figure 6b. Photo of the Jutier corridor in Plombières-les-Bains, excavated in the Roman *opus caementicium* slab (photo by https://remiremontvallees.com/2019/06/12/plombieres-les-bains-et-ses-vestiges-antiques/, viewed 12th June 2019).

shallower springs; while the deeper ones were forced into artesian wells constructed of stacked sandstone cubes, drilled in the centre for a conduit.

The coins discovered at the site mostly date from the period between Augustus and Constantine II, although one dates as early as 57 BC (Bouchet in Michler 2004: 268).

Conclusions

The use of *opus caementicium* layers as a functional element in the installation of thermal structures is not exclusive to the Gallic area, as already highlighted in the introduction (siting the cases of Lugo and Chaves in the Iberian Peninsula). This technique is also present in Italian territories, e.g. Acqui Terme (Scati 1898) and Fordongianus (Taramelli 1903; Serra and Bacco 1998). What makes the sites in Gaul so interesting is the detailed information they have revealed that has allowed us to make early insights into this particular technique.

The descriptions of these sites reveal an extraordinary capacity for project planning on the part of those parties involved in exploiting local thermo-mineral springs, combined with the possibility of committing large sums and manpower to the construction of these facilities.

These examples also show that the first step in exploiting a thermal resource was the careful study of the emergence points of the sources, the soils into which they flowed, and the surrounding landscape.

Once the main points of emergence had been identified, the optimum preparation of infrastructures was undertaken to adapt the waters for use. This involved different solutions, i.e. diverting watercourses (Plombières-les-Bains and Bourbonne-les-Bains) or the systematic excavation of large volumes of rocky substrate (Néris-les-Bains and Évaux-les-Bains). In the latter case, the preliminary work involved excavating large quantities of bedrock, specifically gneiss, and preparing and excavating a trench – *c.* 60m x 60m and several meters in depth. In the absence of data on the actual amount of rock excavated, the time needed for this preparatory work cannot be estimated, but a comparison with similar manual work given in 19th-century engineering manuals provides possible interesting parallels (Pegoretti 1863: 159).

In the presence of marshy terrain, as at Vichy and Bourbonne-les-Bains, the difficulties must have been equally challenging, given the need to drain high volumes of water make large areas of land both stable and accessible. The existence of the continuous inflow of thermal waters increased the complexity of the work, requiring the construction of temporary drains.

Once the inflow of thermal and surface water had been stabilised, layers of *opus caementicium* could be laid. Plombières-les-Bains offers comprehensive insights into understanding the construction technique of these slabs. Observations made at the *Salle des Manoeuvres* indicate that the *opus caementicium* was spread through flows of material 15cm - 30cm thick, within formworks made of beech and oak posts, as we see at the *Bain National*. The development of this technique is common to other Roman-period structures, i.e. for the trophy of Augustus at La Turbie, where the cylinder that forms part of the monument reveals a series of concrete flows (Binninger 2008: 96-98, 102). Palynological analysis of the mortars from the different layers show the presence of pollen attributable to different seasons. This is further proof that the works were carried out at various times of the year, as we might expect for large-scale projects. Such sizable endeavours must have required lengthy construction periods, considering that weather conditions must surely have halted, or at least hindered progress at various times throughout the year.

While concrete was being laid, water wells and pipes were also being constructed. The shapes, construction materials, and dimensions of the wells were varied, depending on the characteristics of each site, e.g. the flow rate of the spring or the physical-chemical properties of the water. However, in every instance it is evident that the Roman engineers sought to ensure the structure's waterproofing and optimise its efficiency.

In our case studies that provided more precise descriptions of the material composition of the concrete pours, it was possible to highlight some aspects of their construction. Given the presence of water and a humid environment, it is logical to assume that these concrete flows were made with mortars that could optimize their watertightness. This would have called for either mixing 'fat lime' and pozzolana, or by combining brick fragments or dust with lime and sand.[13]

To support these observations, specific analysis of the concrete used at Plombières-les-Bains indicated the existence of substances of clay and volcanic origin, as well as fragments of brick and tile. In other locations where no material analysis has been conducted, descriptions of the structures still indicate the existence of brick fragments in the *opus caementicium* of Évaux-les-Bains, Vichy, Bourbonne-les-Bains, and Néris-les-Bains.

As for financing these works, we can point to P. Leveau's article that refers to aqueduct construction being

[13] For a recent study on the quality and importance of concrete composition for Roman baths, see Seymur *et al.* 2023.

supported by the emperor and the community, as well as by donations from private individuals – and that all three sources could coexist in the same project (2001: 85-86). This may well also have applied to facilities providing thermal waters.

The emperor was able to involve himself in construction works via direct contributions of money or by offering labour or specialised personnel – usually drawn from the army. Regarding thermal baths in Gaul, the army's role in the buildings at Bourbonne-les-Bains is indicated by the data gathered there (Sauer 2005: 10-11). Similarities can be seen in several spas in the north-western region of the empire, i.e. Wiesbaden, Baden-Baden, and Aachen, inter alia (Zanetti 2017: 113). The intervention of the army has also been hypothesised for the Lugo thermal site on the Iberian Peninsula (González Fernández and González Soutelo 2016: 129-132). Even clearer evidence comes from the Hammam Essalihine, the ancient *Aquae Flavianae*, in Algeria, where an inscription dated AD 208 recalls the restoration of the structures by a detachment of troops.[14]

Twin monumental inscriptions from Néris-les-Bains refer, on the other hand, to funding by local elites and testify to the construction of structures related to the baths and the spring itself by *Lucius Iulius Equester* and two of his sons (CIL XIII, 1376-1377). Although the inscriptions do not specifically refer to the work of gathering the sources and the early stages of the thermal facility, there is nevertheless clear evidence of the intervention of local notables providing large sums for the improvement of the thermal areas.

Again, within the Iberian Peninsula multiple inscriptions commemorating parties involved in the thermal complex of Archena, near *Carthago Nova*, are of equal interest.[15]

As pointed out above, the lack of data hinders our being able to date accurately, or link these water gathering techniques to a precise period. However, considering that the catchment of the spring was the first priority, and that all sites refer to the late 1st century BC/1st century AD as the time of installation, it seems logical to question whether this technique was specific to this period or not.

As pointed out at the beginning of this contribution, the laying of *opus caementicium* over very wide areas to catch and manage thermal waters was not a technique specific to one area of the empire, and it is possible that further future investigations will reveal its use more widely. It is noteworthy, however, that the use of this technique is found in two important areas in Gaul: the Massif Central, and near the Vosges. Should the contemporaneity of the structures be ascertained, interesting scenarios could play out in terms of the possibility of a reciprocal influence between neighbouring sites, the presence of the same patronage, and the possible use of the same workers.

It is to be hoped that new investigations, or the revision of the previous literature, will provide new insights into this specific construction technique related to the exploitation of thermal waters. Furthermore, the comparison of thermal sites having the same structural characteristics, albeit geographically distant, could open interesting lines of research into the diffusion and transmission of construction techniques related to spas and thermal facilities throughout the Roman world.

[14] AE 1888, 70 = CIL VIII, 17727 = ILS 8916. For the site and structures, see Ibba and Mastino 2017.

[15] CIL II, 3541-3542. For the site and structures, see Matilla Séiquer and Ovejero Ovejero 2017.

Bibliography

Annibaletto, M. 2014. Le stazioni termominerali: tipologie architettoniche e sistemi infrastrutturali, in M. Annibaletto, M. Bassani and F. Ghedini (eds) *Cura, preghiera e benessere. Le stazioni curative termominerali nell'Italia romana* (Antenor Quaderni 31): 129-42. Padova: Padova University Press.

Baraton, S. 2022. Vichy – Parc des Sources. Opération préventive de diagnostic (2021) ADLFI. Archéologie de la France – Informations [En ligne], Auvergne-Rhône-Alpes, mis en ligne le 15 novembre 2022, consulté le 21 novembre 2022, viewed 13 July 2023. http://journals.openedition.org/adlfi/126743.

Binninger, S. 2008. La construction du trophée d'Auguste à La Turbie: l'étude de l'organisation et des rythmes du chantier, in S. Camporeale, H. Dessales and A. Pizzo (eds) *Arqueología de la construcción I. Los procesos constructivos en el mundo romano: Italia y provincias occidentales, Mérida, Instituto de Arqueología, 25-26 de Octubre de 2007* (Anejos de Archivo Español de arqueología, 50): 89-106. Madrid: Consejo Superior de Investigaciones Científicas.

Bonnard, L. 1908. *La Gaule thermale: sources et stations thermales et minérales de la Gaule à l'époque gallo-romaine*. Paris: Plon-Nourrit.

Calmet, A. 1748. *Traité historique des eaux et bains de Plombières, de Bourbonne, de Luxeuil et de Bains*. Nancy: Leseure.

Carneiro, S. 2017. New data from the roman healing spa of *Aquae Flaviae* (Chaves, Portugal), in G. Matilla Séiquer and S. Gonzàlez Soutelo (eds) *Termalismo antiguo en Hispania. Un análisis del tejido balneario en época romana y tardorromana en la península ibérica* (Anejos de Archivo Español de arqueología, 78): 65-94. Madrid: Consejo Superior de Investigaciones Científicas.

Charguéron, C., C. Bertin, D. Rouzaire and P. Vigouroux 2003. *Amélioration de la connaissance des ressources en eau souterraine des sites thermaux en Auvergne. Site de*

Néris-les-Bains (03). BRGM/RP-52470-FR., viewed 14 July 2023, http://infoterre.brgm.fr/rechercher/search.htm.

Chevallier, R. (ed.) 1992a. *L'eau en Gaule, rites sacrés et thermalisme* (Les Dossiers d'Archéologie 174). Dijon: Editions Faton.

Chevallier, R. (ed.) 1992b. *Les eaux thermales et les cultes des eaux: en Gaule et dans les provinces voisines. Actes du colloque, 28-30 septembre 1990, Aix-Les-Bains* (Caesarodunum 26). Tours: Centre de recherches A. Piganiol.

Corrocher, J. 1981. *Vichy antique* (Publication de l'Institut d'Etudes du Massif Central XII). Clermont-Ferrand: Institut d'Etudes du Massif Central.

Corrocher, J. 1982. Les eaux thermales de Vichy dans l'Antiquité. *Revue archéologique du Centre de la France* 21.2: 131-144.

Corrocher, J., M. Piboule and M. Hilaire 1989. *Carte Archéologique de la Gaule: L'Allier 03*. Paris: Académie des Inscriptions et Belles-Lettres.

Courchay, J. and C. Champion 2013. Neriomagus/Aquae Nerii (Néris-les-Bains, Allier): religion, thermalisme et artisanat, in C. Gandini and L. Laüt (eds) *Regards croisés sur le Berry ancien: sites, réseaux et territoires* (Supplément à Revue Archéologique du Centre de la France 45): 57-77. Tours: FERACF.

Coutelas, A. 2012. La planification et le déroulement des chantiers en la Gaule romaine, in S. Camporeale, H. Dessales and A. Pizzo (eds) *Arqueología de la Construcción III. Los procesos constructivos en el mundo romano: la economía de las obras* (Anejos de Archivo Español de arqueología 64): 131-43. Madrid: Consejo Superior de Investigaciones Científicas.

Deman, van, E.B. 1912. Methods of Determining the Date of Roman Concrete Monuments. *American Journal of Archaeology* 16.2: 230-51. https://doi.org/10.2307/497281.

Desnoyers, M. 1982. Néris-les-Bains (Allier), ville thermale gallo-romaine. *Revue archéologique du Centre de la France* 21.2: 145-168.

Dussot, D. 1989. *Carte Archéologique de la Gaule: La Creuse 23*. Paris: Académie des Inscriptions et Belles-Lettres.

Février, S. and Y. Maligorne. 2009. Contribution à l'étude des thermes publics de Bourbonne-les-Bains et de leurs abords immédiats: planimétrie, décor architectonique, chronologie et approche fonctionnelle. *Bulletin de la Société Archéologique Champenoise* 102.4: 33-53.

Forichon, L. 1866. *Monuments de l'antique Néris. Coup de balai aux legends sans cesse débitées sur son histoire*: Néris-les-Bains: Lafont-Marandet, Montluçon: Prot.

Fournier, P.-F. 1947. VIIIe Circonscription. *Gallia* 5.2: 461-465.

Franceschelli, C. 2017. La définition de parcours symboliques dans la ville romaine: le cas de l'allée monumentale du Péchin (Néris-les-Bains, Allier), in C. Franceschelli, P.-L. Dall'Aglio, L. Lamoine (eds) *Spazi pubblici e dimensione politica nella città romana: funzioni, strutture, utilizzazione. Clermont-Ferrand 30 marzo 2015, Bologna 27 ottobre 2015*: 201-24. Bologna: Bononia University Press.

Ghedini, F., M. Marcato and C. Zanetti 2018. Aquae salutiferae nell'Occidente romano, in G. Cuscito (ed.) *Cura aquarum. Adduzione e distribuzione dell'acqua nell'antichità, Antichità Altoadriatiche LXXXVIII*: 63-86. Trieste: Editreg.

González Fernández, E. and S. González Soutelo 2016. La ciudad y el Balneario: los orígenes del Balneario de Lugo en su contexto histórico, in M. Crecente Maseda and S. González Soutelo (eds) *Dos mil años del Balneario de Lugo: un modelo de activación del patrimonio termal*: 122-139. Lugo: Crecente Asociados.

González Soutelo, S. 2014. El original sistema romano de captación y distribución de las aguas mineromedicinales en el Balneario de Lugo: nuevos datos, in *Lucentum: Anales de la universidad de Alicante. Prehistoria, arqueología e historia antigua* 33: 191-200. Alicante: Servicio de Publicaciones de la Universidad de Alicante.

González Soutelo, S. 2015. Systems for collecting mineral waters in Roman Healing spas: a proposal of characterization from Hispania's best documented examples, in J.M. Álvarez Martínez, T. Nogales Basarrate and I. Rodà de Llanza (eds) *Actas XVIII Congreso Internacional de Arqueología Clásica 1*: 289-292. Mérida: Museo Nacional de Arte Romano.

González Soutelo, S. 2016. ¿Cómo era el Balneario romano de Lugo?: hipótesis de trabajo, in M. Crecente Maseda and S. González Soutelo (eds) *Dos mil años del Balneario de Lugo: un modelo de activación del patrimonio termal*: 370-97. Lugo: Crecente Asociados.

González Soutelo, S. 2019. Shall We Go 'Ad Aquas'? Putting Roman Healing Spas on the Map, in *Espacio Tiempo y Forma. Serie I, Prehistoria y Arqueología 12*: 151-89. https://doi.org/10.5944/etfi.12.2019.25939.

González Soutelo, S. 2020. Descubriendo las *aquae*: 40 años de investigación sobre los baños romanos de aguas mineromedicinales en la península Ibérica, in J.M. Noguera Celdrán, V. García-Entero and M. Pavía Page (eds), *Termas Termas públicas de Hispania, Actas del Congreso Internacional Murcia-Cartagena, 19-21 de Abril de 2018* (SPAL Monografías Arqueología XXXIII): 211-34. Sevilla: Editorial Universidad de Sevilla, Universidad de Murcia, Servicio de Publicaciones.

González Soutelo, S. and G. Matilla Séiquer 2017. Inventario y revisión de los principales enclaves de aguas mineromedicinales en Hispania. Un estado de la cuestión, in G. Matilla Séiquer and S. González Soutelo (eds) *Termalismo antiguo en Hispania. Un análisis del tejido balneario en época romana y tardorromana en la península ibérica* (Anejos de Archivo Español de arqueología 78): 495-602. Madrid: Consejo Superior de Investigaciones Científicas.

González Soutelo, S. and L. de Ramón Sánchez 2016. El sistema romano de captación, distribución y uso del agua minero-medicinal en el Balneario de Lugo, in M. Crecente Maseda and S. González Soutelo (eds) *Dos mil años del Balneario de Lugo: un modelo de activación del patrimonio termal*: 320-335. Lugo: Crecente Asociados.

Grenier, A. 1960. *Manuel d'archéologie Gallo-Romaine. 4 Partie, les monuments des eaux*. Paris: Picard.

Greppo, J.G.H. 1846. Études archéologiques sur les eaux thermales ou minérales de la Gaule à l'époque romaine. Paris: Leleux.

Ibba, A. and A. Mastino 2017. Le Aquae Flavianae fra passato e presente, in M. Sechi Dolores and D. Vidal Casellas (eds) *Sistema integrat del paisatge entre antropització, geo-economia, medi ambient i desenvolupament econòmic. Actes dels congressos*: 192-217. Girona: Documenta Universitaria.

Janicaud, G. 1934. Évaux gallo-romain. *Mémoires de la société des sciences naturelles et archéologiques de la Creuse* 25.3: 401-431.

Launay, L. de 1895. Les sources thermales de Néris (Allier) et d'Évaux (Creuse). *Annales des Mines* 9.VII: 563-623.

Leveau, P. 2001. Aqueduct Building: Financing and Costs, in D.R. Blackman and A. Trevor Hodge (eds) *Frontinus' Legacy. Essays on Frontinus' de aquis Urbis Romae*: 85-101. Ann Arbor: The University of Michigan Press.

Liegard, S. and A. Fourvel 1999. Nouvelles données sur les thermes sud de Néris-les-Bains (Allier). *Revue archéologique du Centre de la France* 38: 99-115.

Lintz, G. 1992. Évaux (Creuse), *Ivavnvm (?), Vicus Evavnensis* in *Villes et agglomérations urbaines antiques du Sud-Ouest de la Gaule. Histoire et archéologie. Deuxième colloque Aquitania: Bordeaux, 13-15 septembre 1990* (Supplément à Aquitania): 90-96. Bordeaux: Armedis.

Maniquet, C. 2014. Évaux-les-Bains (Creuse): agglomération secondaire à caractère cultuel ou sanctuaire rural? Nouvelle intervention archéologique sur la galerie couverte menant aux thermes. *Travaux d'archéologie limousine* 34: 27-42.

Marcato, M. 2017. *Il termalismo nelle province romane occidentali: Gallia Narbonense, Gallia Lugdunense, Aquitania, Alpi Marittime, Cozie, Graie e Pennine*. Unpublished PhD dissertation, Università degli Studi di Padova.

Matilla Séiquer, G. and L. Ovejero Ovejero 2017. Archena: el balneario de Carthago Nova, in G. Matilla Séiquer and S. Gonzàlez Soutelo (eds) *Termalismo antiguo en Hispania. Un análisis del tejido balneario en época romana y tardorromana en la península ibérica* (Anejos de Archivo Español de arqueología 78): 222-257. Madrid: Consejo Superior de Investigaciones Científicas.

Michler, M. 2004. *Carte archéologique de la Gaule: Les Vosges 88*. Paris: Académie des Inscriptions et Belles-Lettres.

Morlet, A. 1943. Captage gallo-romain de la source de l'Hôpital. *La Presse Médicale* 30: 445-446.

Morlet, A. 1945. *Captage gallo-romain du Puits Chomel. La Presse Médicale* 9: 113-114.

Oleson, J.P., Ch. Brandon, S.M. Cramer, R. Cucitore, E. Gotti and R.L. Hohlfelder 2004. The ROMACONS Project: A Contribution to the Historical and Engineering Analysis of Hydraulic Concrete in Roman Maritime Structures. *The International Journal of Nautical Archaeology* 33.2: 199-229.

Pegoretti, G. 1863. *Manuale pratico per l'estimazione dei lavori architettonici stradali idraulici e di fortificazione per uso degli ingegneri ed architetti, volume primo* (Biblioteca scelta dell'ingegnere civile XIII). Milano: Galli e Omodei Editori Libraj.

Pelletier, A. (ed.) 1985. *La médecine en Gaule: villes d'eaux, sanctuaires des eaux* (Revue archéologique du Centre de la France 21-22). Paris: Picard.

Ramón Sánchez, L. de and S. González Soutelo 2019. Apuntes sobre los condicionantes hidrogeológicos y las soluciones de captación de las aguas minerales-termales en los balnearios romanos. in S. Reboreda Morillo, S. González Soutelo and I. Souto Castro (eds) *Perspectivas del agua. Modelos de captación de la Prehistoria al Medievo*: 63-82. Madrid: Dykinson.

Roger, J. 2008. Évaux-les-Bains (Creuse): nouvelles données archéologiques sur le vicus, les thermes et l'une des nécropoles. *Travaux d'archéologie limousine* 28: 163-184.

Sauer, E. 2005. *Coins, cult and cultural identity: Augustan coins, hot springs and the early Roman baths at Bourbonne-les-Bains* (Leicester Archaeology Monographs 10). Leicester: School of Archaeology and Ancient History, University of Leicester.

Scati, V. 1898. Della fonte bollente in Acqui e degli edifici eretti intorno alla medesima. A proposito del Mosaico scoperto nel luglio 1898. *Rivista di storia, arte, archeologia per la provincia di Alessandria* VII 23-24: 1-14.

Serra, P.B. and G. Bacco 1998. Forum Traiani: il contesto termale e l'indagine archeologica di scavo, in M. Khanoussi, P. Ruggeri and C. Vismara (eds) *L'Africa romana, Atti del XII convegno di studio, Olbia, 12-15 dicembre 1996*: 1213-1255. Sassari: Editrice Democratica Sarda.

Seymur, L.M, J. Maragh, P. Sabatini, M. Di Tommaso and J.C. Weaver 2023. Hot mixing: Mechanistic insights into the durability of ancient Roman concrete. *Science Advances* 9: 1-13.

Taramelli, A. 1903. Fordongianus. Antiche Terme di Forum Trajani. *Notizie degli Scavi di Antichità*: 469-502.

Thévenard, J-J. 1996. *Carte archéologique de la Gaule: La Haute-Marne 52/1*. Paris: Académie des Inscriptions et Belles-Lettres.

Zanetti, C. 2017. *Il termalismo nelle province romane centrali. Rezia, Germania superiore e inferiore*. Unpublished PhD dissertation, Università degli Studi di Padova.

The Use of Thermal and Medicinal Waters in Aquincum (Budapest, Hungary)

Gabriella FÉNYES
Aquincum Museum of the Budapest History Museum
fenyes.gabriella@btm.hu

Abstract: Around 200 thermal springs spring up around the Roman settlement of Aquincum, in the area now called Budapest. Today, these spas, most of which were founded by the Ottoman Turks, have an enormous tradition and prestige. The use of the thermal-medicinal springs was also mentioned in medieval documents. During some archaeological excavations, 25 sites were identified as Roman baths, although almost all of them appear to be hygienic baths. However, Romans also used medicinal springs and some expressions of their gratitude for the healing they provided were also found. In fact, we consider that medicinal waters were also a very important factor in the construction of the ancient settlement of Aquincum, where three specific groups of hot springs can be distinguished.

The aim of this study is to explore the role of one of them, namely the thermo-medicinal waters gushing from the foot of József Hill. These springs still supply the famous Lukács and Császár spas in Budapest. Roman inscriptions engraved on stone and structures have been documented, as well as remains that were documented in the 19th century and shed light on Roman spa life. This paper examines the following questions: Who visited the ancient spa at the foot of József Hill? Which deities were the Roman altars dedicated to? What did the Roman altars look like in the Roman times? Consequently, we will present an overview of the Roman use of all the spring groups that have been documented in the city.

Keywords: karst springs, altars, building inscription, military camps, civil settlements, 'sleeping nymph'.

Introduction

Evidence for the use of thermal and medicinal water in the Roman city of Aquincum, located in modern-day Budapest, can be found in archaeological and epigraphical data. Such data also sheds light on the role of these springs in the establishment and building of the military fortifications and settlements.[1]

Around 200 thermal springs emerge above ground in and around the Hungarian capital. Today there are famous medicinal baths operating here, some of which were founded by the Ottoman Turks.[2] Use of the thermal-medicinal springs was also documented by medieval writers and charters (Kubinyi 1964: 140-141; Olahus 1938: Caput 5, 14-15). During excavations, twenty-five ruins identifiable as Roman baths have been found so far, almost all apparently used for hygienic purposes.[3] Some inscriptions, however, suggest the medicinal use of thermal waters by Romans in Aquincum. For this paper, I have collected inscriptions and other archaeological finds connected to such exploitation of thermal water resources.

Aquincum – historical background

The territory of Pannonia was conquered by the Romans in the 1st century AD. The occupation was part of a longer process. Aquincum was built on the right bank of the River Danube. Before the Roman conquest, the region was inhabited by the Celtic Eravisci. Their fortified settlement was located on the southern slopes of Gellért Hill. The first Roman military troop, whose name we know, the *ala Hispanorum I* arrived and established its fort there in the middle of the 1st century AD. A civilian settlement (*vicus*) developed around it. The Romans evacuated the Celtic *oppidum* although the *Eravisci* continued to live in smaller settlements lying along the Danube. They gradually became Romanised and assimilated into Roman culture and took up Roman customs. The Romans established a section of their empire's border (*limes*) along the line of the River Danube. Aquincum became a strategically significant place along this fortified border. In AD 73, an auxiliary cavalry fort was constructed six kilometers north of the early fort. In AD 89, the *legio II adiutrix* was moved to Aquincum and was stationed here, with brief periods of intermission, until the end of Roman rule. The legion erected its first fortress next to the cavalry fort. Its permanent fortress was then rebuilt from stone at the beginning of the 2nd century AD. The legionary fortress was surrounded by a civilian town, where the

[1] I would like to express my thanks to my colleagues, Krisztián Kolozsvári, Tamás Lajtos and Sándor Imre-Horváth, for helping me with the drawing of the maps and inscriptions and to Alice Choyke and Bea Mislyenácz for correcting my English text.

[2] About the Ottoman baths of Buda summarized in English: Papp 2018: 77-102.

[3] About the Roman baths of Aquincum summarized: Fényes and Póczy 1997: 67-70. The private bath of the governor's palace is a very interesting bath building not only for its complicated ground-plan and luxurious execution, but also for the thermal springs rushing up in the vicinity of the palace.

relatives of soldiers as well as merchants and craftsmen settled. In the last third of the 1st century AD, a civil town began to develop two kilometers north of the legionary fortress (Figure 1).

Emperor Trajan divided Pannonia into two parts: Upper and Lower *Pannonia*. By AD 106, Aquincum became the seat of the governor of the Roman province of Pannonia Inferior. The first governor was the future Emperor Hadrian. He began to build the governor's palace on the Small Island, a part of Hajógyári (Óbudai) Island in the River Danube.

Aquincum had its first golden age during his reign. The quickly developing civil settlement obtained the rank of *municipium* in around AD 124. The economic prosperity came to an end between AD 167 and 180, when Aquincum suffered from the ravages of the war against the Marcomann, Quadi, Sarmatian and Iazygian tribes. After the war, the border was fortified and renovation and new building projects began.

Aquincum lived its second golden age during the reign of the Severus dynasty. In AD 194, the civil town, the former *municipium*, together with the *canabae legionis* attained the rank of a *colonia*. In AD 214, Emperor Caracalla altered the boundaries between Upper and Lower Pannonia. From that time on, Brigetio, with the *legio I adiutrix*, was part of Pannonia Inferior. The second heyday of Aquincum ended at the end of the thirties of the 3rd century AD, when the conflicts with Quadi, Sarmatians and Roxolans renewed. In AD 260, Pannonia suffered the greatest devastations of the war, the legionary fortress of Aquincum was heavily damaged. In AD 294, Emperor Diocletian divided Pannonia into four parts, and Aquincum became the military center of the new province of *Valeria*. During the reign of Constantinus I, a new legionary fortress was constructed on the eastern side of the earlier fortress. The invasion of the barbarian tribes could not be arrested, so the inhabitants of Aquincum fled to Italy or moved into the late fortress. In AD 433, the province *Valeria* was abdicated to the Huns.[4]

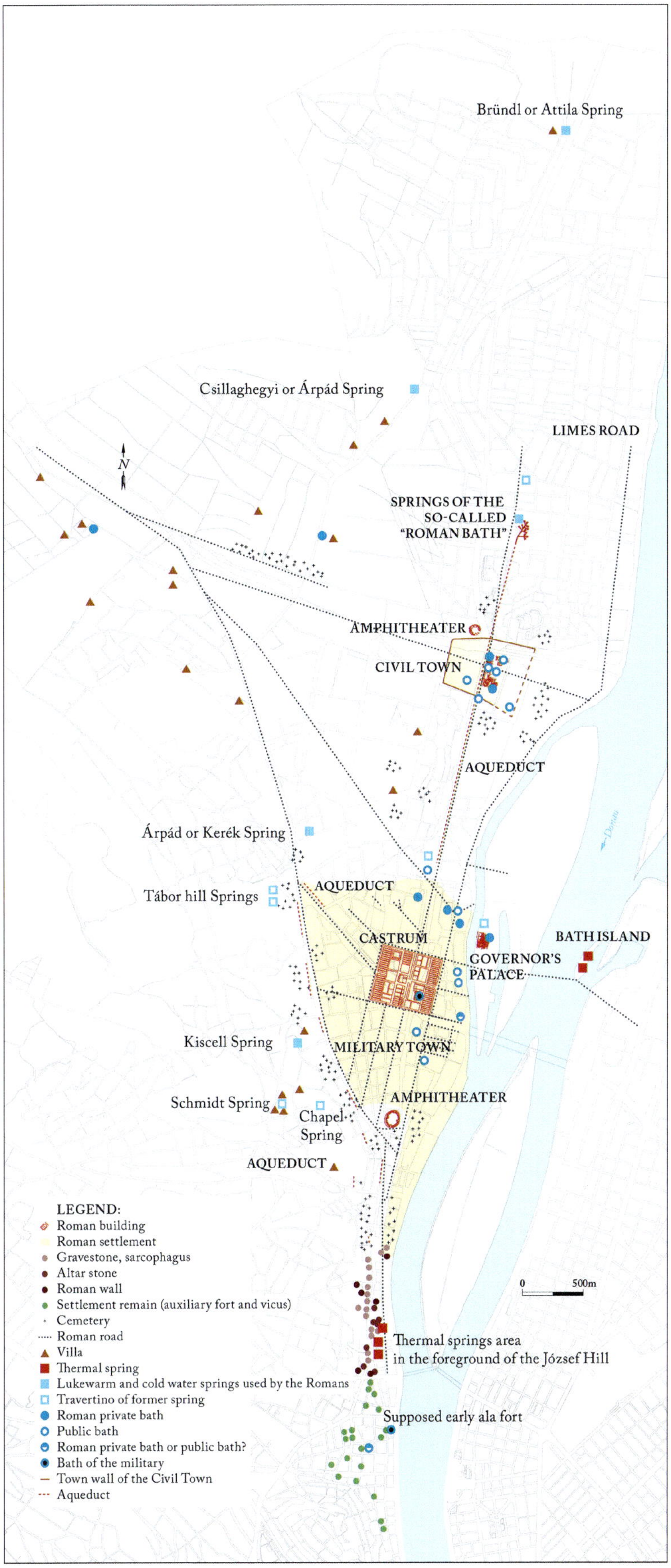

Figure 1. Aquincum in the second and third centuries AD and sites of the springs and excavated baths (Drawing by Krisztián Kolozsvári)

[4] About the history of Aquincum, summarized

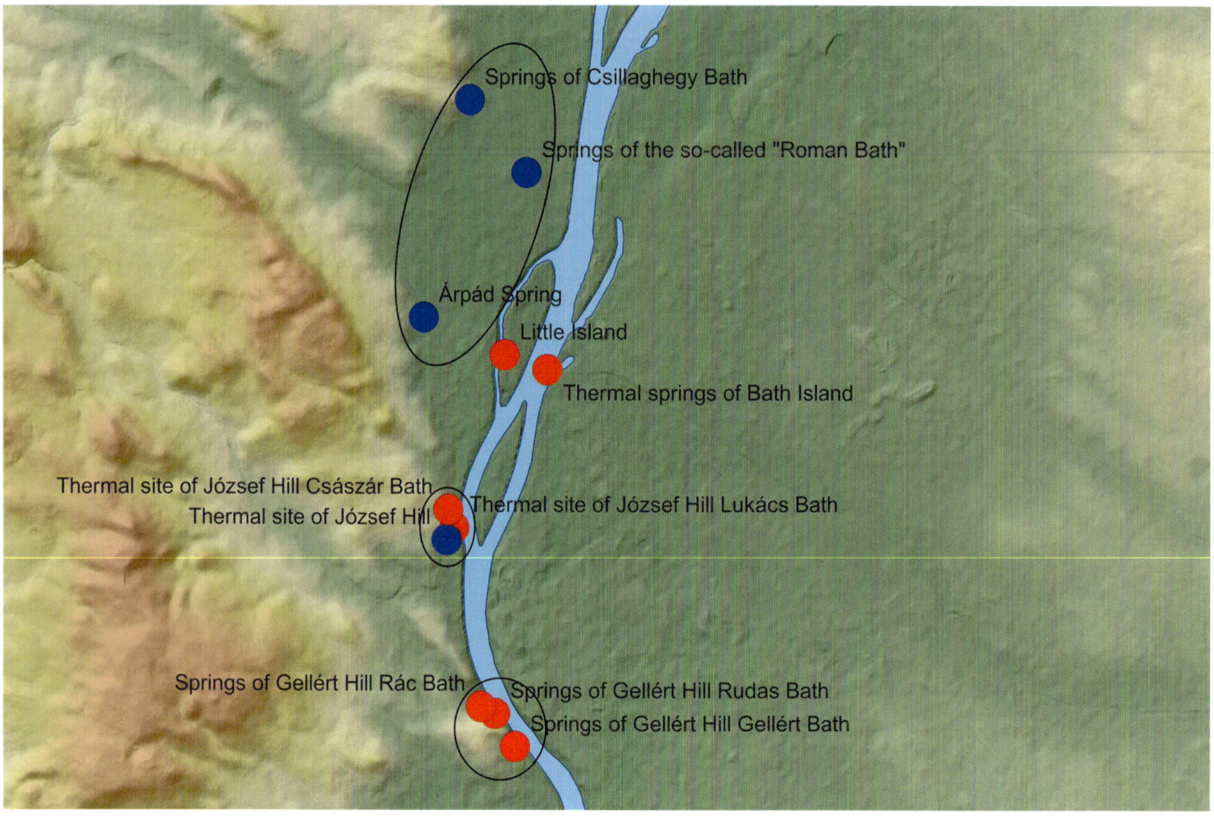

Figure 2. Thermal water springs in Budapest (Drawing by Sándor Imre-Horváth and author)

The thermal water springs of Budapest – geological background

The spring waters of Budapest is primarily karst water, in contrast to other thermal baths of volcanic origin. The territory of Aquincum is part of the Buda Thermal Karst. The geological catchment basin of these springs is probably in the Transdanubian Central Range of Hungary. In the geological past, rainwater percolated downward into the depths, warmed up, expanded, dissolved silicic acid, iron, calcium, barium, sulfur and took up vapors. Under hydrostatic pressure, the water expanded as it warmed underground. Radioactive processes took place, as well. This water came to the surface through fractures in the mountain system. The karst formation, the erosion and the River Danube determined the place and the water composition of the springs. The thermal springs of Buda emerged where the mountains and the plain meet. The thermal waters of Buda rise to the surface from various depths. They vary in temperature and the quantities of minerals dissolved in them. The hot waters of the healing springs cover a long distance underground; therefore they become rich in dissolved minerals. The lukewarm waters of the karst springs come from intermediate flow systems and contain dissolved minerals in smaller quantities. Three specific groups of thermal springs can be distinguished: the springs of Gellért Hill, the springs of József Hill and the North Buda karst springs. There is a thermal water line running across the bank and the islands of the Danube between the József Hill thermal springs and the North Buda karst springs. (Figure 2).[5]

Celtic settlements around the thermal springs of Gellért hill

The springs, which rise up at the foot of Gellért Hill, have hot medicinal water. There is no evidence that the Romans used these springs. But the results from excavations demonstrated the existence of a late La Tène settlement in the vicinity of the springs which rise up by the northern foot of the hill.[6] Celtic pit houses were also excavated in the present-day Rudas Bath, at the east foot of Gellért Hill. The *Eravisci* seemed to have lived in heated pit houses, because these houses were built above the natural underground tunnels of the hot thermal water (Póczy 1959: 66). In 2004, a large quantity of celtic finds came to light during an excavation in Rudas Bath (Maráz 2005: 41). Pits were

recently in English: Facsády 2016: 1-6; Németh 2014: 52-58.

[5] About the hydrogeology of the Buda Thermal Karst recently: Schweitzer 2014: 37-42; Mádl-Szőnyi 2013: 79-83, 34 and 41 Photo table; Goldscheider *et al.* 2010: 1309-1310.

[6] The most recent publication about the last excavation: Maráz 2005: 39-41; Maráz and Papp 2006: 109-112.

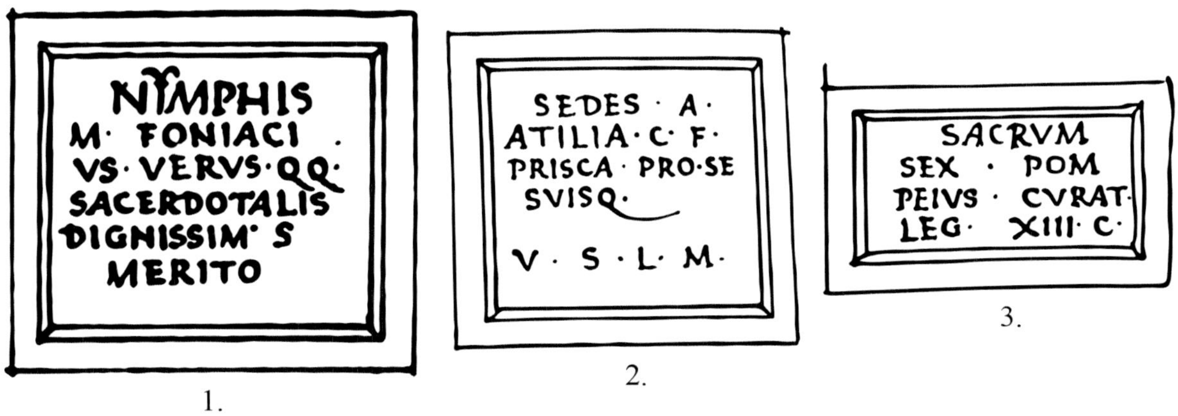

Figure 3. Inscriptions documented by Felice Feliciano from the thermal site at the foot of of József Hill (Drawing by Tamás Lajtos after Ritoókné Szalay 1994: fig. 1)

also found in front of the modern day Gellért Bath, at the south foot of Gellért Hill (Póczy 1959: 63-65).

Roman use of the thermal springs at József hill

Inscriptions from the thermal spring area

From the point of view of Romans, the most interesting groups of springs rush up by the foot of József Hill, along a narrow zone running along the Danube. The springs rose up directly at the foot of József Hill or on the Danube bank. There are springs with hot-medicinal water with temperatures of between 33-65 ºC while others with more lukewarm karst water have temperatures of 24-27ºC (Mádl-Szőnyi 2013: 85; Papp 1942: 70-79; Molnár 1869: 212-219; 1859: 142-165). Medieval charters show that sick people bathed in the thermal waters while a hospital was also founded here because of the thermal baths. Watermills used the lukewarm and hot water throughout the year. A suburb called *Aquae Calidae* existed within the territory and the vicinity of the spring in the Middle Ages (Kubinyi 1964: 123-141; recently: Bencze *et al.* 2023: 52-56; Bencze *et al.* 2020: 25-26). In the sixteenth century, an Ottoman Bath and a gunpowder mill, and in the nineteenth century, two spas, the Lukács and Császár baths were built here.[7] In the nineteenth and twentieth centuries, sick people - after their successful recovery - placed tablets on the wall of Lukács Bath to express their gratitude for being healed.

Roman altars were brought to light next to these healing springs, which also indicate that the thermal water was considered medicinal. In 1479, an Italian humanist named Felice Feliciano made a drawing of an altar dedicated to the nymphs by Marcus Foniacius Verus (Figure 3/1).[8] The inscription reads: *Nymphis / M(arcus) Foniaci/us Verus q(uin)q(uennalis) / sacerdotalis / dignissimis / merito.*[9] It is reasonable to think that the name Foniacius was misread. It should rather be read as Foviacius, since there are three other known inscriptions mentioning the name of Marcus Foviacius Verus. Considering the fact that the name Foviacius is very rare and the inscriptions date to the same period, it appears that two persons, probably father and son with the same name, lived in Aquincum in the second half of the 2nd century AD. Both were high-ranking officers in the *canabae* and the *municipium* and held different priestly positions.[10] According to the first mentioned inscription documented by Felice Feliciano, Marcus Foviacius Verus held the position of a *quinquennalis*, he might be *duumvir quinquennalis* (municipal officer with the function of the censorship) and was for a time

[7] Recently: Papp 2018: 84-90, Lászay-Papp 2008: 63-76.

[8] Felice Feliciano was an Italian humanist who collected Roman inscriptions and was a fanatic of alchemy in the fifteenth century. He travelled to Hungary in December 1479. He accompanied Giovanni d'Aragona, brother of the Hungarian queen Beatrice. It seems that Felice Feliciano described forty inscriptions in Hungary. These inscriptions were compiled in the manuscript of Michael Fabricius Ferrarinus, prior of the Carmelite cloister in Reggio Emilia. His manuscript was used by Theodor Mommsen and his collaborators for the *Corpus Inscriptionum Latinorum*. Theodor Mommsen, since he did not know Felice Feliciano, named the collectors of these inscriptions Antiquus: Ritoók-Szalay 2002: 78-81; 1994: 319, Fig. 1, 321; 1983: 72-73.

[9] CIL III 3488; *TitAq* 291; LUPA 10324. Also published: Szabó 2006: 65-66, Nr. P47; Brelich 1938: 43; Fröhlich 1891, 158, Nr. 17.

[10] One of the three other inscriptions is dedicated to Sol by Marcus Foviacius Verus who was *decurio* of the *municipium* of Aquincum, *duumvir quinqennalis* and former *flamen*: TitAq 347; LUPA 10717; AE 2009: Nr. 1139. The second altar stone was erected to Iupiter Optimus Maximus by Marcus Foviacius Verus Iunior, who was member of the *ordo decurionum* both of the *canabae* and the *municipium* in Aquincum and *augur*: Szabó 2006: 66, Nr. P48a; Szabó-Tóth 2003: 144, Nr. 39. The third inscription was dedicated to Aesculapius and Hygieia by the same person, who was *decurio* in the *canabae* as well as in the *municipium, duumvir quinquennalis*, and former *flamen*: Póczy 1972: 22; 1980: 3, Fig. 2, 18; AE 1972: Nr. 363; Szabó 2006, 66, Nr. P48b; *TitAq* 32. It can be supposed, that Marcus Foviacius Verus, who dedicated his altar to the nymphs, was father of Marcus Foviacius Verus Iunior. Szabó 2006: 65-66, Nr. P47.

sacerdos (kind of priest), when he dedicated his altar to the nymphs. The Italian humanist saw the altar stone in the vicinity of the thermal-mineral springs.[11] The Italian inscriptions collector also recorded that similar stones, with similar inscriptions were removed and taken to the Buda Castle to stand before the apartments of the Hungarian King, Matthias.[12]

Felice Feliciano described two other inscriptions which he saw on the wall of a thermal-lake in *Aquae Calidae*. This is an artificial lake which no doubt existed in the Middle Ages, and which has survived till now. The inscriptions were built into the wall of the lake secondarily. One of them was dedicated to Sedes(?) or Silvanus (Figure 3/2). Probably, the dedication Silvanus is more likely than Sedes because Silvanus was frequently worshiped at springs, and in Aquincum as well.[13] The dedicator was an Italian woman, Atilia Prisca, daughter of Caius, who erected the altar for herself and her family. The altar bears the inscription: *Sedes A(gustae* or *-ugusto?)* or *Si(lvano) De(o) sa[c(rum)]/ Atilia C(ai) f(ilia) / Prisca pro se / suisq(ue) / v(otum) s(olvit) l(ibens) m(erito).*[14]

The other altar was raised in honor of some unknown deity by Sextus Pompeius (or Pomius) (Figure 3/3): *[-----] / sacrum / Sex(tus) Pom/peius curat(or) / leg(ionis) XIII g(eminae).* This legion, was stationed in Pannonia Inferior between AD 194 and 197 AD.[15] These inscriptions are now lost, known only from Felice Feliciano's drawings.

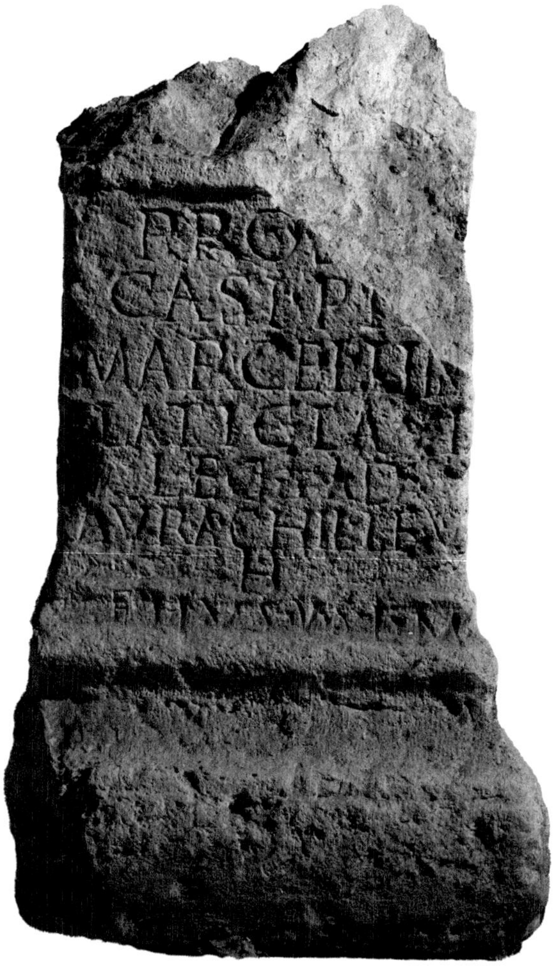

Figure 4. Altar Stone dedicated to an unknown deity by Aurelius Achilleus (Aquincum Museum of the Budapest History Museum, Photo by Ortolf Harl)

In 1891, a further altar was found in the Lukács Bath and transported to the Aquincum Museum (Figure 4). The altar stone is fragmentary and the upper part of the inscription is missing. The inscription reads: --- *] / pro s[alute] / Cas(s)i Pii / Marcellini / laticlavi / leg(ionis) II Ad(iutricis) / Aur(elius) Achilleu/s? // ei[i]us v(otum) s(olvit) l(ibens) m(erito).*[16] The altar was dedicated by *Aurelius Achilleus* to the wellbeing of Cassius Pius Marcellinus, who was deputy commander in the *legio II Adiutrix.* His name is known from other inscriptions, and he might have been the same person who later became governor of Pannonia Inferior, and then nominated consul (*consul designatus*) of the year AD 214.[17]

At the end of the nineteenth century, one more altar stone was brought to light in the vicinity of the Lukács Bath (Figure 5). The inscription reads: *I(ovi) O(ptimo) M(aximo) // C(aius) Iul(ius) Rog/atus mi(les) leg(ionis) / III Aug(ustae) vet(eranus) / leg(ionis) II adi(utricis) / ex voto / ara(m) posuit / libens Gent/iano et Basso // co(n) s(ulibus).* The altar was dedicated to Iupiter by Caius Iulius Rogatus who served first as a soldier in the *legio III Augusta*, and who may have come to Pannonia in a detachment of the troop during the Marcomannic wars between AD 167 and 180 then served in the *legio II*

[11] He described this inscription in front of the Church of the Holy Trinity of *Aquae Calidae*. The ruins of this church came to light in the vicinity of the thermal spring area in 1906: Supka 1907: 98-10.

[12] In 1464 another Italian, Francesco Giustiniani, described another altar dedicated to the nymphs by Iulius Pusinnio, an *immunis* (he was exempted from certain heavy physical duties of ordinary solders) of the *legio II Adiutrix* in the Buda Castle. In fact, the Castle Hill was uninhabited in the Roman period. We do not know where this altar stone was transported from, finding its way ultimately into the Buda Castle. Nevertheless, it may have originally been raised to honour the nymphs of the springs of József Hill: CIL III 3489; *TitAq* 292.

[13] Three altar stones, dedicated to Silvanus, have been found by one group of the North Buda karst springs in the area known today as the so-called 'Roman Baths' (Póczy 1980: 3, 7, Fig. 4-5).

[14] CIL III 3514; *TitAq* 294; LUPA 16632; Fröhlich 1892: 146-147, Nr. 68; Alföldy 1961: 107; Mócsy 1959: 151, 185, 252 Nr. 186/7; Kuzsinszky 1908, 75.

[15] CIL III 3513; *TitAq* 414; LUPA 13670; Kuzsinszky 1908: 75.

[16] CIL III 13371; *TitAq*381; LUPA 5109; Németh 1999: 22, Nr. 41; Kuzsinszky 1934: 216, Nr. 64; Kuzsinszky 1897: 134-135, Nr. 51.

[17] Fitz 1993: 547-549. The house of the deputy commander was excavated in 1977-78 in the legionary fortress, where Cassius Pius Marcellinus had a mithreum made. Kocsis 1989: 81-86.

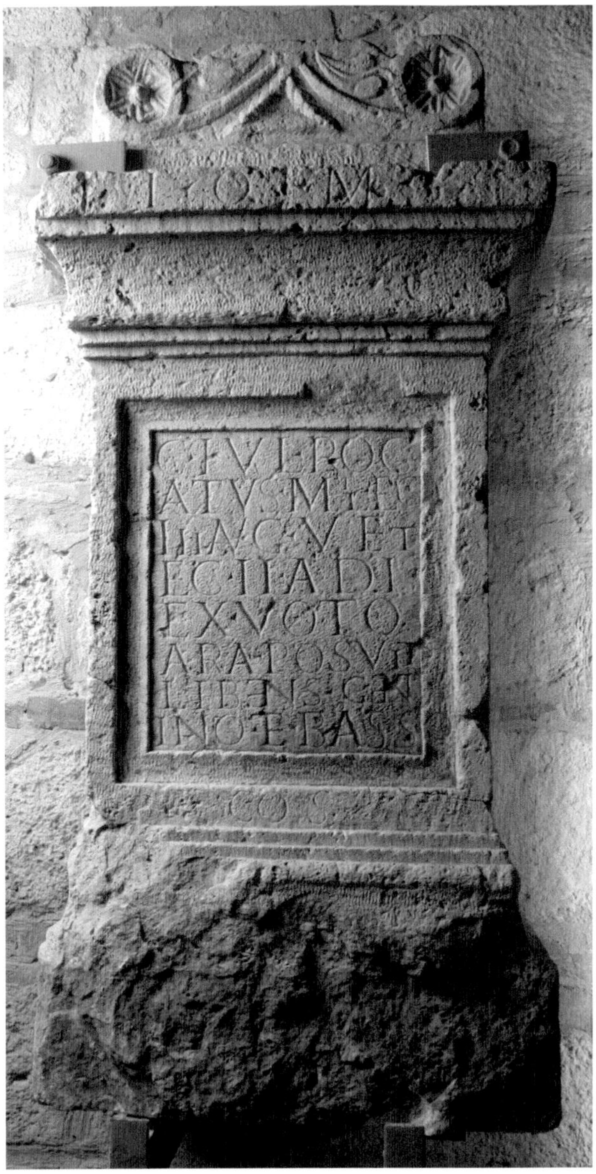

Figure 5. Altar stone dedicated to Iupiter by Caius Iulius Rogatus (Hungarian National Museum, Photo by Ortolf Harl)

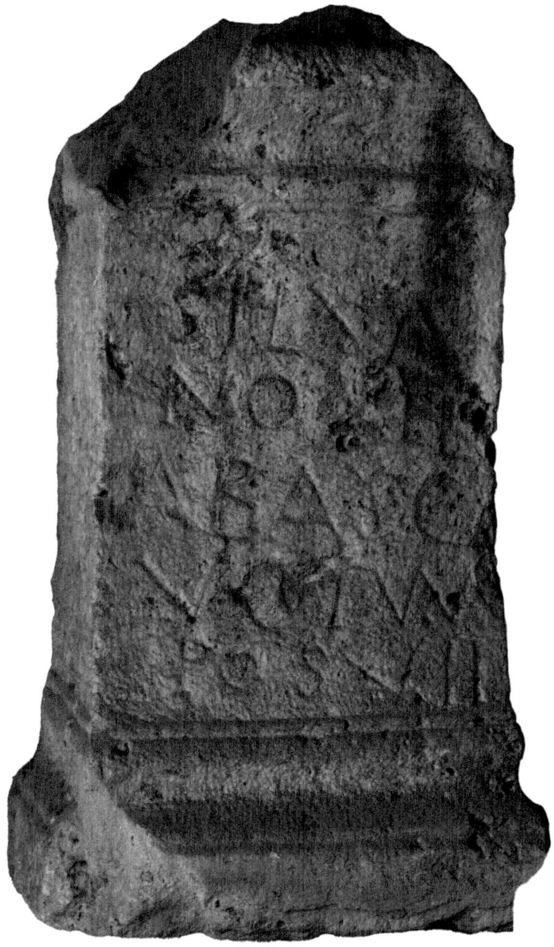

Figure 6. Altar stone dedicated to Silvanus by Abascantus (Aquincum Museum of the Budapest History Museum, Photo by Ortolf Harl)

Adiutrix, which was stationed in Aquincum. He erected his altar in AD 211 based on the names of the consuls.[18]

North of the healing spring groups, a sixth altar was found during sewer construction in 1937 (Figure 6). The inscription reads: *Silva/no Fl(avius) / Abasc(antus) / votum / posuit.*[19] It was dedicated to Silvanus by Abascantus. His name is frequent and is also known from another Aquincum inscription. According to this inscription, Abascantus was the *libertus* (freedman) of Cornelius Paulus who was *primus pilus* (chief centurion) in the *legio II Adiutrix* (Szilágyi 1973: 163-164).

Two more altar stones were documented by Felice Feliciano and other inscription collectors in front of the medieval Church of Saint James, which stood ca. 800m north of the thermal site. Both altar stones were reused in the Middle Ages. One of them bears the inscription '*I(ovi) O(ptimo) M(aximo) / sac(rum) / Aur(elius) Att(a) / v(otum) s(olvit) l(ibens) m(erito)*'.[20] Aurelius Atta was probably of Celtic origin and obtained his Roman citizenship after the period of Marcus Aurelius, most probably as part of the *Constitutio Antoniniana* issued by Emperor Caracalla (Barkóczy 1964: 277-278). The inscription of Aurelius Atta was found again in 1912.[21] The other, now lost inscription, reads: *D(eo) I(nvicto) /*

[18] CIL III 10419; ILS 2318; *TitAq* 117; LUPA 9866; AE 1891: Nr. 64; Frölich 1890: 10, Nr. 11.

[19] *TitAq* 298; LUPA 6514; Kuzsinszky 1937: 126-127, Nr. 47; Kuzsinszky 1934: 163, Nr. 358.

[20] CIL III 3477; TitAq 131; LUPA 5120; Németh, 1999: 51 Nr. 132; Kuzsinszky 1937: 92, Nr. 21; Kuzsinszky 1934: 73 Nr. 332.

[21] About the location of the medieval Church of Saint James: Jankovich 1963: 161.

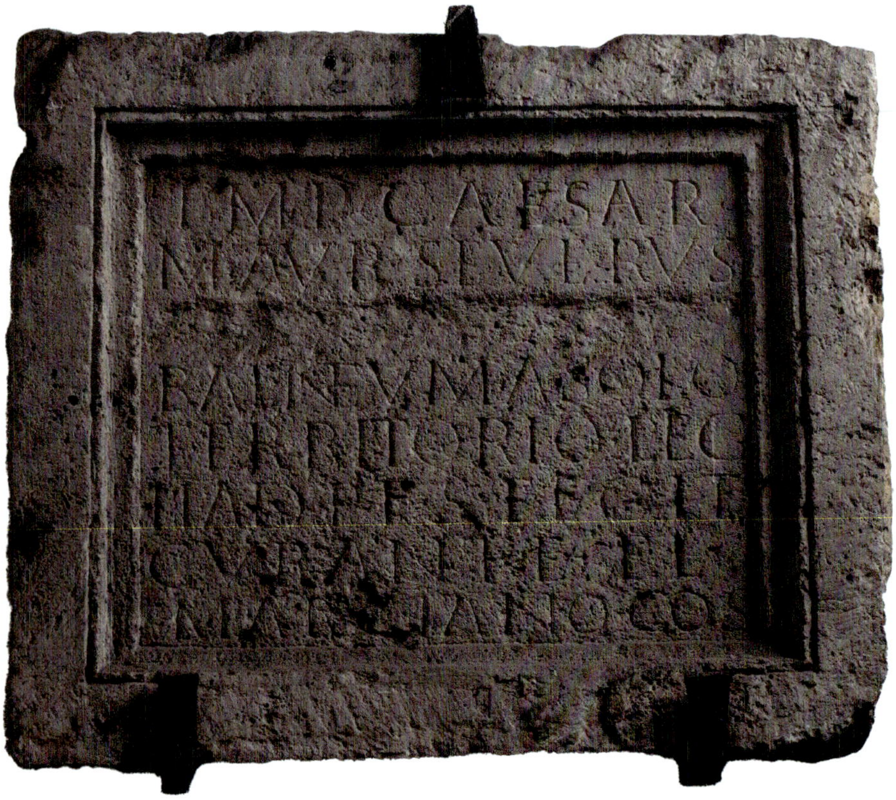

Figure 7. Building inscription of a *balneum* (Aquincum Museum of the Budapest History Museum, Photo by Ortolf Harl)

Allidius / Hermes / v(otum) s(olvit) l(ibens) m(erito). A man with a Greek cognomen dedicated the altar to Deus Invictus Mithras.[22] It is not possible to say where these two altar stones stood originally although they might have been transported from the thermal site or from the so-called governor's villa of the Szépvölgyi Road.[23]

Archaeological ruins in the thermal spring area and its vicinity

Nowadays, the thermal site at the foot of József Hill is divided into two sections by a street, which goes back centuries and may already have existed in the Roman period. Several Roman graves, tombstones and a milestone have been found on both sides of the present-day street (see the map Figure 1). The thermal site has always been inhabited and is still situated in the heart of the modern Hungarian capital. Therefore, there is only scant archaeological evidence available which directly indicates the use of thermal water by the Romans.

In 1859, a famous geologist, János Molnár, noticed that during the cleaning of the catchment of the Lukács thermal spring, terracotta pipes were found incorporated into Roman *opus signinum* (mortar of broken tile fragments) (Molnár 1859: 163). During the last archaeological and wall investigations at the Lukács bath in 2007, a large white Roman marble (door frame?) was found in the remains of the wall of the pulled down Ottoman gunpowder mill (Lászay-Papp 2008: 67). During the latest excavation at the Császár Baths in 2007-2008, two walls dating back to a time before the Middle Ages were also uncovered.[24] In 2019, an excavation was carried out in the neighborhood south of Lukács bath. Although the archaeological remains from the Roman period are scanty, they show that the area around the thermal springs was inhabited by the local Celtic population in the first century AD and by the Romans during the first, second and third centuries AD (Bencze *et al.* 2023: 52-56; Fényes 2022a: 240-246; Bencze *et al.* 2020: 24). A layer containing Roman finds came to light in 1992, below the large, demolished pool of the Császár Baths (Facsády 1994a: 84). On the other side of the modern-day road, Roman settlement features emerged, opposite the Lukács baths: a section of a stone building and a well, were unearthed in 1993

[22] CIL III 3588; TitAq 81; LUPA 13158; Kuzsinszky 1908: 74; Fröhlich 1892: 144, Nr. 61.

[23] About the so-called governor's villa at Szépvölgyi Road see: Póczy 1999: 204; Facsády 2002: 15-20.

[24] Adrienn Papp, personal communication, 10 December 2019.

(Facsády 1994b: 34). These archaeological data also confirm that the territory of the thermal springs was in use during Antiquity.

Building inscription from a bath

In the nineteenth century, a building inscription from a *balneum* was discovered 900 m north of the thermal site (Figure 7). The inscription stone was later reused in the facade of a modern house. The inscription reads: *Imp(erator) Caesar / M(arcus) Aur(elius) Severus / [[Alexander pius felix Aug(ustus)]] / balneum a solo / territorio leg(ionis) / II ad(iutricis) p(iae) f(idelis) S(everianae) fecit / curante Fl(avio) / Marciano co(n)s(ulari).*[25] According to the text, the emperor, Marcus Aurelius Severus Alexander had the governor, Flavius Marcianus, build a bath in the territory of the *legio II Adiutrix*. Since the *legio II adiutrix* used the imperial attribute *Severiana* only from AD 228 onwards, the bath must have been built between AD 228 and 235 (Dobó 1986: 93; Fitz 1994: 1042). Jenő Fitz also thought that the bath was built or rebuilt(?) only after the barbarian invasion was repused in AD 230/231.[26] The name of the emperor was removed from the inscription after the death of Severus Alexander in AD 235 because of *damnatio memoriae* (condemnation of memory).[27]

The famous Hungarian scholar, András Mócsy thought that the stone may have been transported from the area of the thermal springs. He assumed so because the civil town and the military town surrounding the legionary fortress received the rank of *colonia* in AD 194. After that, during the reign of the emperor Severus Alexander, the area of the former military town had been part of the *colonia*, with only the remaining, southern part called *territorium legionis* (territory of the legion) (Mócsy 1972: 138-140). The first military fort(s) at Aquincum was (were) erected only a few hundred meters south of the thermal site, in the first century AD, while the legionary fortress was built 2.5 km north of it, at the beginning of the second century AD. The thermal site was situated between them (see the map Figure 1). The argumentation of András Mócsy is convincing. However, the secondary findspot of the building inscription is the south end of the military town, which is poor in water. The slope of the low hill has no karst water, its springs do not gush forth from deep underground. They are only springs of rainwater flowing through the scree of the hill. Personally I think that the small aqueducts, some sections of which were found along the Bécsi Road, hardly had enough capacity to supply a bath (Fényes 2022b: 118).

The sleeping nymphs

In 1778, the first archaeology professor in Hungary, István Schönvisner, published a book. In the first part of it, he presented the results of his excavation, carried out in 1778, at the legionary baths of Aquincum in the legionary fortress. In the second part of this book, he collected data from the inscribed and relief stones which came to light in Aquincum. He described a relief representing a half-naked nymph in the foreground and other figures in the background sinking into the waves. The heads of the nymph and the bathers are missing (Figure 8). István Schönvisner did not know where the relief stone originally stood. He himself saw it in front of the convent of the Holy Trinity on Kiscelli Hill along with other Roman stones collected there. He supposed that the relief stone was part of the end of an aqueduct, a *nympeum* (fountain), a *natatio* (swimming-pool) or a bath building (Schönvisner 1778: 168, Plate III). He also described an inscribed stone, a building inscription from a fountain (Schönvisner 1778: 169, Plate III). The inscription reads: *C(aius) Iulius Severus ob ho/norem magisteri(i) / coll(egii) fabrum silanum / pecunia sua fecit / Muciano et Fadiano (!) co(n)s(ulibus).* Caius Iulius Severus, who was the *magister* of the association of the craftsmen (*collegium fabrum*) of the military town, had a fountain erected for his election in AD 201.[28] Unfortunately, the relief with the nymph is lost, but the inscription that may have accompanied the relief is still preserved today in the Hungarian National Museum. It is not clear whether the two finds belonged together because their ornamentation was different although their measurements were the same. Margit Németh suggested that the two stones were produced in the same workshop (or group of workshops) in Aquincum at the turn of the second and third centuries AD, belonged to the same establishment and were part of the big building project following the Markomannic wars (Németh 1996: 74-76).

In the sixth volume of the *Corpus Inscriptionum Latinorum*, among the *falsae* (not ancient inscriptions), Theodor Mommsen published an epigram about the sleeping nymph: *huius nympha loci sacri custodia fontis / dormio dum blandae sentio murmur aquae / parce meum quisquis tangis cava marmora, somnum / rumpere sive bibas sive lavare tace.*[29] The renaissance epigram was well known in

[25] CIL III 10489; ILS 2456; *TitAq 5*; Németh 1999: 64, Nr. 178; Kovács 2007: 109-110, Nr. 68; Hable 2002: 267; Rómer 1876: 39, Nr. 27; Fitz 1994: 1041-1042, Nr. 681; Dobó 1986: 93, Nr. 66.

[26] Fitz 1963: 294-295. János Szilágyi was the archaeologist, who suggested that it was not a new building, but an older bath building was reconstructed. However, his hypothesis was not be supported with archaeological evidence: Szilágyi 1956: 11.

[27] Severus Alexander was killed in March 235. After his death the punishment of the *damnatio memoriae* was inflicted on him. He was rehabilitated and consecrated Divus Alexander in May or June 238, after the death of the next emperor, Maximinus Thrax. Groebe 1896: 2538-2539; Christ 2002: 632; Kienast 2004: 177.

[28] CIL III 3580; ILS 7230; TitAq 6; Kovács 2007: 75-76, Nr. 29; Nagy 2007: 119-120, Nr. 126; Fröhlich 1891: 162.

[29] CIL VI/5 3e. „Nymph of this place, these sacred springs I keep, / And to the murmur of these waters sleep; / Ah spare my slumbers, gently tread the cave! / And drink in silence, or in silence leave!" (translated by Barbara Baert)

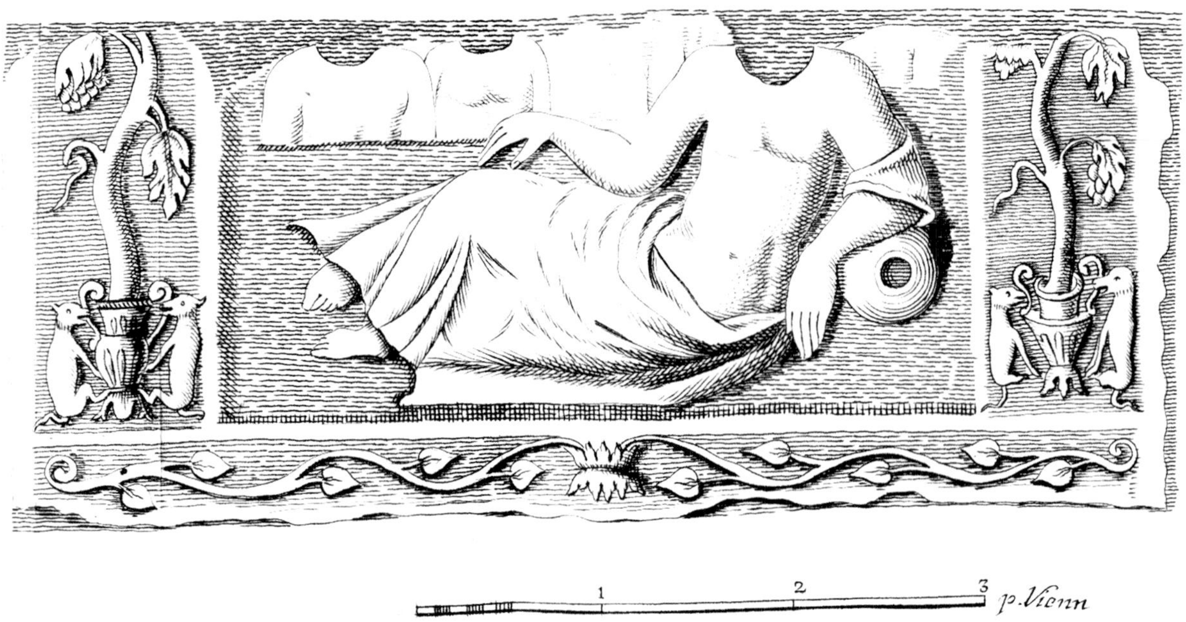

Figure 8. Engraving of a relief depicting a nymph in István Schönvisner's book from 1778 (Aquincum Museum of the Budapest History Museum, Bálint Kuzsinszky Bibliothek)

Rome and Sicily in the fifteenth and sixteenth century as well as in Buda, on the bank of the river Danube.[30] It can be supposed that Felice Feliciano described the epigram on the bank of the Danube, in 1479/1480.[31] Moreover, two Hungarian writers also reported it in the sixteenth century. According to these descriptions the epigram was inscribed under the figure of a nymph on a fountain (Ritoók-Szalay 2002: 90-93; 1983: 67-72).

Collecting antique relics and writing epigrams to the newly discovered sculptures was frequent in Italy in the Renaissance.[32] According to the Italian humanist Bartolomeo della Fonte the author of the epigram *huius nympha loci* was Giovanni Antonio Campano who lived in Rome between 1459 and 1464 and was the member of the *academia* of Pomponio Leto and was patronized by Jacopo Ammanati Piccolomini and Cardinal Bessarion (Macdougall 1975: 358; Pataki 2005: 32-40). The epigram could come to Hungary in different ways. Bartolomeo della Fonte – who collected the epigram in his manuscript – was in correspondence with Hungarian humanists, later he came to Hungary and was the head of the *Bibliotheca Corviniana*. Hungarian humanists studied in Italy and were frequent on diplomatic missions in Italy, for example László Karai went to the pope Paul II in 1470. The pope's secretary was Jacopo Ammanati Piccolomini during that time. In 1474 Giovanni Antonio Campano moved to Naples, and was looking for a livelihood in the court of Ferrante I d'Aragona. The Hungarian king, Matthias Corvinus married the daughter of Ferrante in 1476. Also, the epigram might have come to Hungary via Naples.

It is well known that the Hungarian King of this time, Matthias Corvinus, was enthusiastic about the culture of the Renaissance and invited Italian scholars and artists to his court. The monarch also collected Roman finds, inscriptions and carved stones (Török 1993: 119-120; Ritoók-Szalay 1994: 322). As mentioned above, Felice Feliciano collected Latin inscriptions in medieval Budafelhévíz, *Aquae Calidae*. The altar stone raised by Marcus Foviacius Verus showed that the nymphs were worshipped at the thermal site. Based on medieval written sources, a royal bath, another bath built by the provost of Budafelhévíz, and a third bath next to the hospital of the Holy Spirit stood on the thermal site in the Middle Ages (Bencze *et al.* 2023: 59; Végh 2015: 49-50; Kubinyi 1964: 140-141). It is also known that such ancient stones were frequently reused in the Middle Ages. Roman sarcophagi, for example, were often used as a reservoir for wells (Ritoók-Szalay 1994: 324). It is very likely therefore that the epigram may have decorated a Roman figure, perhaps the very same one

[30] The epigram was accompanied by a description in the *Corpus Inscriptionum Latinorum*: *"Super ripam Danuvii in quo est sculta nympha ad amoenum fontem dormiens, sub figura est hoc epigramma."* (On the banks of the Danube there is a sculpture of a sleeping nymph at a beautiful spring and under the image is also an epigram.) The description came from the manuscript of Michael Fabricius Ferrarinus in Reggio Emilia: Baert 2018: 152-153.

[31] The source of Ferrarinus was Felice Feliciano who came to Hungary in 1479: Ritoók-Szalay 2002: 89-93; 1994: 319-321; 1983: 70-73.

[32] The epigram *huius nympha loci* and the sleeping nymph developed a prototype in the painting and became the subject of artists such as Lucas Cranach the Elder or Albrecht Dürer.

published by István Schönvisner.[33] If that is the case, the original findspot of the relief of the nymph may have been in the area of the thermal spring by József Hill. The relief with the sleeping nymph may have been removed only during the Ottoman era, when the Ottoman bath and the gunpowder mill were built here.

Roman use of the North Buda karst springs

The water of the third group of the springs of Budapest, the so-called North Buda karst springs, is lukewarm and contains dissolved minerals in smaller quantities (Figure 1 and 2). These springs played an important role in the water supply of the civil town, the military settlement and the legionary fortress (Fényes 2022b: 113-114; Póczy 1997: 62-64; 1980: 3; 1972: 15).

The starting point of the north-south aqueduct lay in the area of the so-called present-day 'Roman Bath' (Figure 1). It was also the location of a sacred grove dedicated to the healing gods. The well-houses contained altars dedicated to Aesculapius and Hygieia, Apollo and Sirona as well as others dedicated to Silvanus, Mithras, and Jupiter. Many objects were found on the floors of the well-houses, which may have been votive offerings. It could well be that two shrines and a hospital or inn were built in the sacred grove, as well (Póczy 1980: 3-12; 1972: 18-25).

Aquincum had another aquaeduct of which only sparse remains have been found (Wellner 1973: 179-180, Fig. 3). The starting point of this second aquaeduct was presumably the Árpád, also called the Kerék or Radl spring (Figure 1) (Fényes 2022b: 113-116). Marcus Foviacius Verus dedicated an altar to the nymphs at the thermal site by József Hill, while his son of the same name erected an altar to Aesculapius and Hygieia next to one spring at the starting point of the north-south aqueduct and another to Sol in the vicinity of the Árpád spring.[34] The family of the Foviacii seem to have appreciated the good quality water of the springs of Aquincum.

Roman use of the thermal springs on the Danube river islands

The boundary between thermal-mineral springs and lukewarm springs is associated with a tectonic line running along the islands of the Danube (Figure 1-2). There were some 50-60 thermal springs with temperatures of 51 to 52ºC containing sulfur on the so-called Baths Island (Bél 1737: §VII; Szabó 1857: 250-256; Schweitzer 2014: 42-43). In the 19th century, based on the remains of Roman walls and ceramic finds, it was widely supposed that this was the place the Romans erected their healing spas here (Wellner 1970: 120; Ortvay 1875: 31; Rómer 1873: 323). The island was dredged up between 1872 and 1875 to secure navigable routes on the river. Although an engineer surveyed and made drawings of the pillars of a supposed Roman bridge crossing Bath Island,[35] there does not seem to have been any similar documentation of Roman ruins on the island.

Calcareous, sulfurous springs also sprang up on the Small Island, in the direct vicinity of the Governor's palace (Figure 1-2). There was a private bath comprised of a large oval pool, two octagonal rooms with small niches and other round rooms and apsed chambers in the north wing of the main building. Thermal water might have been piped in from nearby springs (Kérdő 2014: 114-119).

Conclusions

The archaeological evidence clearly shows the fundamental importance of the springs in the everyday life of Aquincum. They may have been a very important factor in the building of the military forts and the establishment of the civil settlements. The Romans consciously exploited the different kinds of water. The first military fort(s) was (were) erected in the direct vicinity of the thermal springs by József Hill, where the flood plain banks of the river Danube first widen out. The legionary fortress and the military town were situated on a broader plain surrounded by lukewarm and hot spring groups. The civil town lay 1 km south of the largest lukewarm spring area, on a higher flood plain in the middle of the marshy alluvial lowlands of the Danube. It can be no coincidence that the private bath of the governor was built in the north wing of the palace where thermal water might have been piped in from nearby springs. The scanty archaeological evidence of the use of hot-medicinal waters can be best explained by the unbroken exploitation of the thermal facilities over subsequent centuries, rather than that the Romans left the curative properties of the springs unused.

Contrary to the traditional hypothesis that Romans built their healing spa on the Bath Island, it seems most likely that they used the thermal-medicinal springs the today supply the present-day Lukács and Császár Baths. Based on the epigraphical and archaeological data it

[33] Margit Németh also studied the question of whether the renaissance epigram decorated the relief with the nymph documented by István Schönvisner. She thought that Matthias Corvinus reused the relief of the nymph in the Buda Castle. Németh 1996: 71, 76. Her hypothesis was based on a brief description from the sixteenth century: Ritoók- Szalay 1983: 67. About the renaissance fountain of King Matthias in the Buda Castle see Buzás 2016: 2-6, and Balogh 1966: 146.

[34] CIL III 3488; *TitAq* 291; LUPA 10324; Szabó 2006: 65-66, Nr. P47; Brelich 1938: 43; Fröhlich 1891, 158, Nr. 17. Póczy 1972: 22; 1980: 3, Fig. 2, 18; AE 1972: Nr. 363; Szabó 2006, 66, Nr. P48b; *TitAq* 32. *TitAq* 347; LUPA 10717; AE 2009: Nr. 1139.

[35] Aquincum Museum Drawings archive Inv. Nr. 272.

seems that the thermal site at the foot of József Hill was used in its natural state. It was a place where according to the dedicatory inscriptions, Jupiter, Silvanus (and perhaps Mithras) as well as the nymphs were honored. Based on the inscriptions from altar stones, people from all social classes used the curative powers of the springs in the 2nd and 3rd centuries AD. If the hypothesis of András Mócsy is correct, a simple bath may have been constructed there in the 3rd century AD. It is also possible that the fountain with the nice relief of the sleeping nymph decorated the thermal site in the Roman period.

Bibliography

Baert, B. 2018. The Sleeping Nymph Revisited: Ekphrasis, Genius Loci and Silence. In: Enenkel, K. A. E. and Traninger, A. (eds) *The Figure of the Nymph in Early Modern Culture*: 149-176. Leiden-Boston: Brill.

Balogh, J. 1966. *A művészet Mátyás király udvarában.* [Arts in the court of King Matthias] Budapest: Akadémiai Kiadó.

Barkóczy, L. 1964. The population of Pannonia from Marcus Aurelius to Diocletian. *Acta Archaeologica Hungarica* 16: 257-355.

Bencze, Z., Fényes. G., Kurunczi, M. 2020. Millenia below Our Feet. Excavation in the Courtyard of the Buda Hospital of the Hospitaler Order of Saint John of God. *Hungarian Archaeology* 9: 21-29. https://doi.org/10.36338/ha.2020.1.4

Bencze, Z., Fényes, G., Gálvölgyi, O. and Daróczi-Szabó, L. 2023. Kétezer év építészeti maradványai és tárgyi leletei a Budai Irgalmasrendi Kórház udvarán. Monuments and artefacts from the past two thousand years, excavated in the courtyard of the Hospital of the Brothers Hospitallers in Buda. *Aquincumi Füzetek* 26: 40-71.

Bél, M. 1737. *Notitia Hunariae novae geographico historica.* Pars Primae Cis-Danubianae. Wien.

Brelich, A. 1938. Aquincum vallásos élete [Religious Life in Aquincum]. in *Laureae Aquincenses I. Dissertationes Pannoniae* 2,10: 20-142. Budapest: A Kir. M. Pázmány Péter Tudományegyetem Érem- és Régiségtani Intézete.

Buzás, G. 2016. Reneszánsz utak – reneszánsz kutak [Renaissance roads – Renaissance wells]. *Archaeologia - Altum Castrum online*: 2-8. https://archeologia.hu/reneszansz-utak-reneszansz-kutak (date of last access 03.09.2023)

Christ, K. 2002. *Geschichte der römischen Kaiserzeit.* München: Beck Verlag 2002.

Dobó, Á. 1986. *Die Verwaltung der römischen Provinz Pannonien von Augustus bis Diocletianus.* Budapest: Akadémiai Kiadó.

Facsády, A. 2016. Summary of the history of Aquincum, in O. Láng and P. Zsidi (eds) *Archaeological Monuments from the Roman Period in Budapest*: 1-6. Budapest: BTM Aquincum Museum and Aerchaeolingua Foundation.

Facsády, A. 2002. Feltárások az úgynevezett "helytartói villa" területén (Budapest III. ker. Szépvölgyi út 41., Hrsz.: 14868). Excavations in the area of the so-called "Governor's villa" (Budapest III, 41 Szépvölgyi Road, Lrn.: 14868). *Aquincumi Füzetek* 8: 15-20.

Facsády, A. 1994a. Nr. 121/6 Frankel Leo u. 35 (Császárfürdő). *Régészeti Füzetek* 1/46: 84.

Facsády, A. 1994b. Nr. 50/1 Frankel Leo u. 30–34. *Régészeti Füzetek* 1/46: 34.

Fényes, G. (in press). Eine neue Badeanlage in der Militärstadt von Aquincum und die allgemeinen Charakteristika der Bäder von Aquincum, in G. Wiplinger (ed.) Bathing Culture in Budapest. International Conference of the Frontinus-Society on the History of Water Management and Hydraulic Engineering Budapest, September 8 - 15, 2022.

Fényes, G. 2022a. Neue Daten zu den weißen Flecken der Topographie von Aquincum, in Bíró, Sz. (ed.) *Pannonia Underground. Proceedings of the international conference held at Szombathely, 25–26 November 2021*: 237–253. Szombathely: Savaria Museum.

Fényes, G. 2022b. Ókori és középkori vízvezetékek Óbudán (Antique and medieval water conduits in Óbuda). *Budapest Régiségei* 52: 113-143.

Fitz, J. 1963. Legati Augusti pro praetore Pannoniae Inferioris. [Governors of Lower Pannonia] *Acta Antiqua* 11: 245-324.

Fitz, J. 1993-1994. *Die Verwaltung Pannoniens in der Römerzeit I-IV.* Budapest: Encyclopedia Kiadó.

Frölich, R. 1890. Római föliratok Alsó- és Felső-Pannoniából. [Roman inscriptions from Lower and Upper Pannonia] *Archaeologiai Értesítő* 10: 1-11.

Fröhlich, R. 1891. Aquincumnak római feliratai. *Budapest Régiségei* 3: 143-164.

Fröhlich, R. 1892. Aquincumnak római feliratai II. *Budapest Régiségei* 4: 125-156.

Goldscheider, N., Mádl-Szőnyi J., Erőss, A. and Schill É. 2010. Thermal water resources in carbonate rock aquilifers. *Hydrogeology Journal* 18: 1303-1318. DOI 10.1007/s10040-010-0611-3

Groebe, P. 1896. M. Aurelius Severus Alexander. in: G. Wissova (ed.) *Paulys Realencyclopädie der classischen Altertumswissenschaft*: 2526-2542. Stuttgart: Metzler.

Hable, T. 2002. Óbuda – Újlak római kori topográfiájának vázlata (Outline of Óbuda – Újlak Roman period topography). *Budapest Régiségei* 35: 267-278.

Jankovich, M. 1963. Újlak és Szentjakabfalva helyrajzi adatai az 1702. évi Zaiger tükrében. [Topographical data of Újlak and Szentjakabfalva in the Zaiger of 1702] *Budapest Régiségei* 20: 155-164.

Kérdő, K.H. 2014. The Óbudai Island in the Roman Period, in K. H. Kérdő – F. Schweitzer (eds) *Aquincum. Ancient lanscape - ancient town*: 111-123. Budapest: Research Centre for Astronomy and Earth Sciences.

Kienast, D. 2004. Römische Kaisertabelle. Grundzüge

einer römischen Kaiserchronologie. Darmstadt: Wissenschaftliche Buchgesellschaft.

Kocsis, L. 1989. Inschriften aus dem Mithras-Heiligtum des Hauses des Tribunus Laticlavius im Legionslager von Aquincum aus dem 2-3. Jahrhundert. *Acta Archaeologica Hungarica* 41: 81-92.

Kovács, P. (ed.) 2007. *Fontes Pannoniae Antiquae in aetate Severorum*. Budapest: Pan Kiadó.

Kubinyi, A. 1964. Budafelhévíz topográfiája és gazdasági fejlődése [The topography and economic development of Budafelhévíz]. *Tanulmányok Budapest Múltjából* 16: 85-180.

Kuzsinszky, B. 1897. Az Aquincumi Múzeum és kőemlékei [The Aquincum Museum and its stone monuments]. *Budapest Régiségei* 5: 96-164.

Kuzsinszky, B. 1908. Magyarországon talált római kőemlékek a vidéki múzeumokban és egyéb helyeken [Hungarian Roman stone monuments held in country museums and other places]. *Múzeumi és Könyvtári Értesítő* 2: 74-112.

Kuzsinszky, B. 1934. *Ausgrabungen und Funde*. Budapest: Hauptstadt Budapest.

Kuzsinszky, B. 1937. Az Aquincumi Múzeum római kőemlékeinek ötödik sorozata [The fifth series of the Roman inscriptions held in the Aquincum Museum]. *Budapest Régiségei* 12: 61-152.

Lászay, J. and Papp, A. 2008. Kutatások a budafelhévízi fürdőkben. Research in the Baths of Budafelhévíz. in J. Kisfaludi (ed.) *Régészeti kutatások Magyarországon 2007, Archaeological Investigations in Hungary 2007*: 63-84. Budapest: Kultúrális Örökségvédelmi Hivatal and Magyar Nemzeti Múzeum.

MacDougall, E.B. 1975. The Sleeping Nymph: Origins of a Humanist Fountain Type. *The Art Bulletin* 57: 357-365.

Mádl-Szőnyi, J. 2013. A Budai termálkarszt rendszer jellemzői, in A. Mindszenty (ed) *Budapest Földtani értékek és az ember. Városgeológiai tanulmányok 2013*: 79-96. Budapest: ELTE Eötvös Kiadó.

Maráz, B. 2005. Budapest - Gellérthegy és környékének késő La Tène-kori településtörténete. (Die spätlatènezeitliche Siedlungsgeschichte von Budapest - Gellért-Berg und seiner Umgebung) *Budapest Régiségei* 39: 39-49.

Maráz, B. and Papp, A. 2005. Régészeti kutatások a Rác fürdő és a tabáni késő La Tène kori fazekastelep területén. Archaeological investigations on the territories of Rác Bath and the late La Tène period pottery workshop of Tabán, in J. Kisfaludi (ed.) *Régészeti kutatások Magyarországon 2005, Archaeological Investigations in Hungary 2005*: 109-124. Budapest: Kultúrális Örökségvédelmi Hivatal and Magyar Nemzeti Múzeum.

Mócsy, A. 1959. *Die Bevölkerung von Pannonien bis zu den Markomannenkriegen*. Budapest: Akadémiai kiadó.

Mócsy, A. 1972. Das Problem der militärischen Territorien im Donauraum. *Acta Antiqua* 20: 133-168.

Molnár, J. 1869. A hévvizek Buda környékén [Thermal springs in the area of Buda]. *MTA Math. és Természettudományi Közlemények* 7: 163-244.

Molnár, J. 1859. A budai Lukácsfürdőről [About the Lukács Baths in Buda]. *A Királyi Magyar Természettudományi Társulat Évkönyvei* 4: 142-176.

Németh, M. 1996. Ein verschollenes Relief aus Aquincum, in: G. Bauchhenß (hrsg.) *Akten des 3. Internationalen Kolloquiums über Probleme des provinzialrömischen Kunstschaffens*. Bonner Jahrbücher Beiheft 51: 71-76. Köln: Rheinland Verlag - Bonn: Rudolf Habelt.

Németh, M. 1999. *Vezető az Aquincumi Múzeum kőtárában* [Guide to the Aquincum Museum Stone monument stores]. Budapest: Budapesti Történeti Múzeum.

Németh, M. 2014. The place and role of the town in the history of Pannonia province, in K. H. Kérdő and F. Schweitzer (eds) *Aquincum. Ancient landscape - ancient town*: 52-58. Budapest: Research Centre for Astronomy and Earth Sciences.

Nagy, M. 2007. *Lapidarium. A Magyar Nemzeti Múzeum régészeti kiállításának vezetője. Római kőtár.* Budapest: Magyar Nemzeti Múzeum.

Olahus, N. 1938. *Hungaria - Athila*. Budapest: K. M. Egyetemi Nyomda.

Ortvay, T. 1875. Hazai és külföldi vegyes hírek [Mixed domestic and foreign news]. *Archaeologiai Értesítő* 9: 30-31.

Papp, A. 2018. *The Turkish Baths of Hungary. Archaeological Remains of the Ottoman Era*. Hereditas Archaeologica Hungariae 2. Budapest: Archaeolingua Foundation.

Papp, F. 1942. *Budapest meleg forrásai* [The hot springs of Budapest] Budapest: Budapesti Központi Gyógy- és Üdülőhelyi Bizottság Rheuma és Fürdőkutató Intézet.

Pataki, Á.Z. 2005. *"nympha ad amoenum fontem dormiens (CIL VI/5, 3e) Ekphrasis oder Herrscherallegorese? Studien zu einem Nymphenbrunnen sowie zur Antikenrezeption und zur politischen Ikonographie am Hof des ungarischen Königs Matthias Corvinus*. Stuttgart: Ibiden Verlag.

Póczy, K. 1959. A Gellérthegy-Tabáni eraviscus telep topográfiájához. [Contribution to the topography of the settlement Eravisci of Gellért Hill - Tabán] *Archaeologiai Értesítő* 86: 63-69.

Póczy, K. 1972. Aquincum első aquaeductusa. [The first aqueduct of Aquincum] *Archaeologiai Értesítő* 99: 15-32.

Póczy, K. 1980. Szent kerületek Aquincum és Brigetio aquaeductusánál. [Sanctuaries at the aqueducts of Aquincum and Brigetio] *Archaeologiai Értesítő* 107: 3-29.

Póczy, K. 1997. Die Wasserversorgung und Bäder von Aquincum. *Schriftenreihe der Frontinus-Gesellschaft* 21: 61-76.

Póczy, K. 1999. Iuppiter Optimus Maximus Teutanus Aquincumban. [Iuppiter Optimus Maximus Teutanus in Aquincum] in: A. Gaál (ed.) *Pannoniai kutatások. A Soproni Sándor emlékkonferencia előadásai (Bölcske,*

1998. október 7.): 201-223. Szekszárd: Wosinszky Mór Múzeum.

Ritoók-Szalay, Á. 2002. Nympha super ripam Danubii. [Nympha on the bank of the Danube] In: Jankovits, L. (ed.) *Ritoók-Szalay, Ágnes Nympha super ripam Danubii. Tanulmányok a XV. - XVI. századi magyarországi művelődés köréből. [Nympha on the bank of the Danube. Essays on 15-16th century culture in Hungary]*: 87-102. Budapest: Balassi Kiadó.

Ritoók-Szalay, Á. 1983. Nympha super ripam Danubii. [Nympha on the bank of the Danube] *Irodalomtudományi Közlemények* 87: 67-74.

Ritoók-Szalay, Á. 1994. A római feliratok gyűjtői Pannoniában [Collectors of Roman inscriptions in Pannonia], in Á. Mikó (ed.) *Pannonia Regia. Művészet a Dunántúlon 1000-1541*: 318-325. Budapest: Magyar Nemzeti Galéria.

Rómer, F. 1867. Kiadatlan római feliratok [Unpublished Roman inscriptions]. *Archaeologiai Közlemények* 10: 24-57.

Rómer, F. 1873. Egyveleg [Miscellany]. *Archaeologiai Értesítő* 7: 223-224.

Schönvisner, S. 1778. *De ruderibus laconici caldariique Romani.* [About the ruins of the Roman sweatrooms and hot rooms] Budae.

Schweitzer, F. 2014. Water-courses and springs in Aquincum and in its environs, in: K. H. Kérdő and F. Schweitzer (eds) *Aquincum. Ancient lanscape - ancient town*: 37-42. Budapest: Research Centre for Astronomy and Earth Sciences.

Supka, G. 1907. A budafelhévizi Szentháromság templom [The Holy Trinity Church in Budafelhéviz]. *Archaeologiai Értesítő* 27: 97-119.

Szabó, Á. 2006. *Pannoniai sacerdotes. A szervezet vallási élet principatuskori vezetői.* [Sacerdotes of Pannonia. The leaders of the religion life in the Principate] Pécs: PTE BTK ÓRT.

Szabó, J. 1857. Fürdősziget Pest és Buda között [The Bath island between Pest and Buda]. *A Magyar Természettudományi Társulat évkönyvei* 3: 250-256.

Szilágyi, J. 1956. "Barbár" betörések és belső harcok Aquincum terében. ("Barbareneinfälle" und innere Kämpfe im Raum von Aquincum) *Tanulmányok Budapest Múltjából* 11: 9-27.

Szilágyi, J. 1973. Kérdéses kőfeliratok Aquincumból [Problems of the stone inscriptions from Aquincum]. *Budapest Régiségei* 23: 159-169.

Török, Gy. 1993. Matthias Corvinus und die Antike, in: Klaniczay, T. - Németh, K. S. - Schmidt, P. G. (eds) Antike Rezeption und nationale Identität in der Renaissance insbesondere in Deutschland und in Ungarn: 119-127. Budapest: Balassi Kiadó.

Végh, A. 2015. *Buda. I. kötet, 1686-ig/ Part I. to 1686.* Magyar várostörténeti atlasz 4. Hungarian Atlas of Historic Towns No. 4. Budapest: Budapest History Museum and Pázmány Péter Catholic University.

Wellner, I. 1970. Az aquincumi helytartói palota építésének kora [The period of the construction of the Aquincum governor's palace]. *Archaeológiai Értesítő* 97: 116-125.

Wellner, I. 1973. Az aquincumi katonaváros nyugat-keleti irányú vízvezetékrendszere [The West to East running aqueduct in the Aquincum Military town]. *Budapest Régiségei* 23: 179-185.

Abbreviations

AE L'Année épigraphique

CIL *Corpus Inscriptionum Latinorum*

LUPA *Ubi erat lupa.* Bilddatenbank zu antiken Steindenkmälern. lupa.at

TitAq Kovács, P. and Á. Szabó 2009. *Tituli Aquincenses*, Vol. I, Tituli operum publicorum et honorarii et sacri, Budapest: Pytheas.

The Role of Statues in the Thermal Springs of the Province of Asia during the Roman Imperial Period

Ahmet YARAŞ
Dr. Prof. Trakya University, Faculty of Letters, Department of Archaeology, TR-22100 Edirne/Turkey, ahmetyaras@trakya.edu.tr

Gamze ÜSKÜPLÜ AKGÜL
Research Assistant, Trakya University, Faculty of Letters, Department of Archaeology, TR-22100 Edirne/Turkey, gamzeuskuplu@trakya.edu.tr

Abstract: During the Roman Imperial Period, thermal springs appeared in various forms depending on the usage factor and healing aspect, and the climatic and social conditions of the different geographical areas.

The scope of this study comprises the thermal springs (for example at Allianoi, Sultaniye, and Çağa) in which statues appear. They were investigated, based on scientific research, publications, and excavation reports. Statues in thermal springs in the provinces of Asia Minor and Galatia were examined, and the places where the sculptures were found in the thermal springs and the conditions under which they were found are described, together with the typology and characteristics of the sculptures used in these thermal springs.[1]

In Turkey, scientific excavation areas are limited, except in the cases of Allianoi, Güre, Hierapolis, Sarıkaya, Çağa, and Sultaniye springs. Investigations were also made regarding where the statues were exhibited in these thermal springs. In line with these investigations, it has been determined that sculptures in thermal springs, which are structurally and functionally similar to Roman baths, are comparable to the areas where they are exhibited in the baths. The places where sculptures are exhibited in thermal springs comprise podiums, pedestals, and square- and apsidal-shaped niches. The features required for displaying the sculptures in apsidal- and square-shaped niches are specified. In the last chapter, the statues and their types found in the thermal springs in the Roman Central Province and other provinces are examined, and their relations with the thermal spring sacred area and with the cities they are affiliated to are mentioned.

Keywords: Imperial Period, Province of Asia, Statue, Thermal Spring

Introduction

During the Roman Imperial Period, some buildings or groups of buildings were constructed near hot water springs to benefit from the therapeutic functionality of hot water springs in the best and most effective way.

Thermal spring structures began to be used as an alternative to medical healing methods because of some architectural innovations and medical advances. Based on their development and architectural features, it is known that thermal springs do not have a specific typological, chronological, or systematic structure like classical Roman baths. However, every thermal spring has a specific system depending on the geographical area where it was established, the region, and the location of the water. Examining the architecture of thermal springs, F. Yegül divided them into three groups based on their structures, architectural sections, and sizes (Yegül 2006: 145).

[1] This paper is derived from the Master's thesis titled 'Roman Imperial Period spas with sculpture findings', prepared under the supervision of Ahmet Yaraş and completed by Gamze Üsküplü Akgül at Trakya University Social Sciences Institute Archaeology Department Master's program. Supported by Trakya University BAP coordinator-ship as thesis project number 2019/161.

Statues in the Asian-Galatian provinces' thermal springs (Figure 1)

Turkey has many different hot water resources due to its geomorphological and geological features. It is known that there are more than 600 hot water springs in total with temperatures higher than 20°C (Özşahin ve Kaymaz 2013: 26).[2] Asia Minor, a region rich in hot water resources, is also important in terms of the number of thermal springs built in antiquity. Since scientific archaeological excavations and research have not been sufficient, studies of the locations, typology, and architecture of these hot springs have remained incomplete. In line with current research, the thermal springs used in the Roman Imperial Period and Late Roman Period in modern day Turkey are as follows: Kestanbol Thermal Spring (Çanakkale), Küçükçetmi (Aphrodite) Thermal Spring (Çanakkale-Ayvacık-Küçükkuyu), Allianoi (Izmir-Bergama), Cleopatra Thermal Spring (Izmir-Bergama), Agamemnon Thermal Spring (Izmir-Balçova), Güre Thermal Spring (Balıkesir-Güre), Ilıca (Balıkesir-Balya), Hierapolis (Denizli-

[2] There are many hot water resources in Turkey that are known but not scientifically recorded. The following list includes hot water resources recorded until 2013 (Özşahin ve Kaymaz 2013: Tab. 2-3).

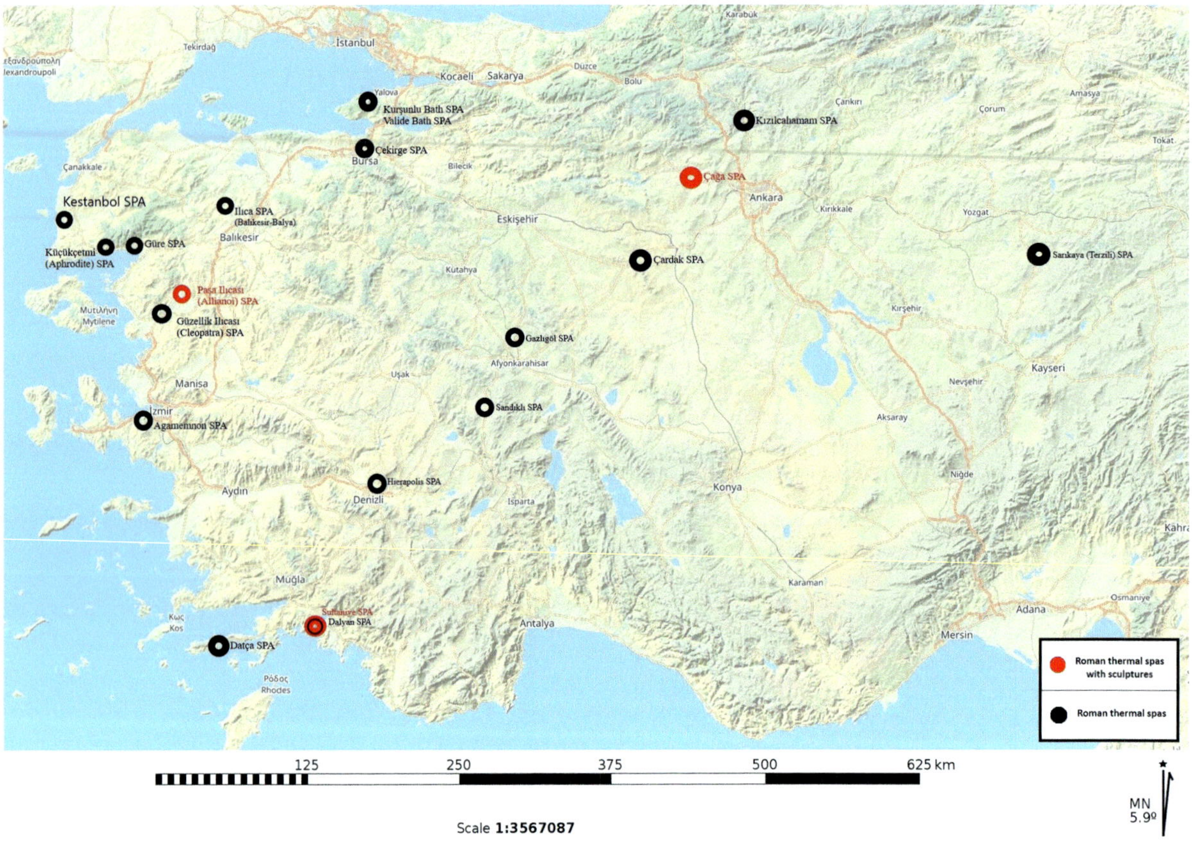

Figure 1. Roman and Late Roman period spas known in today's Turkey. (Edited by G. Üsküplü Akgül, https://caltopo.com)

Pamukkale), Sandıklı Thermal Spring (Afyonkarahisar-Sandıklı), Gazlıgöl (Afyonkarahisar-Gazlıgöl), Sultaniye Thermal Spring (Muğla-Köyceğiz), Dalyan Thermal Spring (Muğla-Köyceğiz), Datça Thermal Spring (Muğla-Datça), Kızılcahamam Thermal Spring (Ankara-Kızılcahamam), Çağa Thermal Spring (Ankara-Güdül), Çardak Thermal Spring (Eskişehir-Sivrihisar-Hamamkarahisar), Kurşunlu Bath (Yalova), Valide Bath (Yalova), Çekirge Thermal Springs (Bursa), and Sarıkaya (Terzili) Thermal Spring (Yozgat-Sarıkaya).

There are few archaeological healing sites studied in Turkey other than Allianoi, Güre, Hierapolis, Sarıkaya, Çağa, and Sultaniye hot springs. The thermal springs in question included in this study are Allianoi and Sultaniye in the Province of Asia and Çağa thermal spring in the Province of Galatia. Statues and statue bases were found during archaeological excavations in these springs.

The hot spring of Paşa (Allianoi) (Figures 2-6)

Allianoi is located in the area called *Pasha Thermal Spring*, approximately 18 km northeast of the Bergama district of Izmir (BAtlas, Paşa Ilıca, 56-E3).

Yortanlı Dam rescue excavations were started in 1998 by Bergama Museum Director Ahmet Yaraş and continued between 2000 and 2007 (Yaraş 1999; 2001; 2002b; 2003; 2004a; Yaraş and Baykan 2005; 2006; Yaraş *et al.* 2008; Müller 2004). Finally, Allianoi was submerged under the waters of the Yortanlı Dam in 2010 when only 20% of the Allianoi site had been excavated.

The fact that Allianoi is close to the ancient cities of *Pergamum* (Bergama) and *Gambreion* (Poyracık) shows that this thermal spring and health centre may have been used frequently by residents. The source of hot water is located on the fault line extending from Paşa village to Çeltikçi village.

Allianoi is a health centre spread over an area of 250-300m in the east-west direction (Yaraş 2002a: 72). The largest building complex in Allianoi is the thermal spa (9700m2). Many sections of the complex were identified, such as the *frigidarium, tepidarium*, and *caldarium*. In terms of its size and well-preserved condition, this thermal establishment is the largest and best-preserved structure containing hot water that has survived to the present day.

During the thermal spring excavations of Allianoi, seven niches were discovered in hall A1 of the northern section. In the north of the hall, there is a section with three niches in apsidal form; the width of this section (on the east-west axis) is 5.80m and the depth is 3.55m,

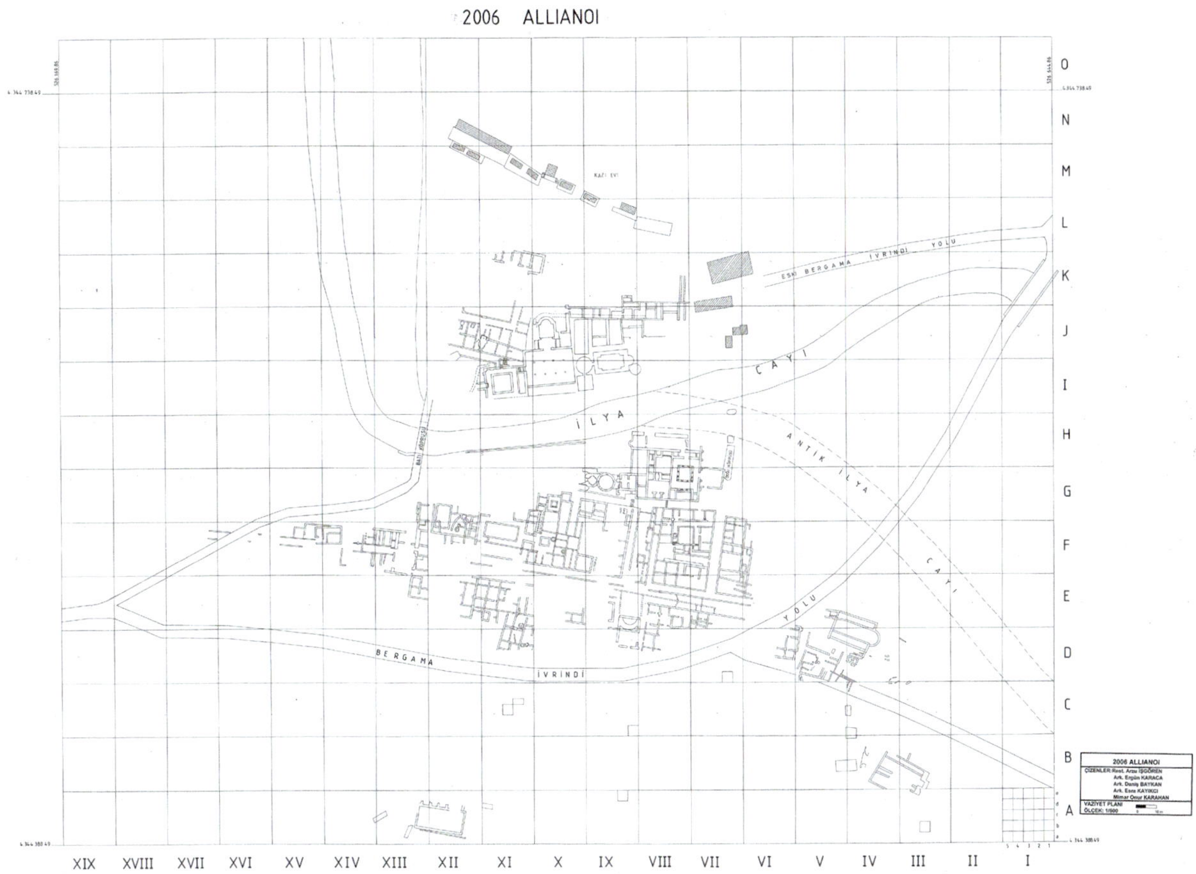

Figure 2. Plan of Allianoi (Archive of Allianoi Excavation)

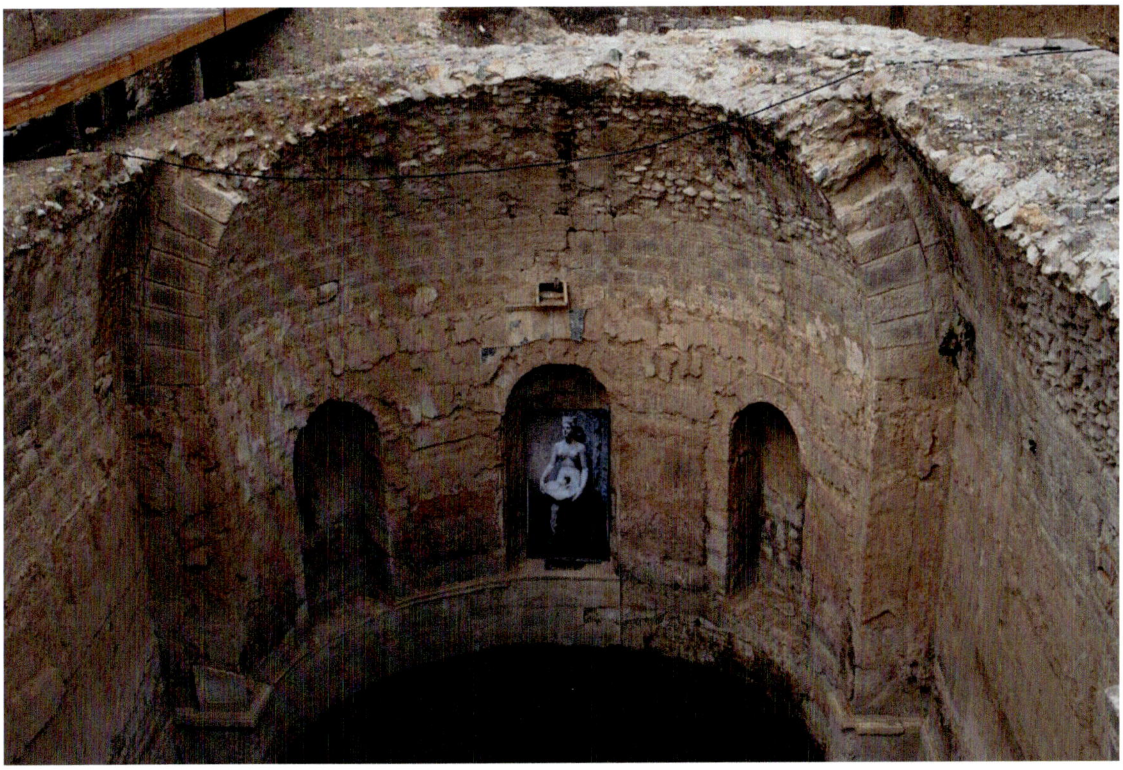

Figure 3. The Northern Thermal Spring of Allianoi - Apsidal Section in the North of A1 Hall (Photo M. Günör)

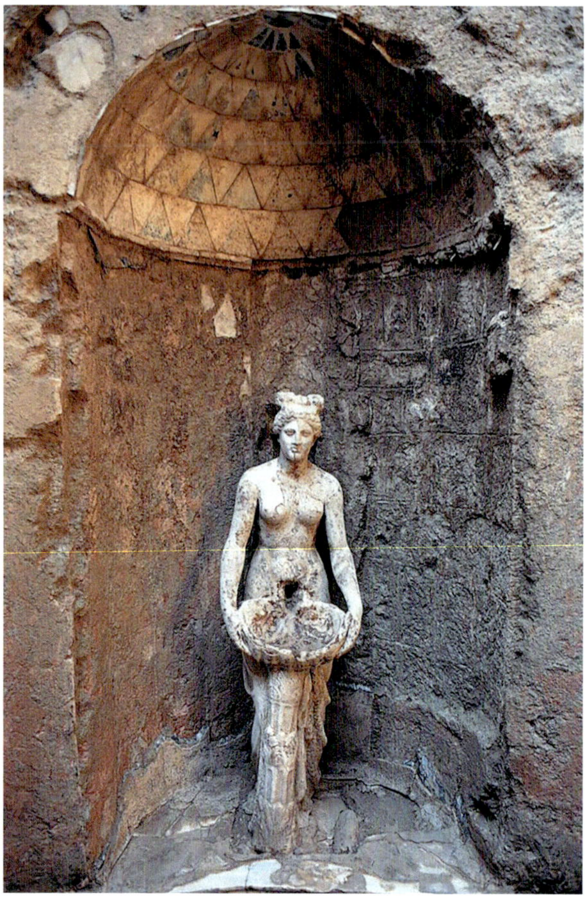

Figure 4. The Northern Thermal Spring of Allianoi - Apsidal Section in the North of A1 Hall (Photo by F. Sayılan)

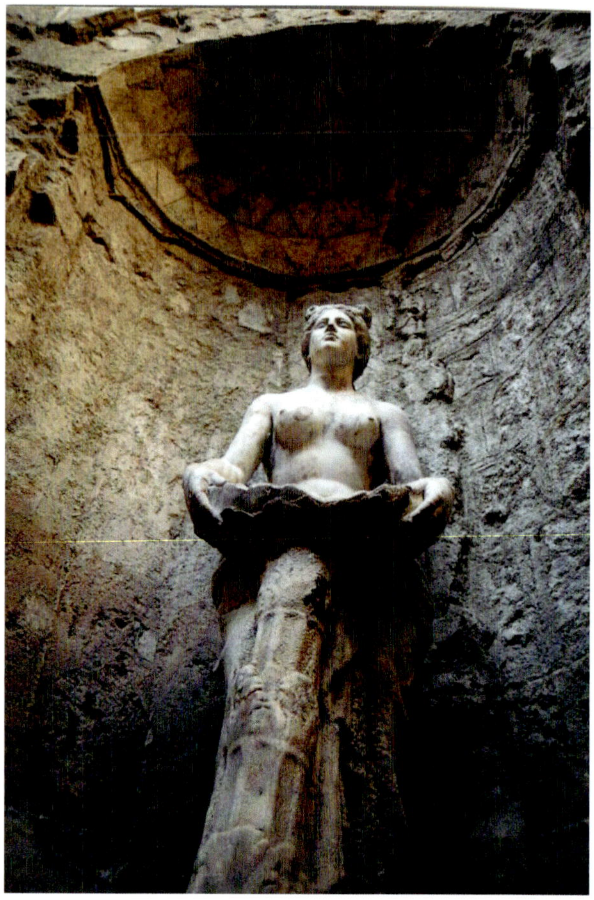

Figure 5. The Nymph Statue found in Allianoi (Photo by A. Yaraş)

up to the inner wall of the middle niche (on the north-south axis) (Yaraş 2004b: 805). The length of the A1 Hall, including the apsidal section in the north is 9.9m in the north-south direction, and its width in the east-west direction is 7.3m. The walls of hall A1 are tiled with a marble coating (Yaraş 2002b: 109). Of the waterspouts found above the three niches, only the one above the niche in the middle has survived to the present day. There are serpentine marble slabs in the form of square plates under this groove. The one in the middle of the three niches has a semi-circular plan, while the ones on the other two sides have a rectangular plan. The ceiling of the middle niche is semi-circular in shape, and this ceiling is triangular in white and green opus sectile style, and its wall is covered with black marble.

In 2000, a fully preserved nymph statue, which holds an oyster, was found *in situ* in the middle of Niche number 1 (Yaraş 2002b: 469). The nymph is depicted standing, leaning slightly forward. The statue is naked up to its lower hips. It is depicted with a himation that curves from top to bottom, starting from under its hips, and then goes down to its feet. The hair of the statue is divided into two from the front in a 'v' shape by a band, and the upper part is less wavy than the lower part. The hair extending from the top and sides to the back comes together and is combined into a stylistic bun at the back. The upper part of its hair is gathered in the front of its head in the form of a double-sided knot called a 'crobylos'. The statue is holding an oyster shell with both hands at the level of its crotch. The oyster shell is decorated with acanthus leaves at the bottom, middle, and top and is supported by a grooved column-shaped foot. The depiction of the statue leaning forward, and the bending of the abdominal lines are masterfully crafted. The hole in the belly of the statue is an indication that it was also used in Late Antiquity. The area where the nymph was located was completely covered with fill soil. For this reason, the surface of the statue is damaged. Apart from the damage caused by the fill soil, the ends of the oyster shell that the statue holds with both hands and part of the plinth are broken and missing.

It is known that there are many representations of a nymph holding an oyster shell in thermal springs (Visconti 1884: Pl. 26, 89, Fig. 101, 561). 'Crobylos', the hair style of the figure, is generally observed on

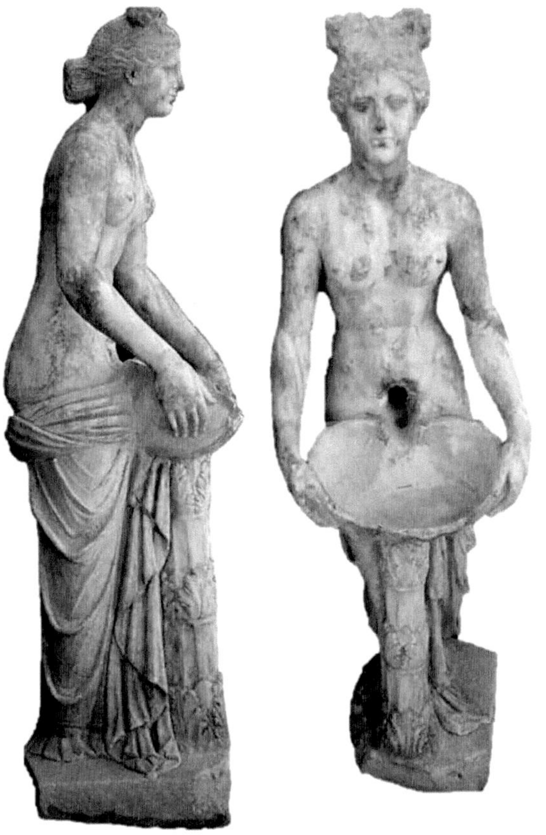

Figure 6. The Nymph Statue found in Allianoi (Photo by M. Güngör)

figures of Venus, the nymph, and Moses (Chauvel and Wuilleumier 1936: 98; Mendel 1912: 328, No. 121)[3].

The Allianoi Nymph has a different place among the statues of this type in terms of both its being *in-situ* and its durability. It is known that the statue was built for the purpose of displaying it in a niche[4].

Apart from the nymph statue found in the Allianoi thermal spa, statues and votive statues have been found in many different buildings in Allianoi. These comprise two Asclepius heads, two female heads, a Pan head, two torsos, 14 statues, votive figurines, and four statue fragments (Yaraş 2004a: 218-235, Cat. No. 1-26, Fig. 1-8).

[3] A similar type of statue head found in Aix-les-Bains is identified as Moses in Mendel's catalogue. Chauvel and Wuilleumier referred to the statue head found in the Faustina Bath of Miletus. For examples like the Allianoi Nymph, see: "Female head found in the Aix Thermal Spring, France" (Chauvel and Wuilleumier 1936: Pl. 2); and the headless and two-armed statue found in Aydın (Tralles), now in the Istanbul Archaeological Museum (Osman Hamdi and Ethem Hamdi 1904; Mendel 2014: 263, Cat. No. 543); the statue found in Crete, now in the Istanbul Archaeological Museum (Yaraş 2004a: 808; Mendel 1914: 303, No. 577); the statue in Ephesus Trajan's Fountain (Yaraş 2004b: 808; Önen 1983: 108); or the Nymph in the South Bath of Perge (Yaraş 2004b: 808-809).

[4] For details on the use and display of the Allianoi Nymph, see Yaraş 2004a: 810-811.

These statues were found outside the thermal spring and therefore were not included in the study.

The Sultaniye thermal spring (Figures 7a-b – Figure 8)

Sultaniye is located 5 km north of the ancient city of Kaunos, within the borders of Köyceğiz district of Muğla province. Since it was in the territory of Kaunos, it was always in interaction with the city. The archaeological excavation of Sultaniye Thermal Spring has just started. All work related to Sultaniye is being carried out by the Kaunos excavation team (Öğün *et al.* 2001: 180).[5] The thermal spring is at the nearest point to Köyceğiz Lake.

In the 1970s, the *Quintus Vedius Capito* monument was found in the harbour agora of the ancient city of Kaunos (Çörtük 2012: 67-78). Since the inscription on this monument and the inscription in the Sultaniye thermal spring are related to each other, the excavation team established the following connection between these two inscriptions:

'The inscription on the post, which was seized here in 2000 and should belong to a large statue group monument, is indirectly related to Quintus Vedius Capito: Titianus, the father of Flavia Maxima, whose statue was erected on this post in the past, was the high priest of the 'Lycian League', and her mother, Vedia Tartulla was the high priestess of the same league. He is known as Flavius on his father's side and Vedius on his mother's side. On the other hand, the names of both his paternal and maternal grandfathers are known thanks to the inscription on the monument of Quintus Vedius Capito. The owner of this monument, Quintus Vedius Capito, is Flavius Maxima's maternal grandfather. Thus, both texts complement each other. The reason why the statue base of Flavius Maxima, the grandson of Quintus Vedius Capito, who was the high priest of the Temple of Leto in the 1st century AD, and Flavia Maxima, who lived at the end of the 2nd century or the beginning of the 3rd century AD, was found here can only be explained as follows: His priestly duty began with his grandfather and it must have been continued by later members of the same dynasty. In this context, it is possible for us to say that the real owner of today's Sultaniye Thermal Spring is the Goddess Leto, who provided healing in ancient times, and the buildings that have been re-planned in almost every period were built here in her name' (Öğün *et al.* 2001a: 178).

According to the findings, the only known statue in this hot spring, which is understood to be dedicated to the goddess Leto, is the statue of Flavia Maxima, the granddaughter of Quintus Vedius Capito, the high priest of the Leto Temple in the ancient city of Kaunos (Marek 2006: 315-317). The existence of this statue is known from the inscription on the statue base made in its name.

[5] On the Sultaniye thermal spring, see Akgül 2019: 34-37.

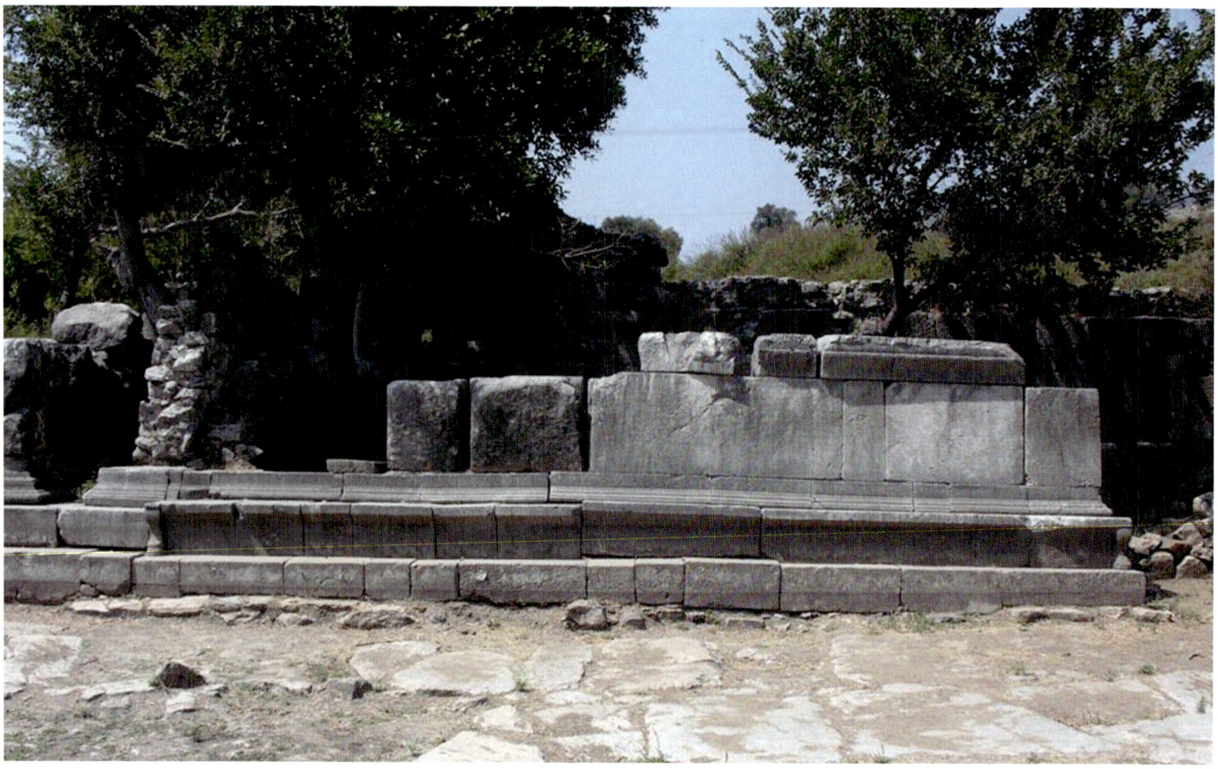

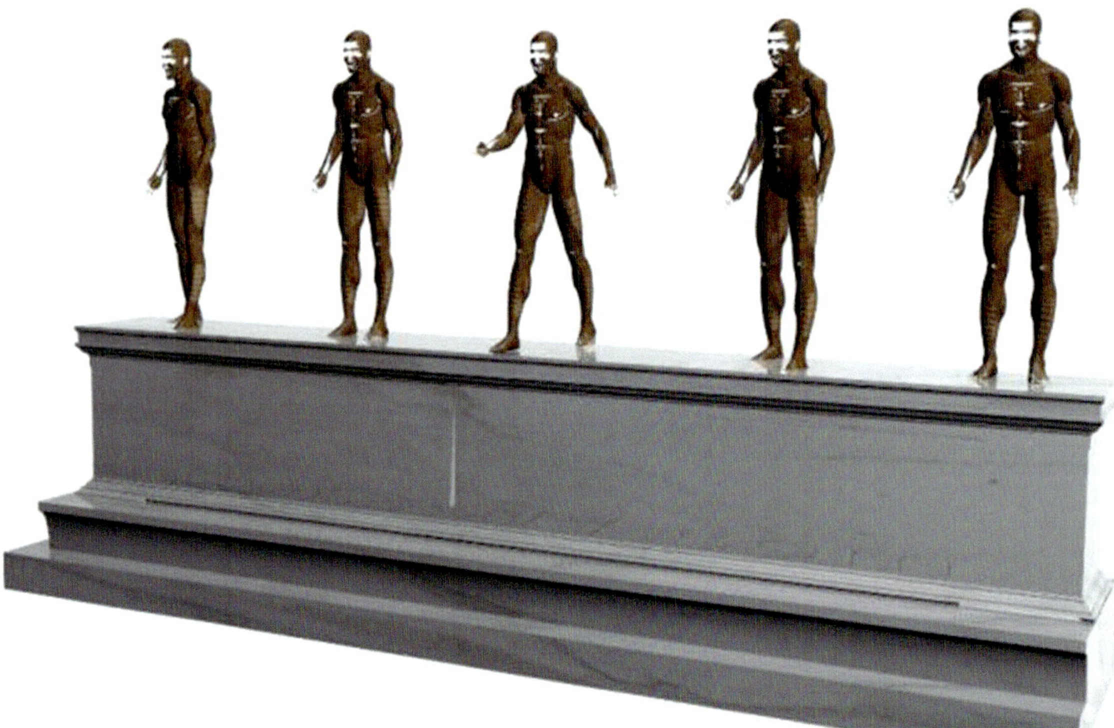

Figure 7 a-b. The *Quintus Vedius Capito* Monument in the Port Agora of Kaunos (Çörtük 2012: Plate 33a - 35e)

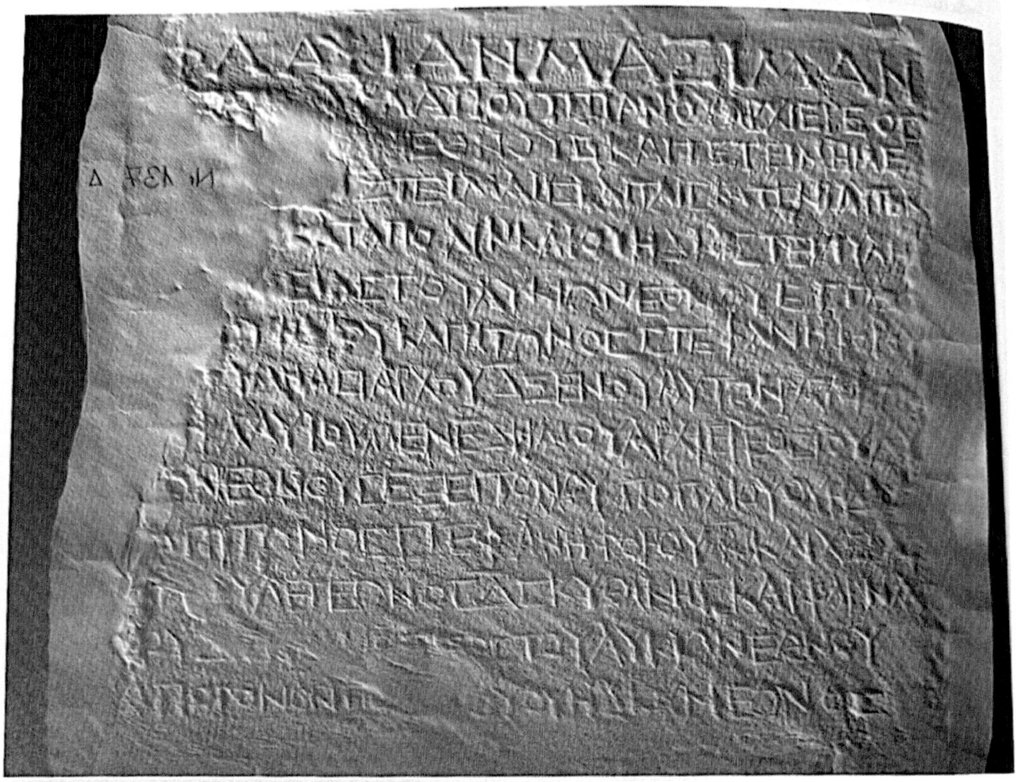

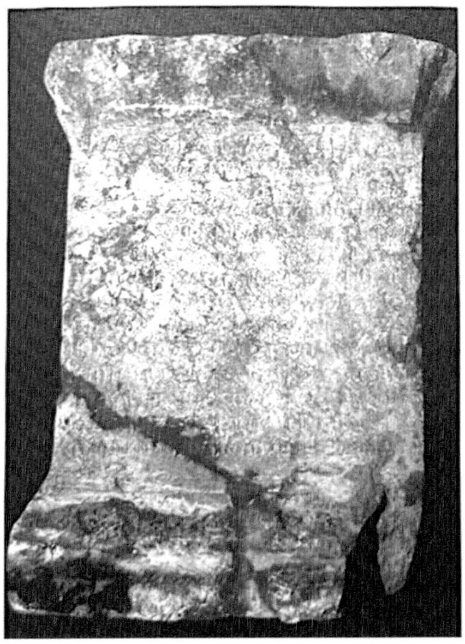

Φλαυίαν Μαξίμαν
[θυ]γατ[έρα]ν Φλαυίου Τιτιανοῦ ἀρχιερέος
[τοῦ Λυκίων] ἔθνους καὶ τετειμημέ-
[νου ταῖς τε] ιζ' τειμαῖς καὶ ταῖς κατ' ἐνιαυτὸν
[τειμαῖς] κατὰ πόλιν καὶ Οὐηδίας Τερτύλη[ς]
[ἀρχιε]ρείας τοῦ Λυκίων ἔθνου(ς), ἔγγον[ον]
[Κοΐντου] Οὐηδίου Καπίτωνος στεφανηφόρου
[..] γυμνασιάρχου δ', ξένου αὐτοκρατόρων,
[καὶ] Φλαυίου Μενεδήμου ἀρχιερέος τοῦ Λυ-
[κί]ων ἔθνους, ἐξέγγονο(ν) Ποπλίου Οὐηδίου
[Κ]απίτωνος στεφανηφόρου β' καὶ χει[λιάρ-]
[χ]ου λεγεῶνος δ' Σκυθικῆς καὶ Φαρνά-
[κ]ου [..... ἀρχιερ]έος τοῦ Λυκίων ἔθνου(ς),
ἀπόγονον Π[οπλί]ου Οὐηδίου Νέωνος

Figure 8. The Statue Base in Sultaniye Thermal Spring (Marek 2006: 315-316)

The Sultaniye hot spring, which is actively used today, was examined by the Kaunos excavation team in 2000, and as a result, it was determined that the hot spring was the sanctuary of Leto (Öğün *et al.* 2001b). Currently, Sultaniye Thermal Spring is the only example in Anatolia of a thermal spring where the healing effect of the goddess Leto is observed. One of the important proofs of the existence of the healing power of the Goddess Leto is mentioned in Homer's *Iliad*[6]. Existence of a Leto statue is not yet known. However, the presence of a pedestal belonging to a statue of one of her priestesses indicates that the thermal site was identified with Leto, and it is necessary to examine it within the context of the sacred area and thermal site relationship.

[6] Homer mentions in his *Iliad* that Apollo brought Aeneas to Artemis and Leto and they healed him, see Hom. *Iliad*, 5.445.

The Çağa thermal spring (Figures 9a-b-c-d, Figures 10a-b-c)

Çağa/Kötü Bath is located at 75 km on the highway between Ankara and Beypazarı. Near to Sarıkaya, it is within the borders of Çağa town in Güdül district. There are still actively used hot water springs around the bath of Çağa/Kötü located in the south of the İlhan Stream (Canik 1973; Alagöz 2013, 2021).

The first excavations in this structure were carried out by the Museum of Anatolian Civilizations in 2003. During these excavations, considering the active hot water springs around the ruins found in Çağa, it was thought that the structure might belong to a thermal spring (Alagöz 2013: 365). Archaeological excavations were continued by the Museum of Anatolian Civilizations in 2012, 2013, and 2014, and geophysical studies were also completed (Alagöz 2013; Sağır and Alagöz 2016; Özen *et al.* 2015; Boyracı 2019).

As a result of the excavations, several main sections of the thermal spring were revealed. A large, longitudinally-shaped pool fed by natural hot water was found. Two apsidal-shaped spaces were found to the north of this pool, and another space with multiple apses was found to the northeast. The sections of the thermal spring, which was built over a large area, have not been fully revealed. A layer of yellow limestone was seen at the bottom of the large pool extending in a north-south direction. The depth of this pool is 1.35m. It is thought that this layer is the sediment accumulated in the pool by natural hot water (Sağır and Alagöz 2016: 47). In this context, it can be said that this is the large pool of the thermal spring which was fed with natural hot water and used for treatment.

There are apsidal and square niches in many parts of the large north-south oriented pool of the thermal spring. The heights and dimensions of the square and apsidal shaped niches in the northern apse unearthed suggest that there may have been statues in these compartments, as in other thermal springs.

During the excavations carried out in the northern part of the large pool, many statue fragments were identified. Apart from the study statue fragments, the head of an Asclepius statue was also found (Alagöz 2021: Res. 7). The detail under the head of the statue shows that it was not made as a monolith with its body. Asclepius' hair is depicted as wavy and parted in the middle. The facial details of the statue are depicted in a simple manner, and its beard is depicted as thick and flat. The statue is broken from the head down and the rest is missing. There is apparently extensive wear-related damage on the surface of the figure[7].

The places of statues in thermal springs

When statues are not found *in-situ*, their locations in the thermal spring structures during the Roman Imperial Period can only be determined by architectural details and the location of the finds.

In Antiquity, the areas where sculptures were exhibited were generally podiums, pedestals, and inside square- and apsidal-shaped niches. The niches in the architecture of thermal springs show that the sculptures here were exhibited in apsidal-shaped recesses and protrusions in areas integrated with the architecture.

The similarity of thermal springs to baths makes it possible that the sculptures exhibited in the baths are similar to the way they are exhibited in the thermal springs. Italy, as the centre of the Roman Empire, is known as the region with the highest number of sculptures unearthed in baths and thermal springs (Manderscheid 1981: 8). The period when baths and thermal springs were intensively built was the 2nd century AD (Manderscheid 1981: 9). Sixty percent of baths and thermal springs were built in this period[8]. The 2nd century AD is seen as the peak period in which sculptures were exhibited in thermal springs and baths, in direct proportion to the peak of construction rate (Manderscheid 1981: 9). According to H. Manderscheid, although this period had 60 percent of construction activities, the proportion of sculptures compared to other centuries was 70 percent or even more (Manderscheid 1981: 9). There are many niches built into the structure of thermal springs and baths of the Imperial Period (Manderscheid 1981: 10). Although the utilisation of apsidal- and square-shaped niches in thermal springs varies, it is generally accepted that these may be areas where sculptures were exhibited. It is possible to observe the niches where sculptures were once exhibited in Çağa and Allianoi. The significant point in constructing niches is to plan the niches for the first statues to be erected in them. If an interior space or a facade is equipped with niches for statues, the statues are expected to be placed there at the end of construction.[9] However, this does not mean that all the

[7] We would like to thank the experts of the Museum of Anatolian Civilizations, who carried out the Çağa Rescue Excavation, and also to the valuable colleague Umut Alagöz, Deputy Director of the Museum, who kindly shared the photos with us.

[8] Manderscheid discusses thermal springs and baths together. He carried out a numerical proportioning of the statues from baths and thermal springs by dividing them into centuries. Manderscheid determined that there were 53 statues in the 1st century, 114 statues in the 3rd and 4th centuries, and 393 statues in the 2nd century, when the most intense construction and sculpture activities were carried out. For more detailed information, see Manderscheid 1981: 8-20. New findings in line with the excavations in baths and thermal springs that continued after Manderscheid's study published in 1981 make it possible to change the distribution of the statues according to centuries.

[9] Manderscheid says that the statues to be placed in the niches were

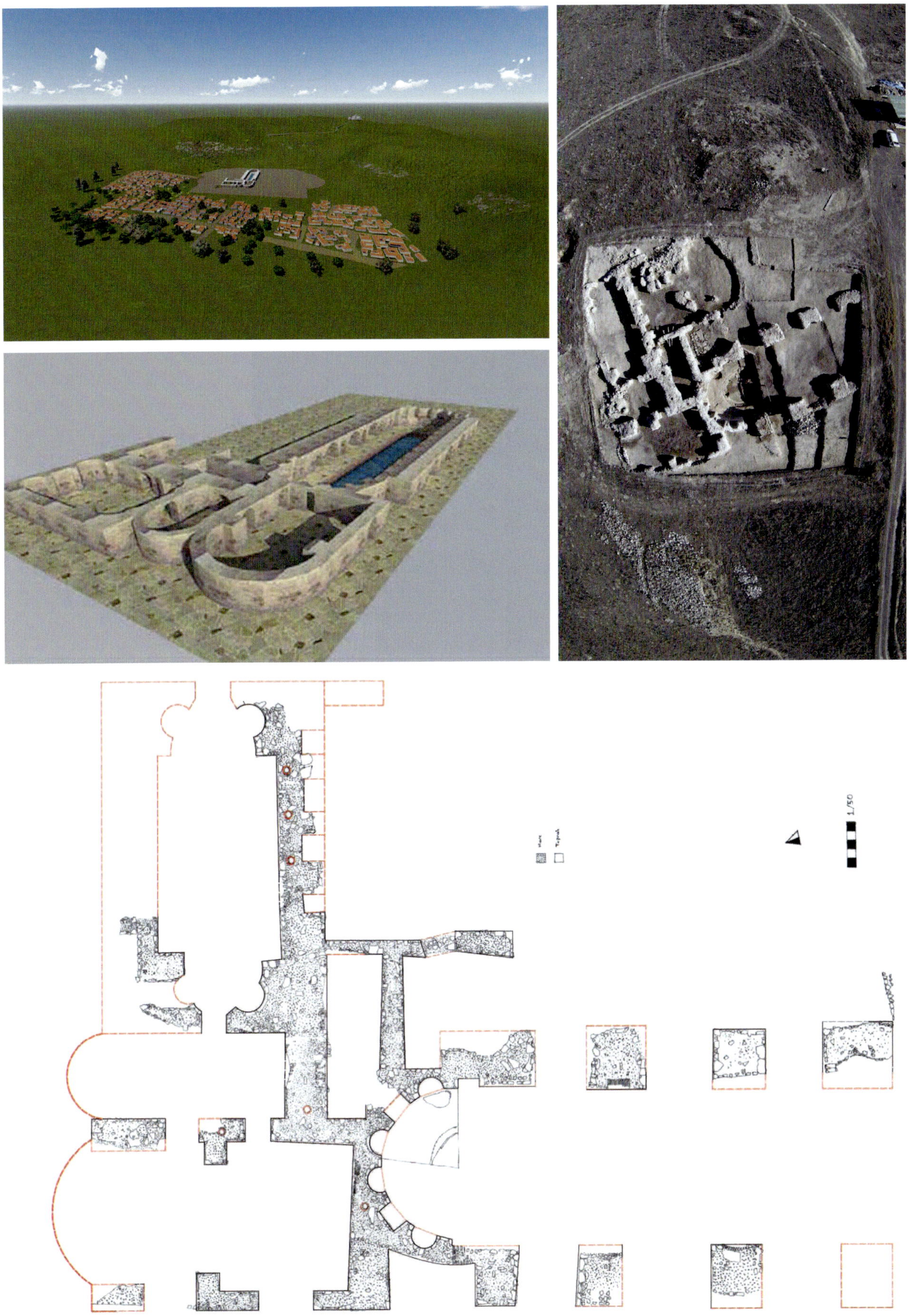

Figure 9 a-b-c-d. Plan and 3D Axonometric Views of Çağa Thermal Spring (Archive of Çağa Excavation) (Sağır and Alagöz 2016: Drawing 1; Sağır *et al.* 2014: Pic. 9)

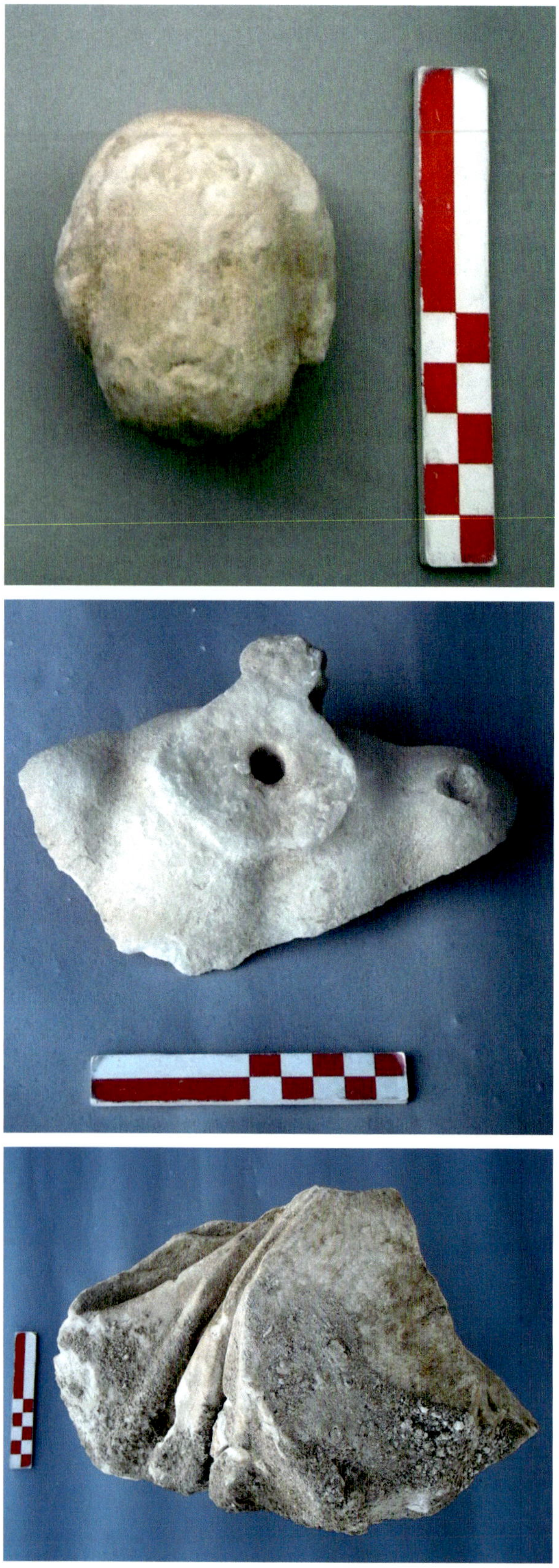

Figure 10 a-b. Sculpture Fragments Found in the Northern Section of the Large Pool of Çağa Thermal Spring (Archive of Çağa Excavation) (Sağır and Alagöz 2015: Fig. 11)

statues in thermal springs were used in niches made during the primary construction period. Such objects may have been donated to the building later, or they may have been used with a different display method. Apart from this, there may also be a secondary use of the statues, resulting from the placement of honorary sculptures in the niches during the repair of the building after a certain period of time following the original construction of a thermal spring (Manderscheid 1981: 10).

The place where the nymph statue was exhibited in Allianoi is in an apsidal-shaped niche. According to the available data, the statue in Sultaniye Thermal Spring is on a high pedestal, in a sacred section related to the thermal spring, or in a high niche by the pool. The statue in Çağa must have been displayed in one of the niches in the northern part of the large pool.

The types of statues used in thermal springs

typological classification of the types of statues found in thermal springs is limited. Although archaeological excavations carried out in hot springs do not show the full inventory of the statues in these structures, they provide some general information.

In the 1st century BC, the Roman architect Vitruvius made suggestions for choosing the right areas for the construction of temples and sacred areas (Vitruvius, 1.2.2). Vitruvius recommended that temples should be built close to water sources, and that temples to be built to healing gods should especially comply with this rule. The natural hot water bubbling from the underground depths always gave rise to a sense of wonder and belief in the unlimited powers of divine spirits (Dvorjetski 2007: 88). Although it was not directly related to cults regarding health, a local god as well as the divinity of the Roman god must have been accepted in most thermal springs. According to archaeological, epigraphic, and ancient sources, including the statues and votive offerings themselves, the gods and goddesses known to exist in hot springs are Asclepius, Hygieia, Apollo, Minerva, Venus, Mercury, Bacchus, Leto and Hercules. (Weiss and Kemble 1962: 11; Croon 1967: 230, 244; Jackson 1990: 5-9; Smith 1922: 393; Fytikas *et al.* 1999: 84-85, 91-94).

In many regions under the hegemony of the Roman Empire, the syncretism of local gods and goddesses, who were previously considered sacred and were worshiped, with Roman gods and goddesses is common. Considering the healing effects of thermal springs, it

finished with the building and the statues were placed in the niches after the construction was completed. He says that these niches would not be placed several decades or centuries later, depending on the purpose for which they were built (Manderscheid 1981: 10).

has been determined that Roman gods and goddesses were located within the building and in temples built as a complex with thermal springs. In the reliefs found in the Aquae Sulis spa-temple complex in Bath, England, Roman and Celtic goddesses are worshiped as a whole in the form of a single goddess. Sulis Minerva and the Roman god Mercury are depicted together with the Celtic goddess Rosmerta (Page 1906: 251). In North Africa, another province of the Roman Empire, a local Asclepius type (Tunisian type) emerged as a result of the syncretism of Eshmun, the local healing god, and Asclepius in Carthage and the lands under its sovereignty (Ploegs 2016: 286). A local Asclepius of this type was found at Henchir el-Hammam (*Aquae Flavianae*) in Kenchela, Algeria (Gsell and Graillot 1893: 512; Christofle 1938: 230); a statue of Hygeia and Asclepius at Jebel Oust (Ben Abed and Scheid 2015: Fig. 5); a Minerva relief found in *Aquae Sulis* Thermal Spring (Page 1906: Fig. 34); a Venus statue in Munigua, Seville, Spain (Mainer 2017: 339); a Venus, an Armoured Venus statue, and a Hermes statue with Small Dionysus in Agnano, Naples, Italy (Macchioro 1912: 284, Fig. 10, 11, 15); a Venus statue found in *Teanum Sidicinum*, located in Teano district of Ceserta province, Campania region of Italy (Gabrici 1908: 410, Fig. 10); the Apollo statue located in Bagni de Vicarello (*Aquae Apollinares Novae*) in Vicarello district of Livorno province, Italy (Sodano 2011: Fig. 12); all these constitute different examples in terms of showing the diversity of god and goddess statues exhibited in thermal springs.

Among the sculptures exhibited in thermal springs, there are also portraits of emperors and empresses. The statue head thought to be a portrait of Constantine found in the Aix Thermal Spring in France (Chauvel and Wuilleumier 1936: Pl. 6) and the portrait of Faustina the Elder, wife of Emperor Antoninus Pius, found in Valchetta / Bagni della Regina (Veio) in Rome (Fusco and Lattanzi 2013: Fig. 257) are examples of emperor and empress portraits exhibited in thermal springs.

It is also common to exhibit nymph statues, which are water nymphs, in thermal springs which were built primarily for different uses of the water. Muses, known as the source of inspiration, as well as Cupido, Ganymedes and Satyr, are examples of different sculptures seen in thermal springs. The nymph statue found in Munigua in Seville, Spain (Blech and Hauschild 1993: Pl. 27c) and the nymph unearthed in Allianoi in the Bergama district of Izmir province are among the examples of statues made to be exhibited in thermal springs. The head of Moses found in the piscine section of Aix-les-Bains in France (Chauvel and Wuilleumier 1936: Pl. II), and the five Moses statues found in Agnano and now located in the Liebieghaus Museum in Frankfurt (Cristilli 2008: Fig. 1-2) constitute examples of Moses statues made to be exhibited in thermal springs. Statues of Cupid or of children holding a goose can also be found in hot springs. Examples include the statues of Cupid with a goose in the *Teanum Sidicinum* (Gabrici 1908: 406, Fig. 5) and in the *Aquae Vescinae* in Lazio, Italy (Giglioli 1912: 48, Fig. 7). The Ganymedes found in Agnano (Macchioro 1912: Fig. 13), the river god mask (Romano 2006: 187-188), and the Satyr statue (Gabrici 1908: Fig. 7) found in *Teanum Sidicinum* are very important as they show the diversity of sculptures used in thermal springs. In addition, based on the statue base from Sultaniye Thermal Spring, it is possible to say that statues of high priests were also exhibited in the thermal springs.

It is very difficult to reveal the relationship of thermal springs with cults, and therefore with gods, goddesses, and other divine personalities, based on the current knowledge and research undertaken so far. The sculpture-reliefs found in thermal springs, such as nymph, Cupid, Moses, and animal and human depictions representing power, must have been used in many public buildings of the Roman Empire due to their properties representing the sanctity of water. Statues such as Hermes with Baby Dionysus, Satyr, and Ganymedes found in thermal springs may have been used to increase the visibility of the building due to the size and fame of the particular thermal spring. The emperor and empress statues and busts found in Roman thermal springs were added during the construction and repair of the thermal spring or for the purpose of administrative representation.

Evaluation and conclusion

In recent years, more studies have begun to be conducted on the nature and function of thermal springs of the Roman Imperial Period. Despite this, there is not yet sufficient research on the details of the sculptures used in thermal springs.

Architectural changes that occur as a result of the continuous use of thermal spring structures can be detected as a result of excavations and research. However, detecting the existence or change of statues is different from architectural structures. Comments on the use of statues remain incomplete due to situations such as destruction or relocation of statues, inscriptions, and other finds.

In general, the thermal springs built during the Roman Imperial Period within the borders of today's Turkey have not been explored as much as the thermal springs in England, Europe, and North Africa, and excavation projects have remained unfinished and incomplete. A number of statues and pedestal findings have been identified in the limited number of thermal springs that have been scientifically studied. These findings have contributed to the research into sculptures used in thermal springs.

The presence of the Leto sanctuary in the Sultaniye Thermal Spring and the presence of a statue of a high priest in the thermal spring-sanctuary complex are innovations in this direction. In fact, it provides extremely important data in the context of the thermal spring-sacred area relationship. On the other hand, we observe that in such thermal springs, instead of common gods with healing powers, various gods of local importance are highlighted. We can say that such thermal springs are generally associated with the city in which they are located.

The statue of a nymph holding an oyster in Allianoi is a typology we are familiar with in baths and water structures. Despite this, the number of examples of the same type found so far in hot springs is small. These sculptures are also named according to their context or where they are exhibited. Statues with similar lines and shapes, whose heads are described as nymph, Venus, and Moses, sometimes cause difficulties when being named. In order to solve this problem, all factors must be examined together, and an evaluation must be made taking into account regional and general factors. This will be an important, albeit small, step towards solving the problem.

The Asclepius of Çağa Thermal Spring shows that the existence of such a cult, which we associate with health in general, also exists in Galatia Province. Apart from highlighting the secondary healing powers of local gods, it is possible to say that the reflection of the therapeutic spiritual power of the Asclepeions of the Roman Empire in hot springs is supported by the presence of the statue of Asclepius.

Bibliography

Akgül, H. 2019. Karia Örnekleriyle Antik Çağ'da Ilıcalar. Unpublished master's thesis, University of Trakya.

Alagöz, U. 2021. Ankara Kırsalında bir Roma Kaplıcası ve Yeni Bir Yerleşim Önerisi. *Byazas* 26: 415–432.

Alagöz, U. 2013. Çağa Roma Hamamı 2012 Yılı Kazı Çalışmaları. *Müze Çalışmaları ve Kurtarma Kazıları Sempozyumu* 22: 365-386.

Ben Abed A. and J. Scheid 2015. Sanctuaire des Eaux, Sanctuaire de Sources, une Catégorie Ambiguë: L'exemple De Jebel Oust (Tunisie), in Centre Jean Bérard (ed.) *Sanctuaires et sources Les sources documentaires et leurs limites dans la description des lieux de culte:* 7-14. France: Collection du Centre Jean Bérard 22.

Blech, M. and T. Hauschild 1993. *Mulva III. Das Grabgebaude in der Nekropole Ost. Die Skulpturen-Die Terrakoten.* Deutsches Archaologisches Institut Madrid, Madrider Beirtage Band 21: Zabern Verlag.

Boyracı, G. 2019. Ankara Güdül-Çağa Roma Hamamı Arkeolojik Kazı Alanı Yakınında Bir Jeofizik Araştırma. Unpublished master's thesis, University of Süleyman Demirel.

Canik, B. 1973. Ayaş İçmece ve Kaplıcasının Jeoloji-Hidroloji Etüdü. *Bulletin of the Mineral Research and Exploration* 80: 137-152.

Chauvel, A. and P. Wuilleumier 1936. Les Thermes Romains d'Aix-les-Bains. *Bulletin Monumental* 95-1: 83-100.

Christofle, M. 1938. *Rapport Sur Les Travaux de Fouilles et Consolidations Effectuées en 1933-1936 par le Service Des Monuments Historiques de L 'Algérie.* France: F. Fontana Press.

Cristilli, A. 2008. Nuovi dati d'archivio sulle "Muse di Agnano" al Liebieghaus. *Napoli Nobilissima* 5-9: 252-257.

Croon, J.H. 1967. Hot Springs and Healing Gods. *Mnemosyne Serie 4* 20-3: 225-246.

Çörtük, U. 2012. Kaunos Liman Agorası Anıtları. Unpublished PhD dissertation, University of Ege.

Dvorjetski, E. 2007. *Leisure, Pleasure and Healing Spa Culture and Medicine in Ancient Eastern Mediterranean*, Supplements to the Journal for the Study of Judaism 116, Boston: Brill.

Fusco, U. and L. Lattanzi, 2013. Via Cassia: Novita Archeologiche dal sito di Campetti a Veio (RM) (Municipio xv ex xx). *Bullettino della Commissione Archeologica Comunale di Roma* 114: 436- 449.

Fytikas M., G.M. Leonidopoulou and R. Cataldi 1999. Geothermal Energy in Ancient Greece: From Mythology to Late Antiquity (3rd Century AD), in R. Cataldi, S.F. Hodgson and J.W. Lund (eds) *Stories From a Heated Earth: Our Geothermal Heritage*: 69–101. Sacramento: Geothermal Resources Council International Geothermal Association.

Gabrici, E. 1908. Teano- avanzi di un grande edifizio termale dell'antico Teanum Sidicinum, scoperti in contrada Santa Croce. *ATTI Della R. Accademia Dei Lincei* NSc 5: 399-416.

Giglioli, G. 1912. Note Archeologiche Sul Lativm Novvm Aqvae Vescinae. *Avsonia* 6: 39-87.

Gsell, St. and H. Graillot 1893. Exploration Archéologique en Algérie, Ruines Romanies au Nord de l'Aures. *Mélanges de l'École française de Rome* 13: 461-541

Homeros, 1896. *Iliad:The First Six Books of Homer's Iliad.* Classic İnterliner Trans., New York: Arthur Hinds and Company Press.

Jackson, R. 1990. Waters and Spas in the Classical World, *Medical History* 34/10: 1-13.

Macchioro, V. 1912. Le Terme Romane di Agnano, *MonAnt* 21: 224- 284.

Mainer, V.P. 2017. El culto de Venus en Hispania. Estudio y análisis de las fuentes documentales y arqueológicas en la Península Ibérica. Unpublished PhD dissertation, University of Madrid Complutense.

Manderscheid, H. 1981. *Die Skulpturenausstattung der Kaiserzeitlichen Thermenanlagen*. Monumenta Artis Romanae 15, Berlin: Gebr. Mann Verlag.

Marek, C. 2006. *Die Inschriften von Kaunos*. Münih,: C.H. Beck Press.

Mendel, G. 1912. *Catalogue des Sculptures Grecques, Romaines et Byzantines I*. Constantinople.

Mendel, G. 1914. *Catalogue des Sculptures Grecques, Romaines et Byzantines II*. Constantinople.

Müller, H. 2004. Allianoi. Zur Identifizierung eines Antiken Kurbades im Hinterland von Pergamon. *Istanbuler Mitteilungen* 54: 215-225.

Osman Hamdi Bey and Ethem Hamdi Bey 1904. Fouilles et Découvertes a Tralles. *Revue Archéologique, Quatrième* Série 4: 348-362.

Öğün, B., C. Işık, A. Diler, B. Schmaltz, C. Marek and A. Zäh 2001a. Kaunos 2000. *Kazı Sonuçları Toplantısı* 23/2: 365-372.

Öğün, B., C. Işık, A. Diler, O. Özer, B. Schmaltz, C. Marek and M. Doyran 2001b. *Kaunos Kbid*. Antalya: Orkun ve Ozan Medya Hizmetleri A.Ş.

Önen, Ü. 1983. *Ephesos Ruinen und Museum, Die Stadtgeschichte in Kunstwerken*. İzmir: Duyal Press.

Özen, L., İ. Elyıldırım, Ö. Çokdoğan and A.R. Çakır 2015. Ankara Güdül Çağa (Kötü) Hamamı Restorasyon-Konservasyon Çalışmaları. *Müze Çalışmaları ve Kurtarma Kazıları Sempozyumu* 24: 33-42.

Özşahin, E. and Ç.K. Kaymaz 2013. Türkiye'nin Termal Su Kaynaklarının Coğrafi Açıdan Değerlendirilmesi. *Atatürk Üniversitesi Edebiyat Fakültesi Sosyal Bilimler Dergisi* 50: 25-38.

Page, W. 1906. *Romano-British Somerset: Part 2, Bath*. A History of the County of Somerset I. London: Victoria County History.

Ploegs, G.E. 2016. *The Impact of the Roman Empire on the Cult of Asclepius*. Published PhD dissertation, University of Warwick.

Romano, I.B. 2006. *Classical Sculpture: Catalogue of the Cypriot, Greek and Roman Stone Sculpture in the University of Pennsylvania Museum of Archaeology and Anthropology (Museum Monograph)*. Philadelpia.

Sağır, E. and U. Alagöz 2016. Çağa Roma Hamamı 2014 Yılı Kazı Çalışmaları. *Müze Çalışmaları ve Kurtarma Kazıları Sempozyumu* 24: 43-56.

Smith, J.R. 1922. *Springs and Wells in Greek and Roman Literature Their Legends and Locations*. New York: G.P. Putnam's Sons Press.

Sodano, C. 2011. La valorizzazione dei dei beni culturali, L'Apollo di Vicarello, un'opera restituita al suo territorio. *Kermes Istituzioni e Strutture* 83: 41-50.

Talbert, R.J.A. 2000. *Barrington Atlas of the Greek and Roman World*. Princeton: Princeton University Press.

Vısconti, C.L. 1884. *I Monumenti del Museo Torlonia Di Sculture Antiche*. Roma.

Yaraş, A. 1999. 1998 Yortanlı Barajı Kurtarma Kazısı. *Bergama Belleten* 9: 44-49.

Yaraş, A. 2001. 1998-1999 Bergama Yortanlı Barajı Kurtarma Kazısı. *Müze Çalışmaları ve Kurtarma Kazıları Sempozyumu* 11: 105-118.

Yaraş, A. 2002a. Bakırçay Havzası'nda Asklepios Kültü ve Paşa Ilıcası-Allianoi. Unpublished PhD dissertation, University of İstanbul.

Yaraş, A. 2002b. 2000 Yılı Allianoi Kazısı. *Kazı Sonuçları Toplantısı* 23/1: 463-478.

Yaraş, A. 2003. 2001 Allianoi Kazısı. *Kazı Sonuçları Toplantısı* 24/2: 373- 384.

Yaraş, A. 2004a. 2002 Yılı Allianoi Kazısı. *Kazı Sonuçları Toplantısı* 25/2: 217- 228.

Yaraş, A. 2004b. Allianoi Nymphesi, in T. Korkut (ed.) *60. Yaşında Fahri Işık'a Armağan Anadolu'da Doğdu, Festscrift für Fahri Işık zum 60. Geburstag*: 803-815. İstanbul: Ege Yayınları.

Yaraş, A. 2005. Die Therme Allianoi. *Archeologische Ainzeiger* 2004: 71-74.

Yaraş, A. 2006a. Wasser in der Heiltherme von Allianoi, in G.Wiplinger (ed.) *Cura Aquarum in Ephesos: Proceedings of the Twelfth International Congress on the History of Water Management and Hydraulic Engineering in the Mediterranean Region, Ephesus/Selçuk*: 443-452. Leuven-Paris: Dudley, MA.

Yaraş, A. 2006b. Antik Çağ'da Ilıcalar. *Doğal Şifa Kaplıcalar* 2: 26-28.

Yaraş, A. 2006c. Allianoi: Chronique des Fouilles de 2005. *Anatolia Antiqua* XIV: 363-367.

Yaraş, A. 2011. Antik Sağlık Merkezi Allianoi ve Hastanesi, in E. Önen, M. Mutluer and N. Çetin *Uluslararası Bergama Sempozyumu (07-09.04.2011 Bergama)* Vol.1: 372-387. İzmir: Lamineks Press.

Yaraş, A. and D. Baykan 2005. 2003 Yılı Allianoi Kazısı. *Kazı Sonuçları Toplantısı* 26/2: 51- 62.

Yaraş, A. and D. Baykan 2006. 2004 Yılı Allianoi Kazısı. *Kazı Sonuçları Toplantısı* 27/2: 297-310.

Yaraş, A., D. Baykan and E. Karaca 2008. 2006 Yılı Allianoi Kazısı. *Kazı Sonuçları Toplantısı* 29/2: 71-84.

Weiss, H. B. and H.R. Kemble 1962. *They took to the waters; the forgotten mineral spring resorts of New Jersey and nearby Pennsylvania and Delaware*, Trenton: Past Times Press.

2. Healing Spas in Context.
The Role of Bathing Establishments in the territory

Banja Bansko (R.N. Macedonia). Through Time and Space

Vane P. SEKULOV
NI Institute for protection of cultural monuments and the Museum of Strumica
v.p.sekulov@gmail.com

Abstract: Banja Bansko is located at the foot of the dominant Belasica Mountain, 12 km southeast of the town of Strumica in southeastern Macedonia. Coins previously discovered at the Parilo spring, which identified it as a sacred spring, were quite logically contextualised with objects from the cave sanctuary, including the Grotto, the Temple of Hermes and the Great Bath.

The most important part of Banja Bansko is the Parilo spring, located 60 metres southwest of the complex which was supplied with its thermo-mineral water. The sacred Parilo spring was revered and people were aware of its divine power. Offerings were deposited at the spring long before the 4th century BC, the period from which the first coins discovered at the spring date, in order to obtain the favour and blessing of the gods.

The cult continued in the cave formed from the water of the thermo-mineral spring and where a sanctuary was built where the nymphs were probably worshipped. The sanctuary has two distinct sections that together occupy a total of 135m^2: a cave on the southwestern side and a walled area on the northeastern side.

The Banja Bansko enclosure also includes a temple dedicated to Hermes on the western side. Marble statues or fragments of marble statues, marble pedestals and small bronze figurines dedicated to Hermes were discovered among the ruins of the temple. The Great Bath has 11 rooms with 2 large and 2 smaller pools, with a total usable area of 623 m^2. The bath was built in 3 phases, starting in the 3rd century AD and existed until the mid-5th century AD.

Keywords: Banja Bansko, sacred spring, grotto, Temple of Hermes, The Great Bath

Introduction

The southeastern Macedonian village of Bansko, which borders Greece and Bulgaria, is situated 12 kilometers southeast of Strumica (Figure 1). The locals refer to the eastern section of the village as Parilo or Parillo ('steaming'), where the thermo-mineral water spring is located. The spring has a 42 liters per second flow rate, and the water temperature is 72°C.

In terms of orography, the territory of the village belongs to the northern slopes of the east-to-west-oriented Belasica mountain. The geological structure of the soil consists of Old Paleozoic, Neogene, and Quarter strata. The Belasica mountain, which length is 45 km in the east-west direction and inclined to the north at an angle of 65°, is part of the Macedonian-Serbian tectonic massif and it is rich of cataclasites and mylonite's structures. Taking into account all these aforementioned elements, it is not unusual that all these circumstances led to the development of significant geothermal springs.

The thermal bath in the Bansko village was noted by the Turkish explorer Hadji Kalfa in the 17th century (Матковски 1991: 394). According to his notes, 'the village is located in the area of Strumica, close to the city of Strumica (...). Here in the cherry season gather all traders from land and sea, of all seven climates of the world (...) they erected thousands of tents'. Feathered, human, and lion milk were all marketed, and women openly traded their secrets. In this location, 'many hot springs, as well as a few cold ones, flow under the brim of the mountain... In the bath beneath the stone archway, hot water runs from three small springs, with water so hot, you can boil an egg.'

Petar Janković, a geographer who traveled also to this area in the summer of 1901, described the geological phenomenon as well as the physical and topographical features of the Strumica region in his book *Der Plauš und die Strumica*: 'Every natural manifestation is present here, including extraordinary fertility, an abundance of water, and a warm Mediterranean climate that promote the growth of all kinds of crops, making the area of Strumica the most stunning and alluring location in Macedonia. There is a very hot and powerful thermal bath close to Bansko in the crevice beneath Belasica. An enormous spring spouts water with the temperature of 75°C. The water is unusually hot, slightly sulfurous, and located under the crest of Teće-baša' (Janković 1908: 176). The top of the spring is coated with a plaster and measures 2m length and 1m width. The water spouts in such an enormous amount that it pours out of the spring like a torrent, with only a small portion entering the hammam while the majority overflows into the plain, forming ponds and marshes. These indicators confirm that the thermal bath is hotter and more potent compared to all the others in Macedonia.

Due to the construction of the hotel, 70m north of the Parilo spring, in 1978 geostatic surveys were conducted.

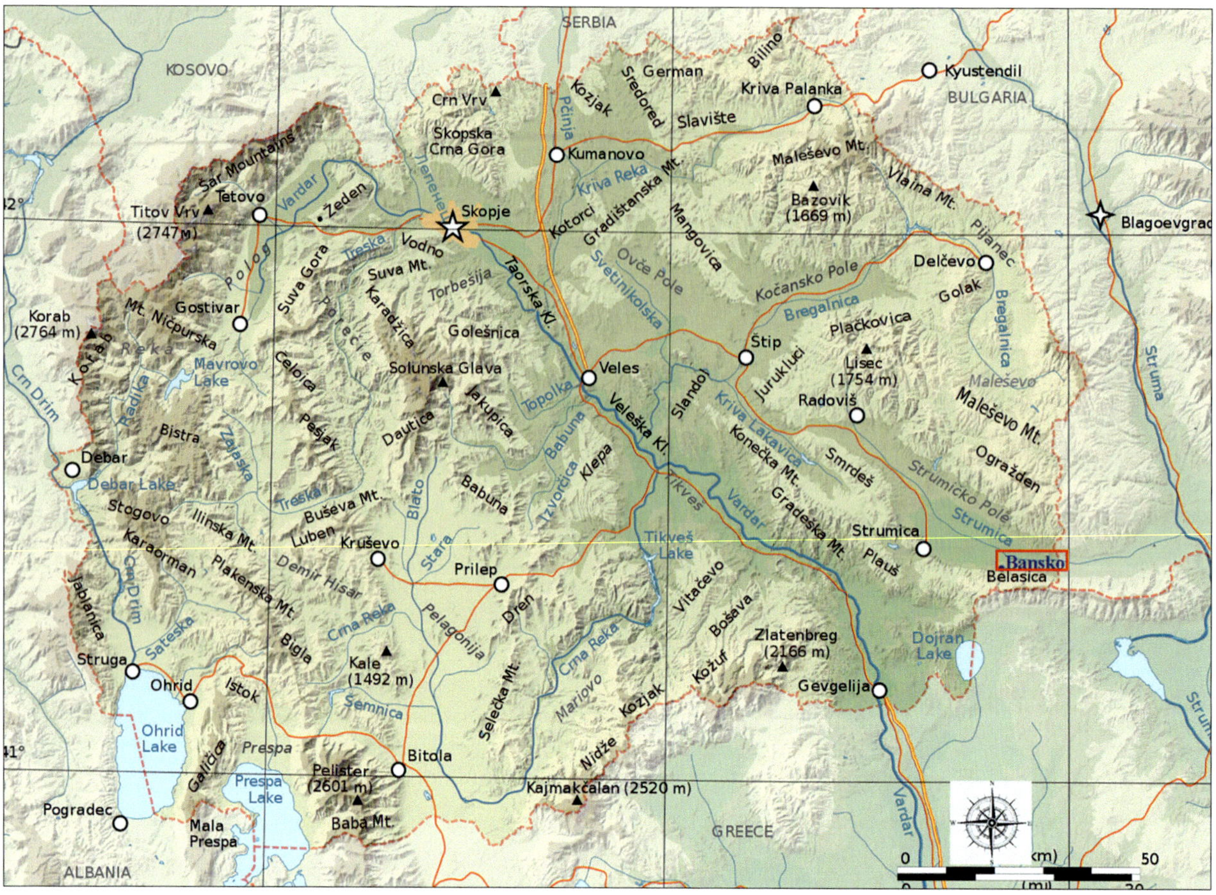

Figure 1. Localisation of Bansko in the R.N. Macedonia.

During this investigation, only a few meters below the surface, researchers discovered a solid structure that bears a resemblance to some kind of remains of a building. Soon after this discovery, archaeological excavations took place and in the forthcoming period a sophisticated network of buildings, that have been hidden beneath the earth's surface for more than 15 centuries, were revealed.

The previously discovered coins in the Parilo spring, which is designated as a holy spring, were quite logically brought into context with the cave, including the Grotto, the Temple of Hermes, and the Great Bath. Together with the recently discovered necropolis, they are organically connected parts of the Banja Bansko monumental complex, which is situated at the foot of the dominant Belasica mountain (Figure 2).

The sacredness and beneficial aspects of the thermal waters were in all aspects preserved, and ten centuries later, a few baths from the Ottoman era were built over the Roman buildings.

In this paper, I shall try to represent the intricate content that evolved across time and space on the area of Banja Bansko.

The sacred spring Parilo

The most fundamental part of Banja Bansko is the spring Parilo, which is located 60m southwest (Figure 2, marked with a yellow arrow). This is the spot from where the entire complex had been supplied with thermo-mineral water.

The spring formerly occupied an area of about 20m^2, but in 1968, without any prior examination or archaeological monitoring, it was almost destroyed and enclosed inside a concrete shaft to satisfy the needs of the local agricultural economy.

According to what is said in the *Book of Genesis*, 'the water existed before the Earth, darkness covered the deep, and the Spirit of God hovered over the water.' Water is a metaphor for the whole of all virtuality; it is the foundation of all potential existences and the source of all shapes, forms, and creations. Water always signifies regeneration and new birth, and it is an inevitable element of death and rebirth. In the aquatic cosmogony, a second death is suffered or endured during a general or sporadic flood, not to the eventual annihilation of humanity, but to a certain temporary arrival. A fresh creation, a new life, and ultimately a new human being

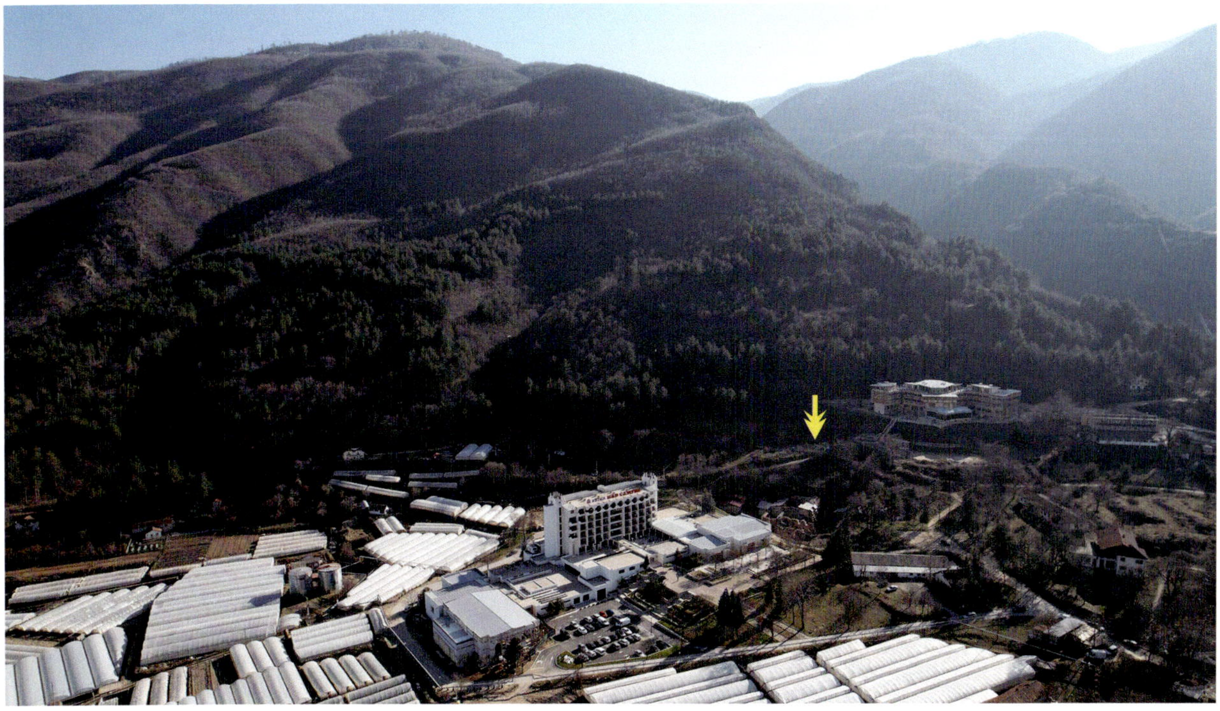

Figure 2. Banja Bansko monumental complex, which is situated at the foot of the dominant mountain of Belasica. Photo: Aleksandar Donchev.

are the effects of the return. Water is a crucial and constant element in all features of religious structures because it dissolves crimes, molds them, washes them away, cleans them, and eventually restores life (Eliade 2002: 80). Water and spiritualism have a lot in common, and water's ability to purge and to cleanse is a perennial issue. Therefore, it is not a surprise that many cultures hold the belief that water has heavenly, life-giving, purifying, and therapeutic powers. Thus, it is possible to observe how water plays a part in the concepts of medicine and spirituality. Eventually, life near natural hot springs, where these springs are viewed as heavenly gifts, has elevated toward the spiritual aspect of water.

Without a doubt, Banja Bansko's thermal and mineral springs have attracted visitors for centuries. They ascribed to the hot mineral water divine, nutritious, unadulterated, and therapeutic powers. The spring was admired for many centuries, and people acknowledged the sanctity of the place. Therefore, in order to obtain the gods' favor and blessing, ancient people bestowed gifts in the spring long before the 4th century BC, according to the earliest numismatic evidence.

Affording to some unofficial information, concerning the circumstances of the building procedures of modern structures, it is possible to conclude that the workers, who were involved in this process, collected hundreds or maybe thousands of ancient coins. Unfortunately, nowadays these coins are not documented and eventually lost, and only a small portion of 70 coins have been recovered and kept at the Archaeological Museum in Skopje. The remaining coins are dated between the 4th century BC and the 4th century AD.

But, also, during the first archaeological excavation of the spring area, carried out in 2022, remnants of a structure were discovered.

Grotto

The cultic and divine power of the place sustained and expanded its presence into the cave that was formed by the thermo-mineral water spring. In the inner structure of the cave, according to archaeological finds, a sanctuary dedicated to the nymphs was created (Figure 3).

The sanctuary has two distinct sections and encompasses a total size of $135m^2$: a cave on the southwest side and a built area on the northeast (Figure 4).

There are also at least two sections in the sanctuary's cave portion, although only the western one has been excavated. Part of this section, that was excavated, was destroyed by an earthquake in March 2015. This event assisted as an indicator that the cave's vaults are fragile and unsteady. As a result of this condition, further archaeological exploration of the entire cave was postponed.

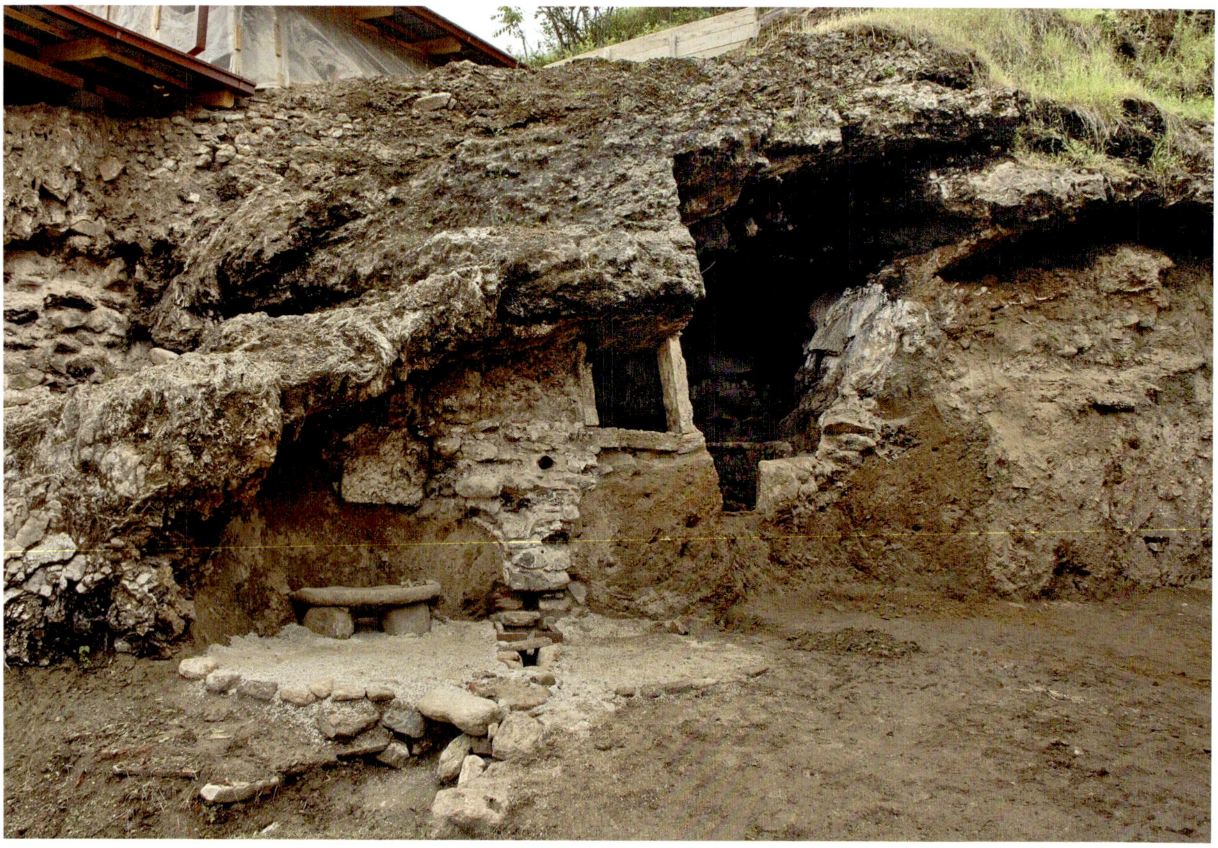

Figure 3. Grotto, northeast side. Photo: by Author.

The cave's newly found structure is roughly 30m^2 in size and reaches a height of 4m. The holy basin occupies a bigger portion of this space and offers ideal circumstances for direct communication with the deity through the water. The water in the holy basin is heated to an ideal temperature for the devotee's body and spirit.

This structure has pentagonal shape with a size of 15m^2, and up to 1.10m depth. The stone structure is covered with hydrostatic mortar and the bottom is paved with large, substantial, and asymmetrical stone slabs that perfectly complement the surrounding environment. There are seating benches on three levels that are parallel to the southeast and a portion of the southwest side.

Numerous coins were discovered at the bottom of the pool, but the aggressive thermo-mineral water had severely damaged them, rendering them illegible.

Indeed, a grotto is a natural or artificial cave that has been utilized by people as a place of worship since ancient times, and they are often little caverns with natural streams or mineral springs. For example, the four great oracular sanctuaries of Apollo, at Delphi in Greece, and at Didyma, Claros, and Patara in Asia Minor, two of those (Delphi and the one at Claros) were related to the divine power of the cave because the prophetic priests attained inside a grotto (Ustinova 2009: 2). However, the wet caves are typically referred to as *nymphaea*, like residences for nymphs called Naiads, divinities that preside over fountains, wells, springs, streams, brooks and other bodies of fresh water.

The cult to these nymphs is usually represented in votive reliefs. A group of three nymphs is frequently depicted in these offerings, showing various positions. Nymphs can also be represented alone, but in the company of other deities too. One of them could be the goddess Aphrodite, whose terracotta figurine was found in the cave in Bansko; and the second one is the god Hermes, whose several marble and small bronze figures were found in the immediate vicinity. As an example, out of 113 known reliefs that depict nymphs, 52 of them are accompanied by Hermes (Laferrière 2018: 31).

A walled structure was erected next to the eastern side of the cave by the end of the first century AD (Figure 5). The building is orientated southwest-northeast along the longer axis. The complex has two levels with four sections and a functional space of 104m^2. The larger, lower-placed room was a linking point between the visitor and waters, while the two smaller, higher-

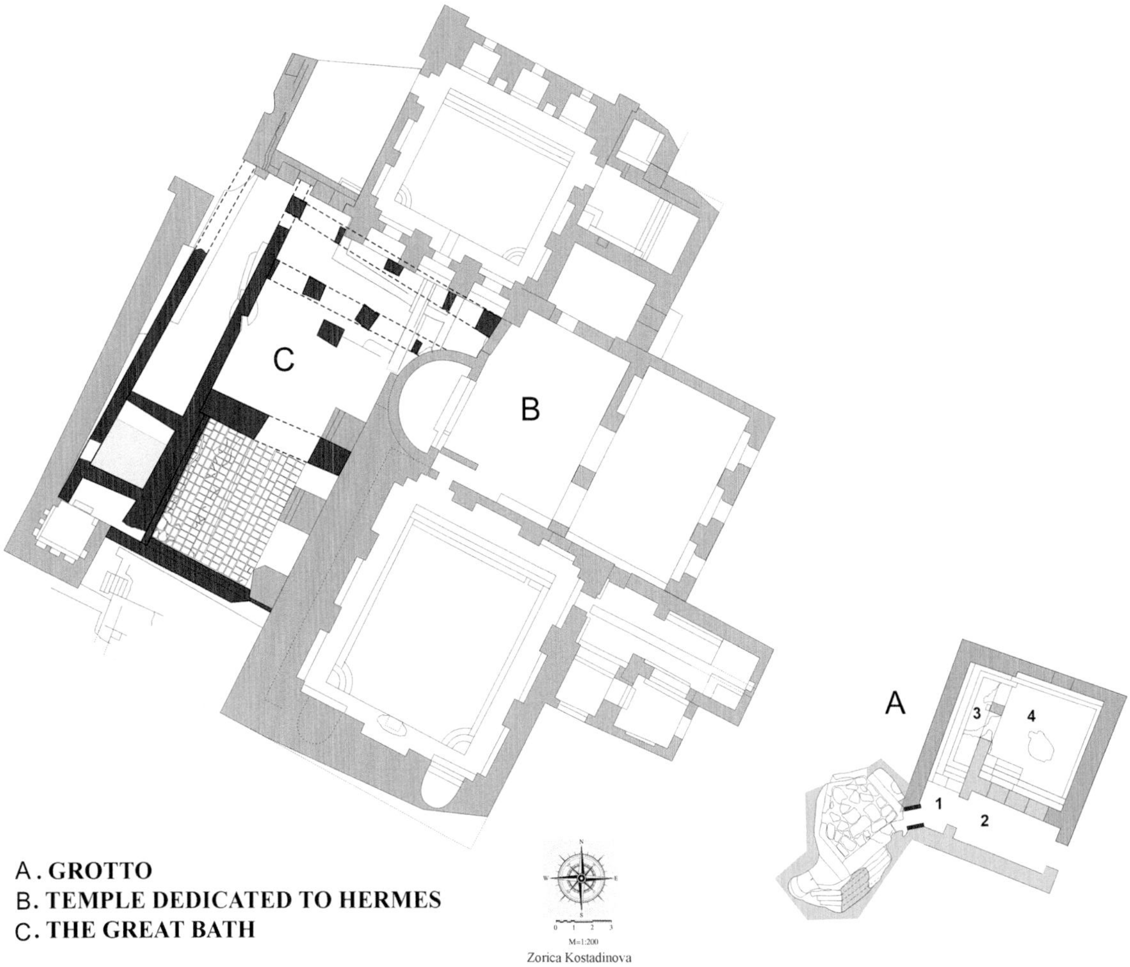

Figure 4. Plan of the archaeological site described in this article. Plan: Zorica Kostadinova.

placed rooms served as dressing-rooms. All four rooms were vaulted but only room nº3 preserved its original, undamaged vault. The vault on room nº4 was retrieved when the building was abandoned, albeit eventually collapsed as well.

The vault on room nº3 measures 1.85m in width, 3.0m in height above the ground, and 6.70m in length. It is oriented southwest-northeast. Bricks are made particularly for use in trapezoidal vault construction. Floor of room nº3 and room nº4, is decorated with tiles arranged in the technique of *opus spicatum.*

Ceramic pipes installed under the vault of room nº4 provided water to both sides (Nº3 and 4). Through a wall channel, water flows from the Holy spring toward the roof of the building.

Temple dedicated to Hermes

The general belief in ancient times was that the thermal springs and the structures built around them were guarded by nymphs and gods, and that one needed the blessing from gods in order to receive healing from these enchanted waters. Typically, they referred to the gods associated with health, such as Asclepius and his daughter, the goddess Hygeia.

Last but not least, Vitruvius advised that only locations with hot springs should be chosen for the worship of water-related gods and these are the places for planning and building temples dedicated to them, especially those related to health: 'The correct form will come from nature, for example, that all temples should choose the healthiest places and suitable sources of water, in places where the gods have erected them to be the most ill' (Vitruvius 1997: I, 2).

On the western side of the complex at Banja Bansko a temple dedicated to god Hermes was created. From the point of architectural design, there isn't much to say about the temple itself. The major portion of the temple is located beneath the structures that were later built on its ruins, particularly the Great Bath. What is now visible is a lengthy, enclosed passage pointing southwest to northeast. In addition, there

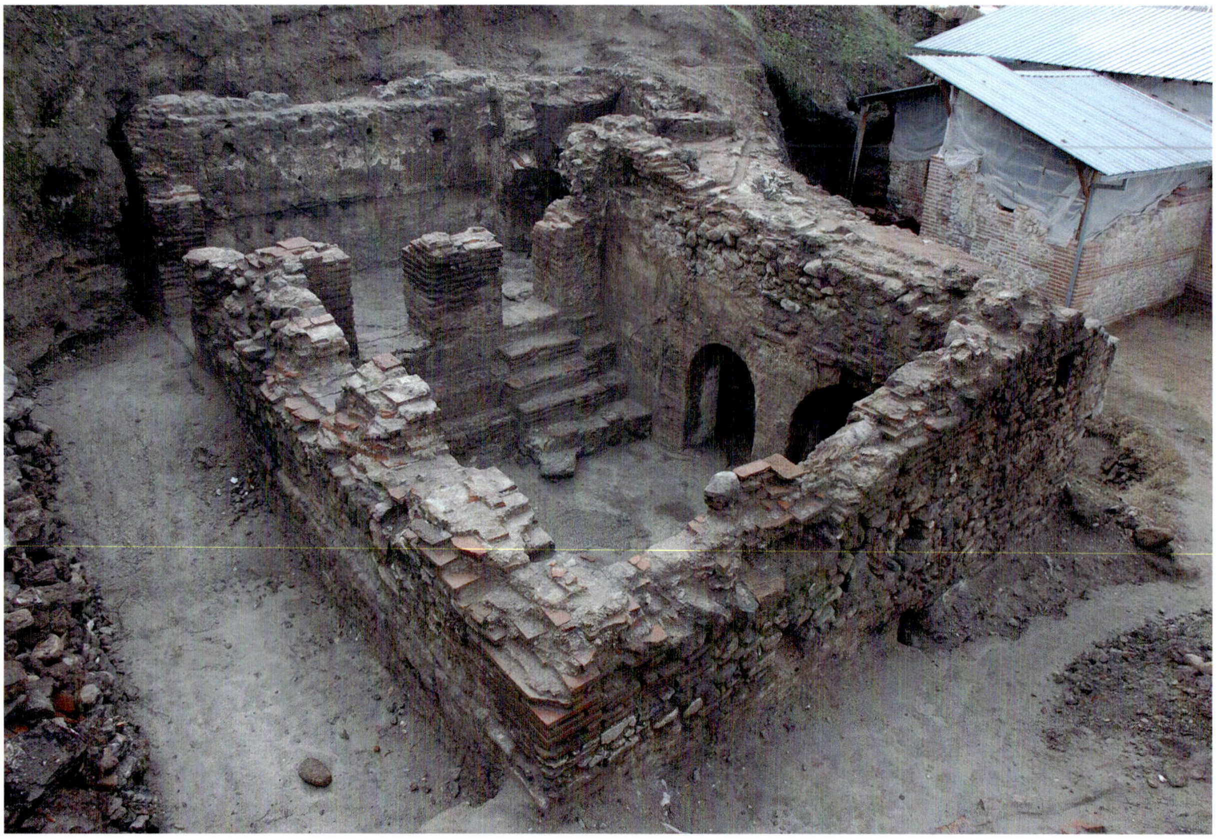

Figure 5. A small building next to the eastern side of the cave Grotto, Photo: by Author.

was a long, open porch running from the southwest corner toward the southeast. Judging from the porch's substantial stone base, the porch had a colossal roof supported by wooden beams. Along with other artifacts a heavily damaged portion of the altar was discovered in this area. This is the place where aggressive thermal mineral water continued to flow long after downfall of the temple. There is a bigger premise that has been excavated and is partially hidden beneath the northwest wall of Premise no. 3 of the Great Bath on the opposite side, to the southwest, which ends in the same way as the southeast. Hydrostatic mortar was frequently used to cover the walls and the substantial gaps between the bricks that were used for the floor because this kind of masonry's structure was proficient for retaining a water. Without any doubt, this was the central place of the temple. Once more one should consider that the holy water of Parilo spring was transferred toward the sacred basin where, through bathing, persons could interact directly with the deity. It was a place for prayer, seeking help, expressing appreciation, and leaving special gifts.

In the ruins of the temple were found some marble statues or fragments of them, and small bronze figurines (Figure 6).

On one of the marble plinths in front of this area (Figure 7) has a Greek inscription that reads as follows:

> Οὐαλερία Διο[- - -]η ἡ ἀρ-
> χιέρεια τὸν Ἑρμ[ῆν].
>
> 'Valeria Dionike, the High-Supreme Priestess, dedicated the statue to the god of Hermes' (Babamova 2010: 39).

Another marble pedestal with an inscription had been discovered during archaeological excavation conducted in 2016; however, this marble pedestal has been severely damaged, and the only thing that can be read is the name of the donor: Python's cognomen. The sculpture may be dedicated to the god Hermes once more, or it could be to the goddess Hygeia, who was also honored in this temple and whose tiny marble sculpture was discovered during the 2016 archaeological excavations.

In that context, the identification of the marble egg-holding palm or more precisely to which deity this artifact belongs, that was discovered during the excavations in 2002, is ongoing dilemma. Namely, previously it was assumed that the hand belongs to the sculpture of Asclepius or perhaps even Sabazios, but

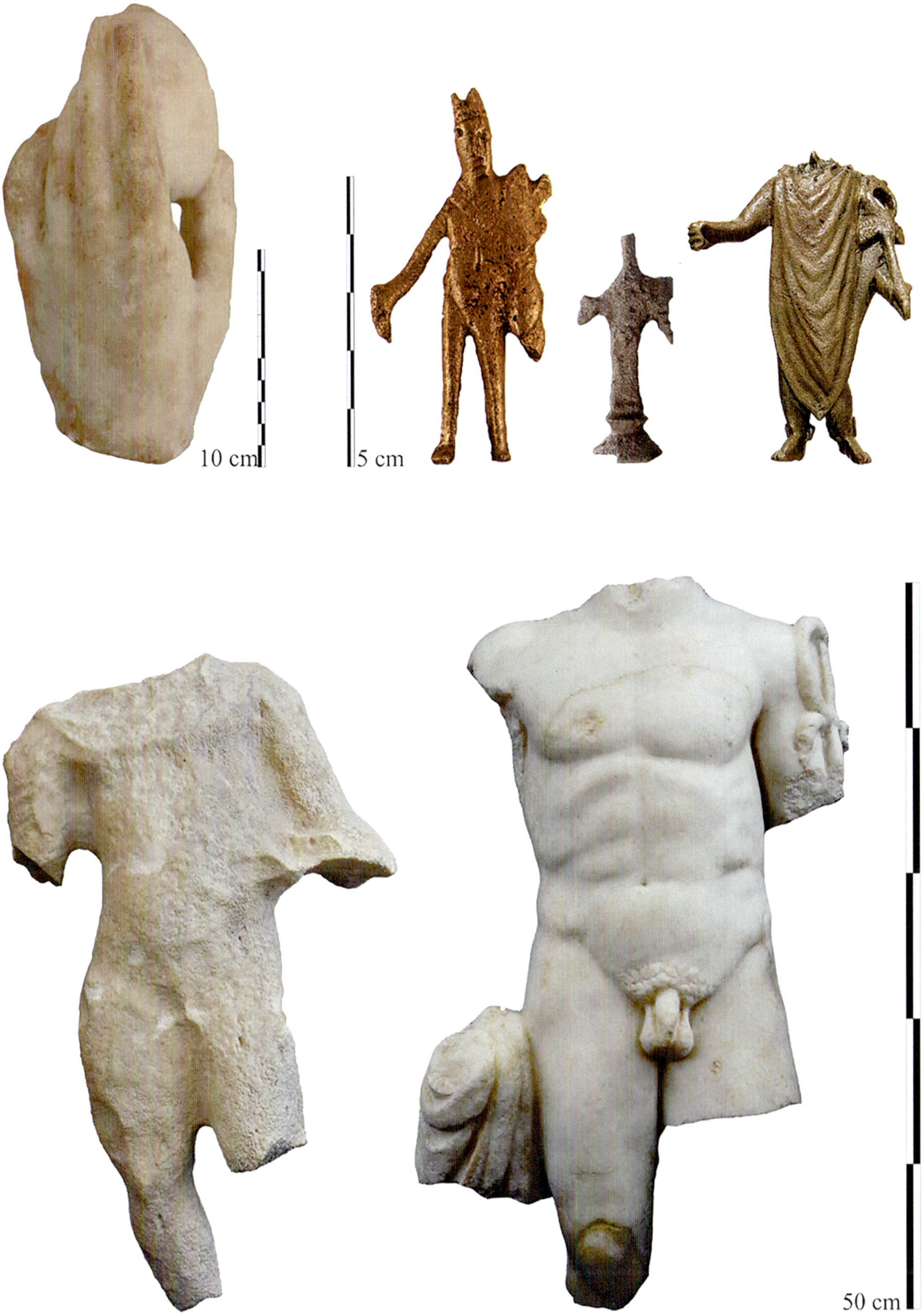

Figure 6. Photos of the marble statues and the small bronze figurines located in Temple of Hermes. Photo: by Author.

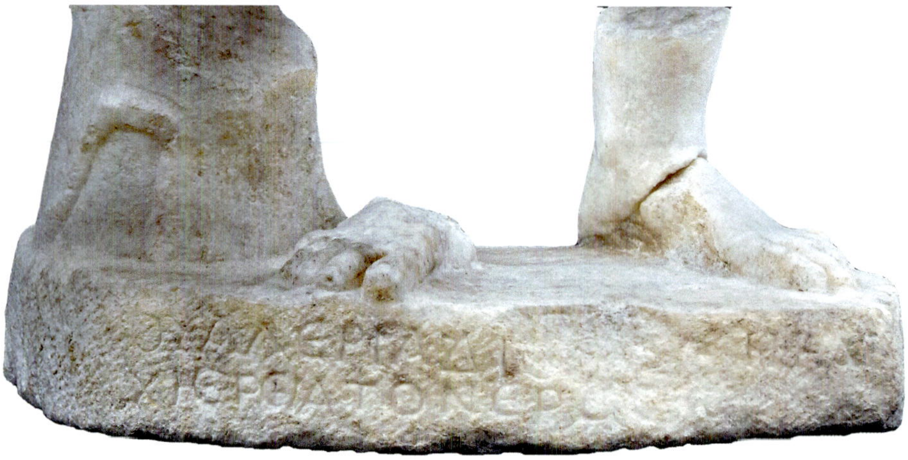

Figure 7. The marble base of Hermes with inscription. Photo: by Author.

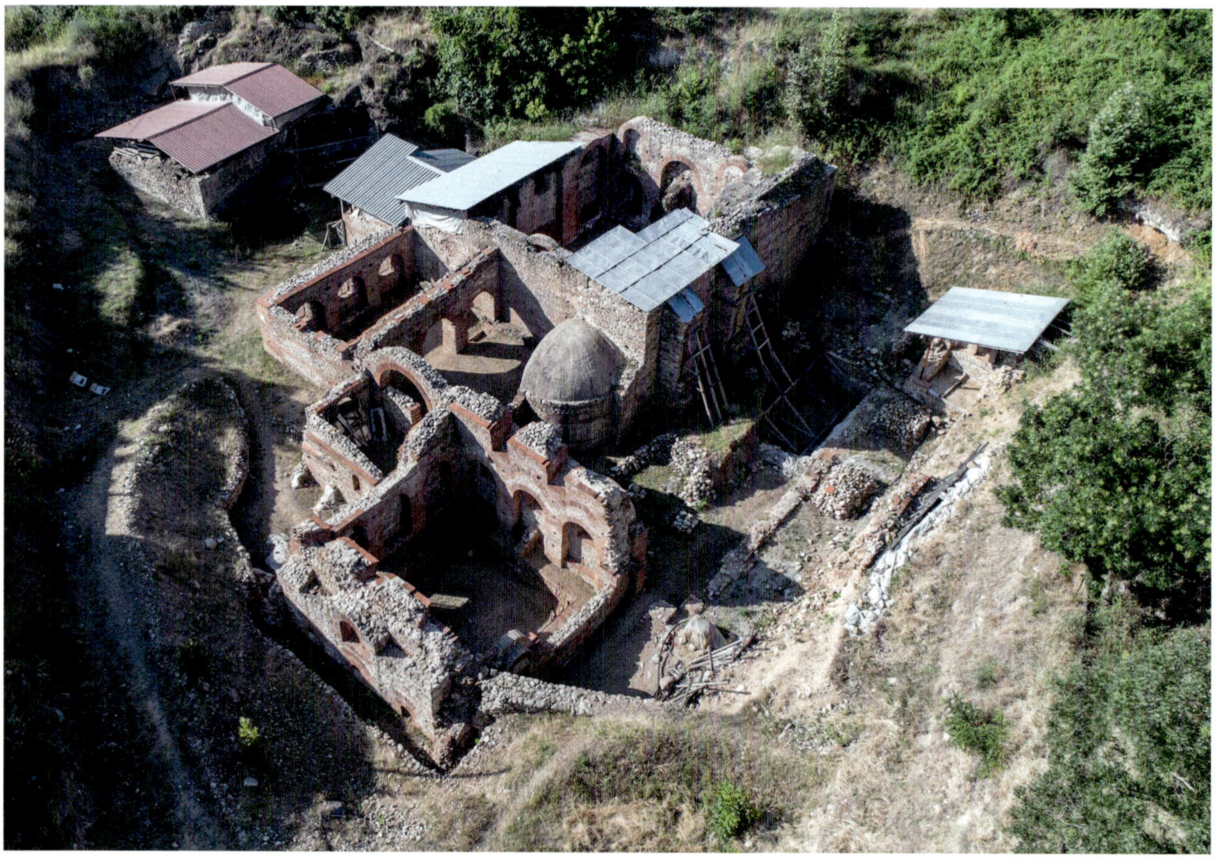

Figure 8. The Great Bath. Photo: Aleksandar Donchev.

now there is a possibility that it actually belonged to the sculpture of Hygeia.

The Temple of Hermes was completely destroyed in the first decades of the third century AD and the sculptures and pedestals were demolished and used as building material in the construction of the Great Bath and other buildings.

The great bath

Built in three basic phases of the Great Bath, 11 rooms have been discovered so far, 10 of which have been fully excavated (Figure 8) with a total usable space of 623 m2 (Figure 9).

Romans carefully developed thermo-mineral baths, in the territories they conquered. They were drawn

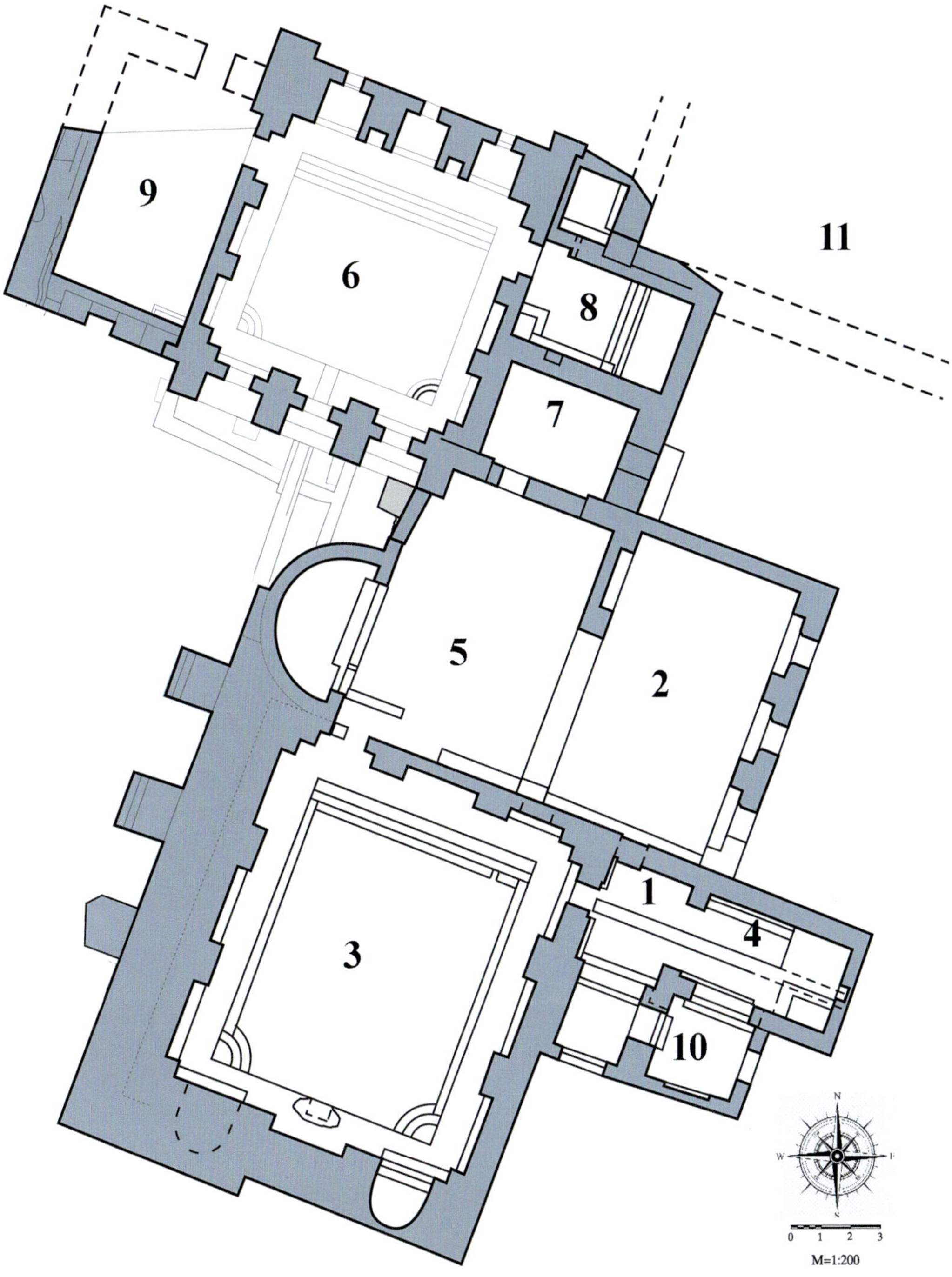

Figure 9. The Great Bath. Plan: Zorica Kostadinova.

by the therapeutic effects of the thermal springs, and whenever they came across them in conquered provinces, they frequently resided close to them and constructed exquisite baths.

Only three rooms made up the bath's basic layout in the first phase: an apodyterium, a sizable room with a pool, and a two-part sweat room.

Most of the original apodyterium is below the floor level of the second phase building and only the southwest wall is preserved.

The sudatorium and the central pool area were accessible through the western door, which was located on the southwest wall between the apodyterium and the rest of the bath.

The central room nº3, which includes a pool, served as the hub around which the first and second sections of the bath complex were constructed. This room is 137m2 in size. The center of the space is taken up by the 90.95m2 pool or *natatio?*. It ranges in depth from 1.30 to 1.5m. The pool's perimeter walk is 1.05m wide.

Room nº3's walls are intact, reaching a height of 8m. The foundation of the wall pedestal for the fountain is still in the center area of the southwest wall, between the two bathtubs. There is a niche above the pedestal. This room has a semicircular vault over it.

The small door in the east corner led to the sudatorium, and the north door of the room acted as an exit.

The sudatorium (nº1 and 4) consists of two rooms that are 30m2 in total, connected by a sizable arched entryway. The heating system with an arching design is in the middle of the room. The core element of the heating system is the central channel that runs along the middle of the sudatorium.

The sudatorium is 9.50m long, 0.45m wide, and 0.70m deep. The hot vapor was supplied continually by a little amount of hot water. Through three apertures in the southeast side of room nº3, a canal that carries hot water into the sudatorium was used to supply the complete heating system.

The semicircular vault in the arched sudatorium rises to a height of 3.80m. Up to 4 meters from the southeast wall, only the first sections of the semicircular vault have been preserved.

Without any doubt, the apodyterium quickly after the bath's construction proved to be useless, therefore it was destroyed, the communications were cut off, and a new one was constructed on top of it. The second stage of the bath's development has now started.

A new, larger apodyterium (72.42m2) was constructed right over the old one (room nº2). Some of its walls, up to 5.70m, have been maintained. The two enormous arched doors on the northwest side are used to enter the frigidarium. The space featured vaulted ceilings that extended from the northwest to southeast walls. The floor was paved with bricks.

Northwest of the apodyterium is the frigidarium (room nº5). The room has a floor made of brick tiles, a surface area of 70.65m2, and walls that have been preserved up to a height of 6.10m (Figure 10). The primary entrance to the spa was in the northeast wall of the central premise, which also had an entrance in the west corner leading to the one with the pool. Even if there are no visible indications of the roof's construction, the scale of the rooms indicates that it was vaulted. The northwest wall contains the semicircular bathtub or piscina, with a semi-dome. The 1.15m deep bathtub has a 3.40m diameter. There was no hot water provided for it.

In addition to these newly built rooms, in the second phase of construction of the Great Bath were added other, smaller buildings that increased and supplemented its functionality. Another premise with a tub for bathing (room nº10) was built for the needs of the sudatorium. The new facility covered an area of 9.60m2 with a preserved height of the walls of 3 m.

A new facility (room nº7), located in front of the central entrance to the bath, was also added. It covers an area of 17.50 m2, with a preserved height of the walls of 4.50m. The floor formed a tub with a drain, covered by means of and a finely smoothed dual-layer of mortar of an intense red colour, which continues along the walls forming an arch. The building phases of this premise follow its renovations and constructions. Judging by the remains of the vaulting construction of the south-eastern and north-western wall, the roof of this premise represented a vault.

Shortly after the second phase ended, the bath seemed to have gone through some type of crisis. There were statics problems as well, which were most evident in the pool area of the main room where the dome pressed up against the walls and they could not hold its weight.

The windows on the southwest wall and the bathtub in the west corner were raised, and a new wall from outside was erected to the northwest wall to strengthen it. When the additional buttress didn't have the anticipated results and the bath's problems were evident, the older part of the room had to be shut down totally. The front door was locked, and there were new structures being built close by. In fact, a new, independent wing was built and managed separately.

The main point of the third phase is once more the swimming pool (room nº6), which has an area of 83.6m2 and walls that were kept up to a height of 6.15m. The pool is 56.88m2 in size. The range of its depth is 1.21 to 1.38m. The three recesses on the northeast wall of the space held the bathtubs, completing the function of the pool. A brick vault that ran the length of the premise's north-eastern to south-western walls served as the roof structure.

Northwest of the room with a pool is the new apoditerium - room nº9. The dimensions of the premise are 7.35 x 5.05m, on an area of 37.12m2. The floor is paved with brick, and throughout the north-western wall is the canal for water supply of the baths and of the main pool in the central premise. This premise is connected with the central premise by means of an entrance from the eastern corner. The entrance to the

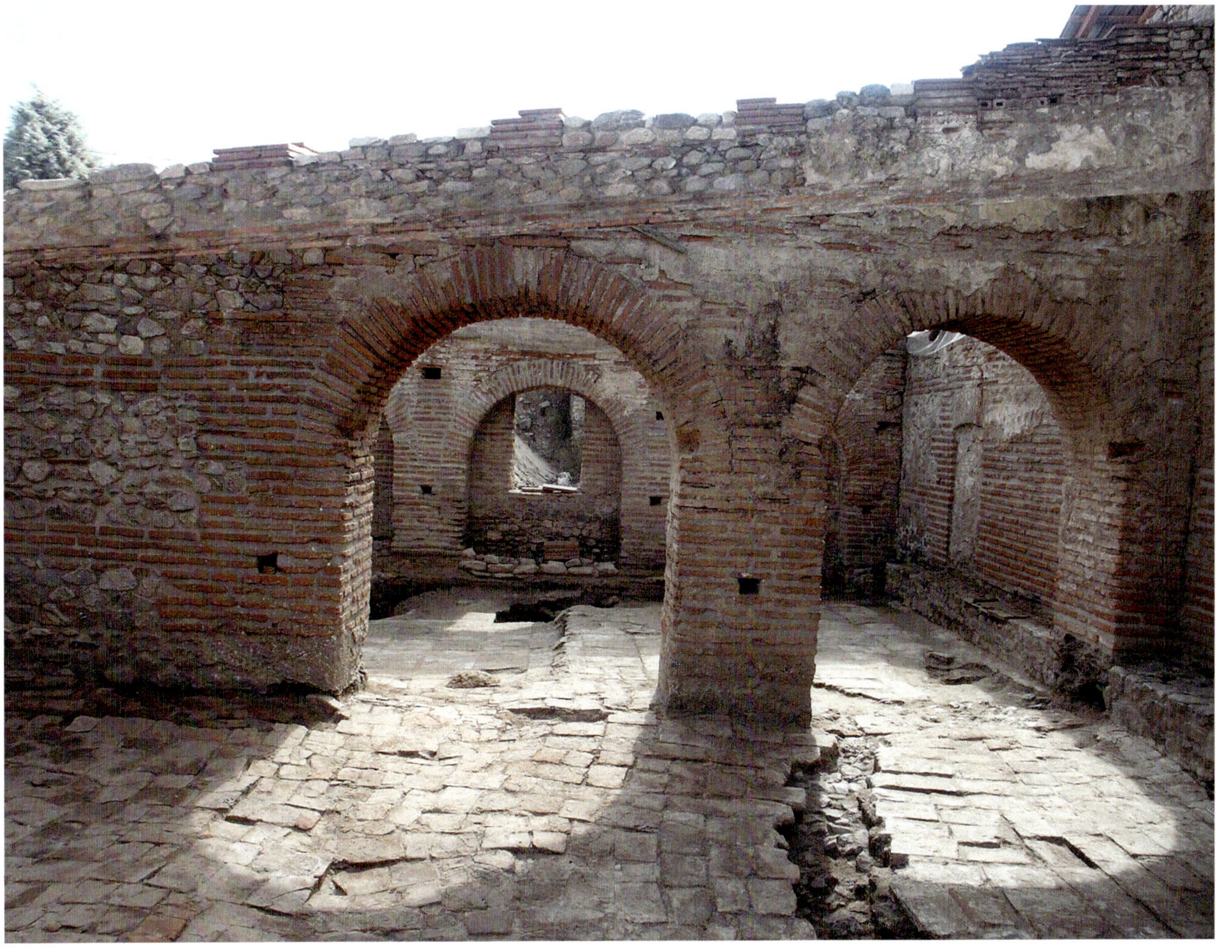

Figure 10. The communication between the frigidarium and the apodyterium. Photo: by Author.

apoditerium, as well as the entire complex of the third phase, is located on the south-western wall. The floor is completely preserved and is paved with properly arranged bricks. The roof construction of this premise is unknown due to the insufficient preservation of the walls and the lack of data related to vaulting.

To the southeast of the structure housing the pool, there was a door leading to another location (room nº8). It actually consists of three smaller rooms connected logically by one another. A bathtub and a brick-and-mortar floor connecting the walls to the floor are features of the southeast location. The northwest corner of the structure is brick-paved, and there is a little shaft in the west corner. A canal that ran along the southwest wall of the smallest of the three premises, on the north, was used to drain wastewater from the pool into this area. It had a mortared floor.

Parts of two walls that make up the western corner of another room, nº11, have been found northeast of these three rooms. It is a wide and expansive hall from the third phase of the Great Bath based on the width of the found walls, which is 1.40m. Furthermore, we can conclude that room nº11 marks the ending of the third phase of the Great Bath's growth over time and space based on the present archaeological excavations.

Undoubtedly, the thermal mineral springs of Banja Bansko have been attracting people who inhabited the area for centuries. They recognized that the spring's healing and divine power came from a god, and they worshipped them. In order to express their thanks or to obtain gods' favors, they donated gifts and other expressions of gratitude starting well before the fourth century BC. The chronology of the place was determined after the examination of the earliest coins in the spring. The water of the thermal mineral spring Parilo forms the cave which was another cult place and sanctuary dedicated to the nymphs. They were either guided there by Hermes and by Aphrodite.

It is believed that Hermes' temple was constructed in the second century AD, including cults to Hygeia and other deities who protected people's physical and mental health. It was renowned and considered

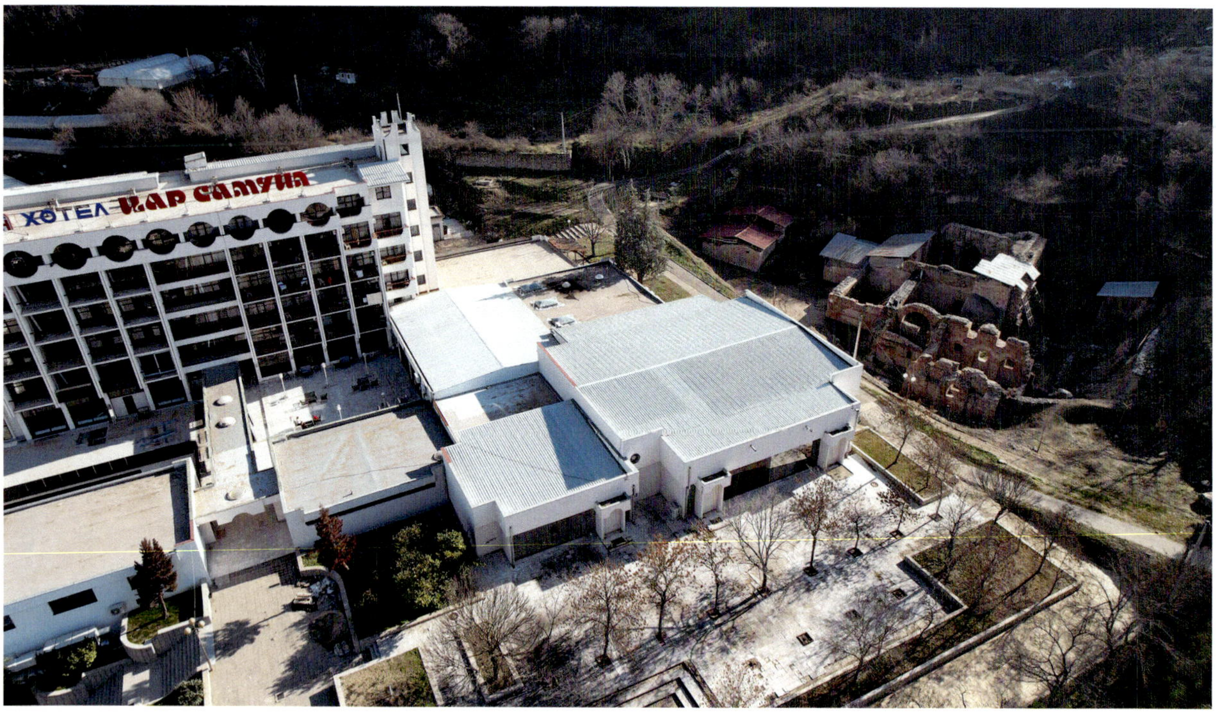

Figure 11. Car Samuil Hydrothermal Medical Center, sited close to the Roman thermal spa. Photo: Aleksandar Donchev.

as a sacred site with therapeutic water. The temple dedicated to the god Hermes was destroyed in the first half of the third century AD.

In the pool of the first phase, a coin of Alexander Severus (231-235 AD) and a memorial coin with representation of Alexander the Great were discovered. A coin of Valerian I (253-260 AD) was discovered in the built-up niche. The coin of Maximinus Thrax 'the Thracian' (235-238 AD) was discovered during some conservation works in the main room of the first phase; particularly, it was discovered under a brick of the pathway around the pool, in a location that had been reserved just for it. It is evident that this coin was placed there to symbolize both the emperor's rule and the period when the bath was built.

In the pool of the third phase, coins from Maximian I (dated 295-296 AD), Diocletian (dated 295-298 AD), and Licinius (dated 320 AD) have been found. An interesting fact is that in the rooms of the second phase, were not discovered any coins.

If we consider Maximinus Thrax coin (235–238 AD) as a chronological benchmark, The Great Bath could be dated to the fourth decade of the third century AD.

The second phase of the construction probably started in the third quarter of the third century AD when the small apodyterium was demolished and a new, much larger one, was built, including a newly built frigidarium, they made a common spatial entity.

Most likely, the third building phase took place during the substantial restorations carried out in the final decade of the third century, or maybe at the start of the fourth century AD. According to current information and evidence, the Great Bath was in use until the middle of the fifth century AD, like it is confirmed by a coin struck by Theodosius II to honor his three-decade rule.

Nevertheless, it should be emphasized that there are still chances to uncover new structures and buildings because there are carried out continuous archaeological excavations. In addition to this assumption, on the western side of the site, a 23m long perimeter wall of a building is visible and should be excavated in the near future.

With the spread of Christianity, especially from the fifth century AD, Banja Bansko began to lose its significance and declined into obscurity. Another important factor is that the whole architectural complex was completely covered with soil. This condition was unchanged until Ottomans arrived at the end of the fourteen century AD. They constructed four smaller baths above the level of the cave sanctuary and the Great Bath, and unintentionally carried on the custom of using the waters from the sacred Parilo spring, which they shared with people in the pre-Roman and Roman times.

Whether by accident or not, a new religious site was created here, a shrine in the form of a tomb, for an unidentified Ottoman saint.

A new phase in the promotion of the thermal mineral waters of the Parilo Spring began at the end of the 1970s, and during the following years, four hotels were constructed around this place. The main intention for this building activity was to reanimate and revitalize the complex of sanctuaries and baths.

It is The *Car (Tzar) Samuil* Hotel, which was built next to the existing structures and this hotel is the legitimate heir of the Roman thermal bath. Namely, this building preserved the allure of employing thermal-mineral water for medical and therapeutic purposes (Figure 11).

The fundamental principle has not altered, even though the circumstances have been updated to fit contemporary times and technologies. Car Samuil Hydrothermal Medical Center has developed into a modern and urban thermal treatment facilities, to restore the tradition and magnificence of the ancient temple of health and wellness.

People who continue to benefit from the virtues of thermo-mineral water are still enthralled by the enchantment of the Parilo spring's water, which has been known since antiquity.

Time flows, and the spring is still here.

Bibliography

Бабамова, С. 2012. Нови антички натписи од Македонија (Babamova, S. New Ancient Inscriptions from Macedonia), *Živa Antika Monographs*, 10, 27-50. Скопје.

Burket, W. 1985. *Greek Religion*. Maiden, MA: Blackwell Publishing Ltd. and Harvard University Press.

Dvorjetski, E. 2007. *Leisure, Pleasure and Healing, Spa Culture and Medicine in Ancient Eastern Mediterranean*, Boston.

Eliade, M. 2002. *Sveto i profane (Sacred and profane)*, Zagreb.

Janković, P. 1908. Der Plauš und die Strumica. *Grundlinien der Geographie und Geologie von Mazedonien und Alt-Serbien. Nebst Beobachtungen in Thrazien, Thessalien, Epirus und Nordalbanien von Dr. J. Cvijić*, 175-178, Gotha.

Laferrière, C.M. 2019. Hermes Among Pan and the Nymphs on Fourth-Century Votive Reliefs, *Tracking Hermes, Pursuing Mercury*, 31-48. Oxford University Press.

Матковски, А. 1991. *Македонија во делата на странските патописци*. Скопје. (Matkovski, A. *Macedonia in the works of foreign travel writers*. Skopje.)

Vitruvius 1997. *Deset knjiga o arhitekturi* (*Ten books on architecture*). Institute of Civil Engineering of Croatia. Zagreb.

Taseva, S. and P.V. Sekulov 2017. *The great bath of the late Roman thermal spa in the village of Bansko*, Skopje.

Ustinova, Y. 2009. *Caves and the Ancient Greek Mind: Descending Underground in the Search for Ultimate Truth*, Oxford.

Ceremonial Buildings at Thermo-Mineral Springs: The Example of Via Scavi at Montegrotto Terme

Maddalena BASSANI
Iuav University of Venice, Department of Architecture and Arts, Associate Professor of Classical Archaeology, Palazzo Badoer, San Polo 2468, 30125 Venezia (Italy)
mbassani@iuav.it

Abstract: This article proposes a new interpretation of the lesser-known structure known as the 'Polylobate building' in the thermal area of Viale Stazione-Via degli Scavi in Montegrotto Terme, near Padua. Although this building was interpreted as a residential building in the past, no conclusive data has ever been presented to support this hypothesis. In essence, the available information was very limited and most of the articles in which it was cited never attempted to understand the typology and structure of this monument.

Thanks to an in-depth analysis of data from excavations carried out in 1970, and a comparative study with other similar buildings attested both in Italy and in other thermo-mineral healing structures, this paper will offer new documentation useful for understanding the relationship with the buildings in the archaeological area of Montegrotto Terme and with analogous structures normally interpreted as nymphaea.

Consequently, this research offers new insights to attempt interpret the so-called polylobate building as a nymphaeum with a sacred-ceremonial function to be found within the thermo-mineral area of *Aquae Patavinae*, but also in other healing contexts attested throughout the Roman Empire, from Italy to the eastern and western provinces.

keywords: thermalism, Montegrotto Terme, archaeological area, *nymphaeum*

Introduction

The archaeological area of Via Scavi is in the center of the present-day town of Montegrotto Terme, whose salty-bromine-iodine waters which can reach 86°C, are used today both for therapeutic bathing in case of joint and skin problems, and, through vapors, for inhalation cures against breathing disorders. Furthermore, the treatments in the Euganean area with thermal mud are very famous to cure joint and skin diseases.

The archaeological context, excavated during the 18th and 20th centuries (Figure 1), presents three pools for therapeutic bathing (letters A-C) with rooms for treatments (no. 1-7), a small theatre (E) and a so-called polylobate building (D). Furthermore, a complex water system (G) and two *noriae* (water wheels, H), that probably used thermal waters from a Roman reservoir (M) under the present Viale Stazione, served the pools and the theatre in its late phase (perhaps a fountain was built in the middle of the orchestra in the 3rd-4th century AD). To the late phase pertain the specular small rooms (F), perhaps service buildings.

The structures date between the mid-1st century BC and the 3rd-4th centuries AD, with restoration and rearrangement work as early as the 2nd century AD, possibly due to landslides and subsidence of the geological substrate. The remains were part of an extensive settlement called *Aquae Patavinorum* or *Patavini Fontes*: it consisted in several settlements, only partly visible today and was not far from *Patavium*, on which it depended administratively from the second half of the 2nd century BC to the full imperial age.

On the archaeological area of Via Scavi several contributions have recently been proposed for the baths and the theater,[1] while to date there is a lack of a study specifically devoted to the so-called 'polylobate building' considered a *therma* or *nymphaeum* in a few limited syntheses works (Tosi 1987: 188) that have not sufficiently developed effective arguments for understanding its function and relationship to other structures and infrastructures. To attempt to overcome this gap in studies, I have recently published a pertaining article,[2] thanks to the archive dataset of the Archaeological Superintendency and new interpretive hypotheses. I want to present here additional elements concerning the structure and its relation to

[1] Many articles are included in the proceedings of the Conference *Aquae patavinae* 2011 (Bassani, Bressan and Ghedini 2011) and *Aquae patavinae* 2012 (Bassani, Bressan and Ghedini 2012), with bibliography; for a general overview see Ghedini *et al.* 2015 and Bassani *et al.* 2021.

[2] Bassani 2022. I would like to thank the colleagues of the Archaeological Superintendence of Padua for their availability, in particular Chiara D'Incà, Carla Perazzini, Cristina Vallicelli, Alessandro Facchin, Francesco Bighin. The study of the polylobate building has been carried out during the Horizon European Project rurAllure (www.rurallure.eu, no. 101004887).

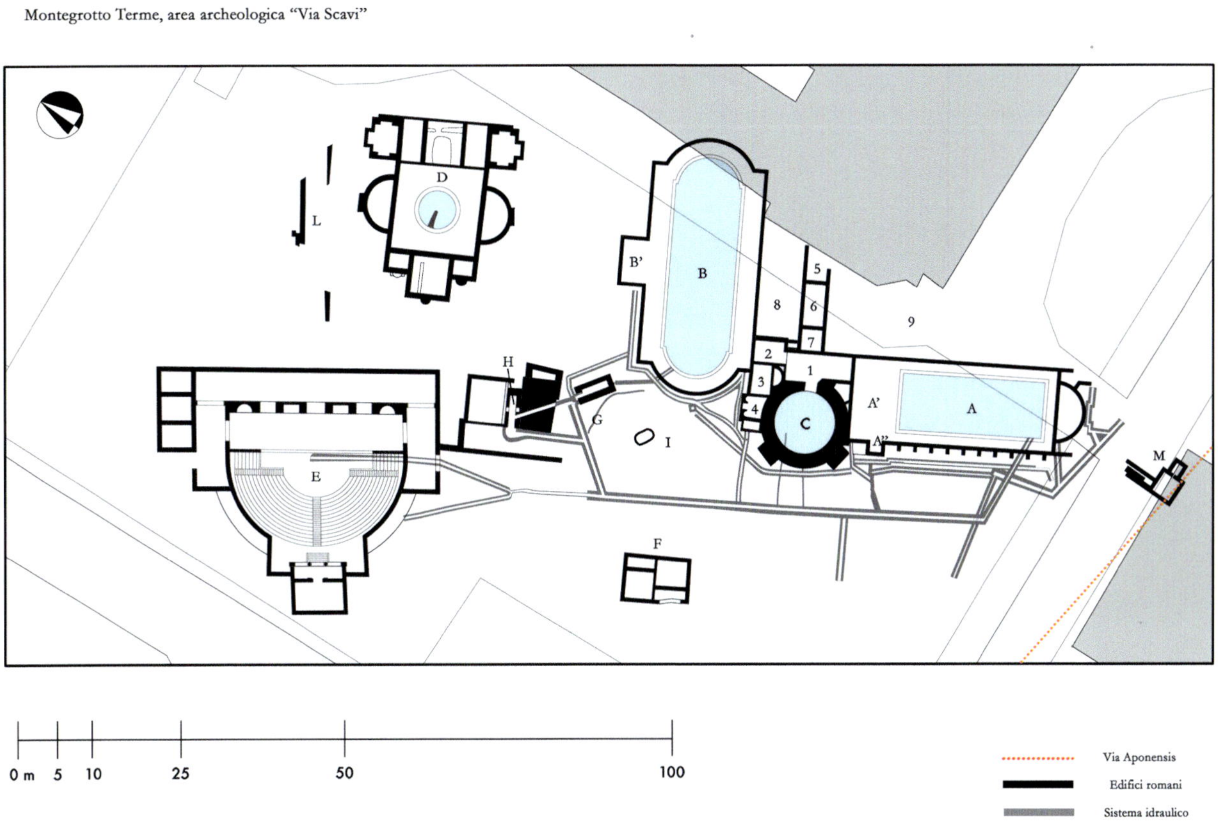

Figure 1. Montegrotto Terme, Viale Stazione/Via Scavi (Veneto region, Italy). Plan of the Roman archaeological area: A-C, thermal pools; D, polylobate building; E, small theatre; F, late buildings for service uses; G, water network; H, water wheels; I, small water basin; L, corridor; M, thermal cistern (by L. Catana and M. Bassani).

the topography and pilgrimage routes related to the *Patavini Fontes* in Antiquity.

The polylobate building

In the archaeological area of Via Scavi there has been a succession of excavations and restoration works, of which those implemented in the 1980s heavily impacted on the ancient structures: in some cases, the restoration involved the massive use of concrete and new stones or bricks that caused considerable alterations to the ancient masonry, thus preventing a full understanding of its functioning. In other cases, it was the construction of buildings for tourists that caused obliteration of part of the two major thermal pools, as was the case with the Montecarlo Hotel erected in the 1960s and now in complete disrepair: it destroyed parts of the large Roman pools and ancient remains close to them (Bassani and De Venanzi 2024).

The excavation of the so-called polylobate building follows the period of resumed investigations of Via Scavi, between the 1950s and 1970s, conducted by the Archaeological Superintendency: unearthed in the summer of 1970, very little excavation data remain of the building, but I have been recently able to track down some images of those works in the photographic archives of the Superintendency.

Placed northeast of the small Roman theater and north of the three pools, the building occupied a total area of 672m2 (see Figure 1): it was therefore of considerable size, and, in terms of volume, it must have been a monumental construction. From vestibule 1 (6.3x5.3m) two pairs of identical and symmetrical rooms, 2-3 and 4-5, were reached to the north and south, although it cannot be ruled out that the latter had independent external entrances. The dimensions of the elongated rectangular rooms 2 and 4 measure 6.6x3.4m, while the multilinear rooms 3 and 5, in their maximum measurements, are 4.4x5m: the latter have three rectangular exedras, which enclose to the north and south this first group of rooms.

The core of the building should be recognized in a large central room 6 with a square floor plan (12.70x12.80m = 43x43 *pedes*), provided with a circular basin A (5.6m) that was served by a pipeline (for adduction water?)

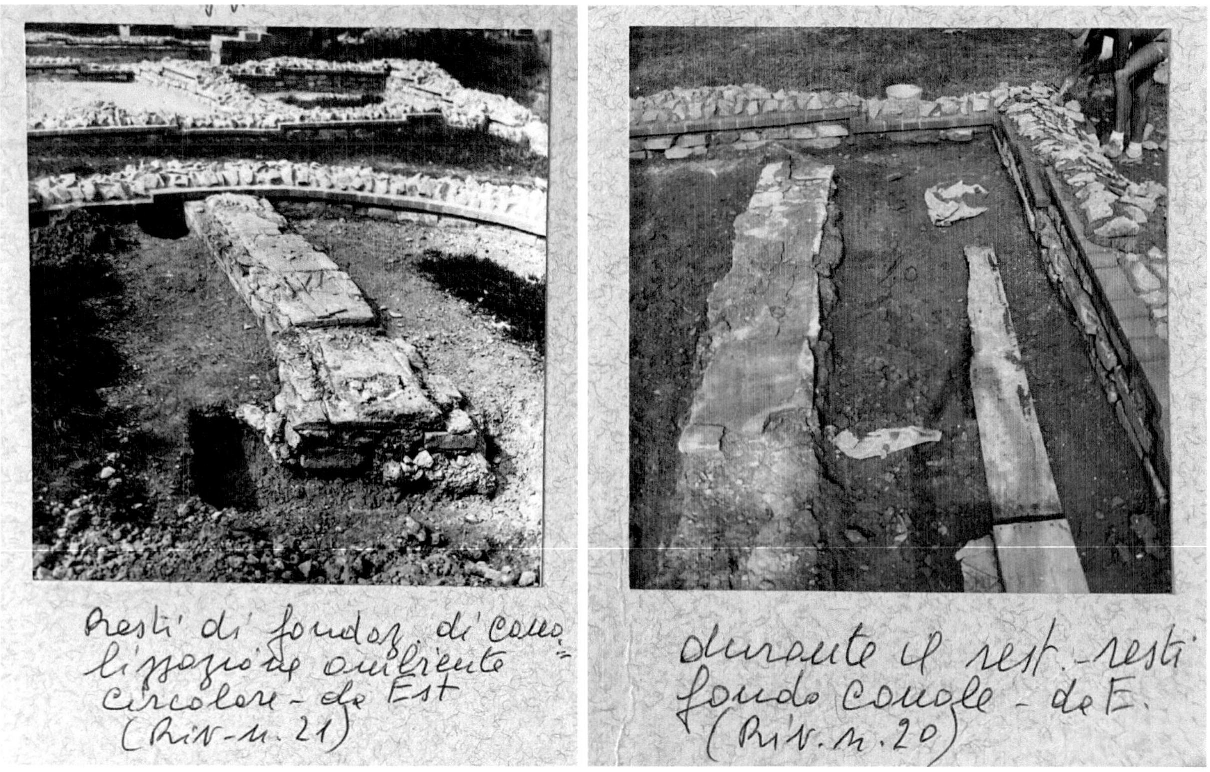

Figure 2. Montegrotto Terme, Viale Stazione/Via Scavi, polylobate building (Veneto region, Italy). A: View of the coverage of a channel in basin A of room 6 (from Bassani 2022: 108, fig. 11A); B: view of the coverage of a channel in room 9 (from Bassani 2022: 109, fig. 12).

clearly recognizable in the photo preceding the heavy restorations carried out here and indicated in the related caption: 'Remains of foundat[ion] of canalization [in the] circular room' ('Resti di fondaz. di canalizzazione ambiente circolare' Figure 2.A). Now the culvert cover looks like a simple wall, but thanks to archival photos, the coverage beneath it is clearly recognizable. Furthermore, two large exedras, i.e., apsidal rooms 7-8 (diam. 7.3m, prof. 3.3m), opened onto this room to the north and south, provided with a rectangular niche at the bottom of each apse, recognizable only from the foundations.

Finally, in the innermost western portion of the building complex and aligned with the vestibule are the three rooms 9-11, all of which open eastward and are accessible from room 6: room 9, larger in size than the other two (5.5x5.4m, 19x19 *pedes*), does not appear to have had side doors to access the two rooms 10-11, which are smaller in size (room 10: 2.1x3m; room 11: 2.2x2.9m) and have apses at the bottom. Although In a 1971 map a wall is indicated inside room 9, it could be the cover of a conduit from the west perimeter of the room, that runs eastward and has the same orientation as the conduit present in pool A of room 6 (Figure 2.B). This would be confirmed by a photo of the archive of the Archaeological Superintendence and by the related caption, which reads: 'during the rest.[oration] remains [of the] channel bottom' ('Durante il rest. [auro] resti fondo canale'): thus attesting, during the restoration work, the presence of a channel with the same orientation as the one in the basin. It could have been, then, a fountain or water feature clearly visible from the entrance.

Finally, three partition walls were found parallel to the long northern perimeter side, with an east-west direction (see Figure 1, L), possibly pertaining to a corridor. Given the shortage of information, it is impossible to say whether there was a symmetrical one to the south as well, between our building and pool B, or whether it was limited only to that sector of the health resort: we could certainly interpret it as a service compartment, to reach/separate the buildings.

According to the excavation records and as a result of various inspections, it seems clear, despite the heavy changes made during the restoration, that the building technique is *opus latericium*, similar to that used for other buildings: the chronology should therefore be placed in the late 1st-2nd century AD.

Looking at the building from a general point of view, it is evident how it was articulated around basin A in room 6, which should be interpreted as a fountain and not as a bathing pool since there are no steps to access it. It is also difficult to clarify whether the water main that served basin A had a connection to the water network (G) behind the large healing pools (see Figure 1) and whether it was the same one that served the probable canal in Room 9 as well.

In addition to the Roman cistern M with thermal water indicated during excavations in the 18th century, a careful study of hydrological maps related to Montecarlo Hotel clarified that the latter from the 1960s-1970s used for its therapeutic pools springs present right next to the polylobate building (Bassani 2022). Hypothetically, therefore, it is possible to imagine that the polylobate building drew water from one of these springs, which over the centuries may have been depleted because they were subject to constant and massive use by the hotel facilities. Indeed, one might speculate that the polylobate building was built just above an important spring, monumentalized in the circular basin A.

As for the decorative apparatus and roof system, very little is known. The 1971 plan within entrance room 1 indicated 'remnants of a marble slab floor' within a rectangular box drawn in the room and shown on the plan. It is possible that the rest of the building was also decorated with marble, but everything has been removed, perhaps already in the Medieval age.

Finally, it is most astonishing that, as reiterated in the few documentary notes in the Superintendency Archive, no artifacts were found during the excavation, whereas many fragments of decoration and artifacts were recovered during the excavation of the rest of the archaeological area (in the pools and in the theatre) in the 18th and 20th centuries, as well as during the investigations that led to the discovery of the small theater in 1965. Does this mean that it was totally despoiled as early as ancient or Medieval times because it constituted an irresistible quarry of precious objects and building materials?

This question I cannot answer, while I think one can try to explain the function of this building by comparing it with some known examples in Italy and elsewhere. The building, in its morphology, size and internal organization, recalls examples of *nymphaea* for ceremonial-worshipping use and not structures intended for therapeutic uses such as *balnea*. The connotative elements in this sense are:

- The centrality of water due to the presence of a large central circular pool, into which one could not descend but at most walk around.
- The symmetry of the mixtilinear (and not just polylobate) compartments, arranged in pairs following a precise axiality from the entrance to the bottom room 9, itself, perhaps, provided with a water pipe.
- The proximity to one of the main thermo-mineral springs in the therapeutic area, later exploited by Montecarlo Hotel until its water vein was exhausted.
- The autonomy of the so-called polylobate structure from the area of the baths and theater, i.e., its separation from the curative circuit.
- The orientation and access of the polylobate building from the east in the direction of one of the Roman roads that served the health resort.

These features mark, in my opinion, a peculiarity of the building compared to other buildings present, but more importantly they are the same as those found in other examples of *nymphaea*, on which it is now worth dwelling.

Nymphaea in thermo-mineral contexts: some examples

To attempt to understand the function of the supposed *nymphaeum* of Via Scavi and its relation to the rest of the curative structures in the archaeological area, I think it is useful to recall, firstly, the known types of *nymphaea* attested in Roman times, and secondly, to analyze some particularly illustrative cases found in thermo-mineral contexts.

From a general point of view, the Roman *nymphaea* consist of a rectangular chamber (subterranean or semi-subterranean: Type I) with spring/fountain and collection basin, sometimes provided with niches and small side recesses (Mingazzini 1955; Neuerburg 1965; Settis 1973; Lavagne 1988; Gros 2011: 252-260). The building type derives from Hellenistic *nymphaea* related to the worship of springs and Nymphs, as widely demonstrated. This rather simple version, which finds several exemplifications throughout the Italic territory, then underwent an evolution in the Flavian-Trajanic period, which corresponded to a rectangular hall with an apse, usually semicircular and with a barrel vault: it was often flanked by mixtilinear/polylobate rooms useful to create a space in which several deities could be worshipped and with whom members of the imperial court could sometimes be associated (Type II). During architectural development, which would later lead to true 'water exhibits', such as the *Septizodium* of the Severans alongside the *Palatium* on the Palatine, the strongly cultic aspect toward the spring and the Nymphs, which these buildings had maintained over time, seems to wane in favor of their predominantly monumental connotation, although in some cases water-related rituals may have continued into later times.

It should be emphasized, however, that the *nymphaea* of types I and II considered in the aforementioned works were often connected to aqueducts or freshwater veins, which served cities and/or private estates. Similar compartments or structures are also present, however, in health resorts, where the water was mineral and indeed played a fundamental role from a sacrate, therapeutic, and therefore also economic point of view: their nature as places to practice devotion was pervasive and enduring, since the religious value recognized to that medicinal water remained constant over time, patronized by Nymphs and/or other deities. Examples of this can be found both in the Italic Peninsula, which has been reported in some previous studies, and in the Provinces.

Simple rectangular chamber or apse nymphaea within health resorts

Two *nymphaea* caves pertinent to type I are known in Latium and Umbria, at Ponte di Nona and Cesadoro respectively, both locations characterized by therapeutic mineral waters.

The first case is a context not far from *Praeneste* and close to the Via Prenestina and Tivoli, where the presence of cold springs with a relevant component of dissolved magnesium salts is documented (Potter 1989; Bassani 2014: 165): around them a settlement was organized, equipped with a *mansio*, a shrine and an adjoining enclosure rich in votive offerings including anatomical votive objects, and other structures of uncertain function, with a private building in the imperial age (Figure 3).

Among the structures is a rock-cut *nymphaeum* on the northwestern slope, with two niches and ducts carved into the rock that were reported by Rodolfo Lanciani in the early 20th century: the sacred purpose of the *nymphaeum*-cave could be confirmed by the discovery, inside it, of a fragment of polychrome glass *patera.* It should also be pointed out that although included in a complex settlement area, the *nymphaeum* was separate from the *mansio* with baths and the temple area, as if to mark its topographical and functional autonomy from the other constructions for civil and cult use. Finally, while the date for the shrine goes back as early as the 4th-3rd centuries BC, the *mansio*, the *nymphaeum* and other buildings date from the 1st century BC to the 1st century AD.

Moving to Umbria, another cave *nymphaeum* was discovered in the province of Perugia (Cesadoro-Collazzone, Umbria) in 1734-1735, following diggings carried out in an area of probable sacred nature (Figure 4) (Sensi 2006; Bassani 2014: 177-178). The latter was connected to a cold sulfur water spring that still gushes out inside the cave, which was about 2 mt high at the time, and then flows into a small stream that joins the Saragano river. Inside the *nymphaeum*, whose dimensions are not known to date, many sacral-type artifacts were found, including a marble statue of a male figure with cornucopia, smaller than life-size (0.9m), another of Hercules of small size as well as a relief with Harpocrates. That sacred ceremonies were practiced in the *nymphaeum*/grotto is attested by the recovery of a rectangular trapeze/altar and a circular pedestal with a hole at the top, which could be identified with a cylindrical altar provided with an upper cavity for officiating at sacrifices. Furthermore, the ritual practices are attested by the finding of a great many other objects, including oil lamps, small containers, a pinecone and many hen and peacock eggs, as well as more than four hundred coins from the age of Domitian to Antoninus Pius. Indeed, even in this case the *nymphaeum* is dated between the 1st-2nd centuries AD, not unlike the mixtilinear building in Montegrotto Terme.

A similar chronology is finally recorded in the Type II *nymphaeum* at the *Aquae Cutiliae*, in the province of Rieti, characterized by cold mineral water flowing from two springs, one sulfidic-carbonate, the other bicarbonate-sulfate-alkaline-earthy (Alvino and Leggio 2006) (Figure 5). Here, on the northern side of the very large pool (60 x 24m) dug into the rocky bank and 1.8m deep, stands the large apsidal chamber *nymphaeum* 2 (7.20 x 6.35m, diam. apse 4m), to which were associated both the two specular rooms B, and the long corridor that led to the court above, reached by staircase H. To the Flavian age is dated a remaking of the upper part of the apse of the *nymphaeum*, which involved the addition of eight water outlets and the related water system behind, to which corresponded the creation of a niche (2.20m) below which a basin was placed. It seems important to note how in this case, as well as at Ponte di Nona, the position of the *nymphaeum* appears rather secluded from the other rooms facing the rectangular courtyard of the pool. Its separation from the bathing circuit visible both on the ground floor and on the upper floor seems intentional and not accidental. It could underline a precise desire to divide the places frequented by bathers where cures and therapies were carried out, from a 'sacred' and cultic place such as the *nymphaeum*.

This separation between bathing circuits and the ceremonial places sacred to the Nymphs is equally well evident in the *Aquae Flaviae nymphaeum* at Chaves (Portugal), the subject of recent investigations (Carneiro and González Soutelo 2019) (Figure 6). It coincides with a monumentalized well-fountain (1x1.35m, prof. 1.7m) placed within a semicircular exedra and provided with a tympanum above the cavity, where there was

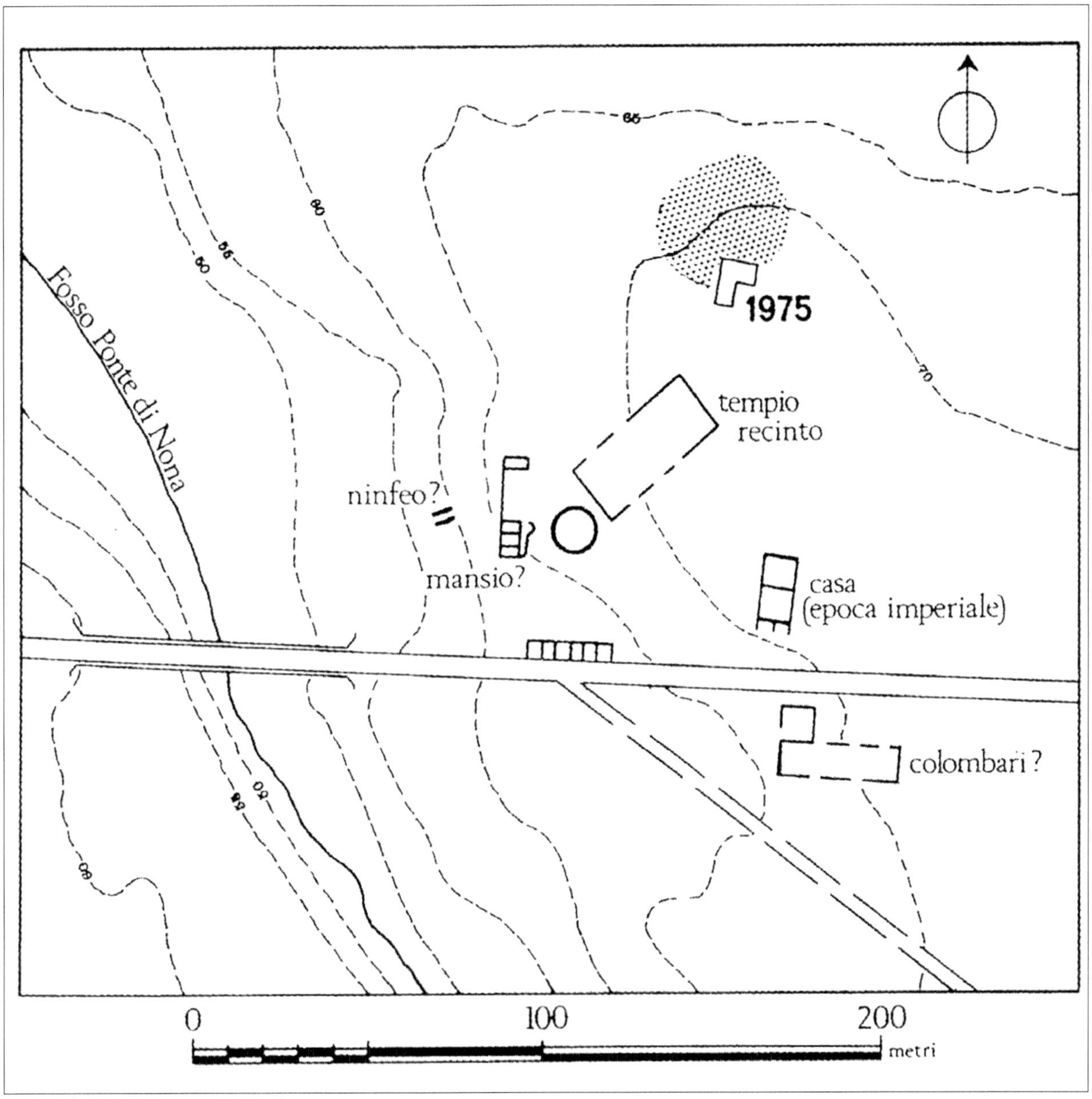

Figure 3. Ponte di Nona, Preneste (Latium region, Italy). Plan of the archaeological area with the *mansio*, the *nymphaeum*, the shrine and other Roman buildings (from Quilici 1974: 92, fig. 80).

spring water collected for sacred-ceremonial uses. The *nymphaeum* was indeed included in the therapeutic station but, as has been appropriately pointed out, it was designed to reproduce an underground cave sacred to the Nymphs, that was not directly accessible except by following a route distinct from that used to reach the two baths and the treatment rooms next to them.

If, therefore, the cases briefly presented here show the presence of *nymphaea* of type I even in mineral areas where, indeed, medicinal spring water was the protagonist of the installations themselves, it may now be useful to consider the two most significant examples of *nymphaea* comparable to that of Montegrotto Terme (Type II), with which analogies are indeed surprising and, in my opinion, interesting.

Nymphaea as multilinear buildings: the case of the Aquae Apollinares Novae and Baños de Fortuna

The most significant curative context that offers useful comparisons for the supposed Euganean *nymphaeum* is that of the most important Roman spa near Lake Bracciano: the present-day location of Vicarello coincides with the *Vicus Aurelii*, which in ancient times was famous for its numerous springs called *Aquae Apollinares Novae*, mentioned together with the *Aquae Apollinares Veteres* of Stigliano in the *Tabula Peutingeriana*

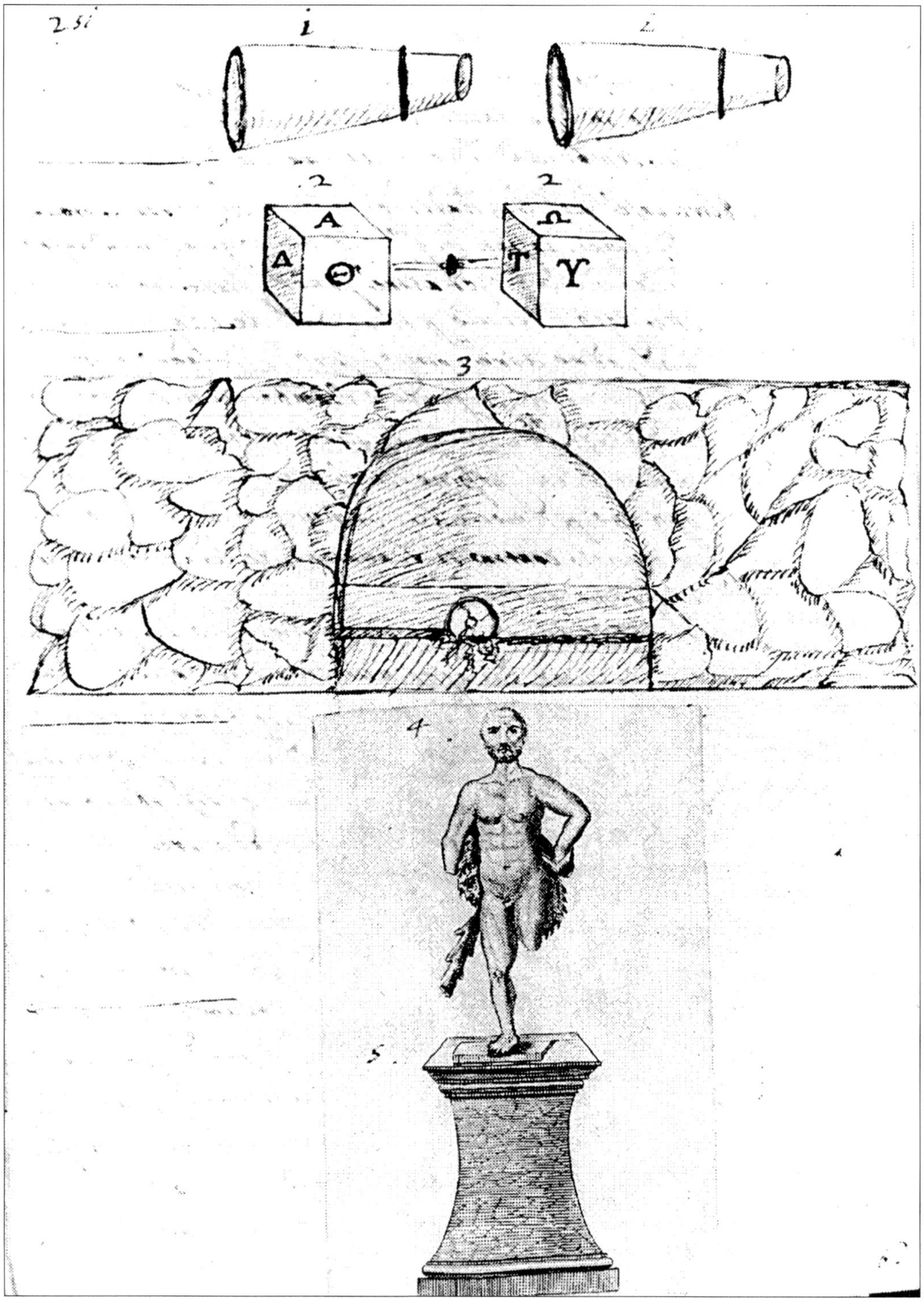

Figure 4. Cesadoro-Collazzone, Perugia (Umbria region, Italy). The archaeological objects found in the grotto/*nymphaeum* in a drawing of the 18th century (from Sensi 2006: 334, fig. 7).

(Colini 1979; Cordiano 2003; Cordiano 2011; Bassani 2014: 162-163) (Figure 7.A).

A number of springs are known in the area, some with radioactive bicarbonate-sulfate water at 50°-59°C, others oligomineral, slightly alkaline, flowing out at 16°C. Already frequented in prehistoric and protohistoric times, in Roman times the site presented two main springs in the curative area, to the east and west: the first near the building interpreted as a *nymphaeum*, the other served the thermal core that was used and remodeled between the 18th and 19th centuries, and in which was found the famous *stipe* with thousands of votive offerings.

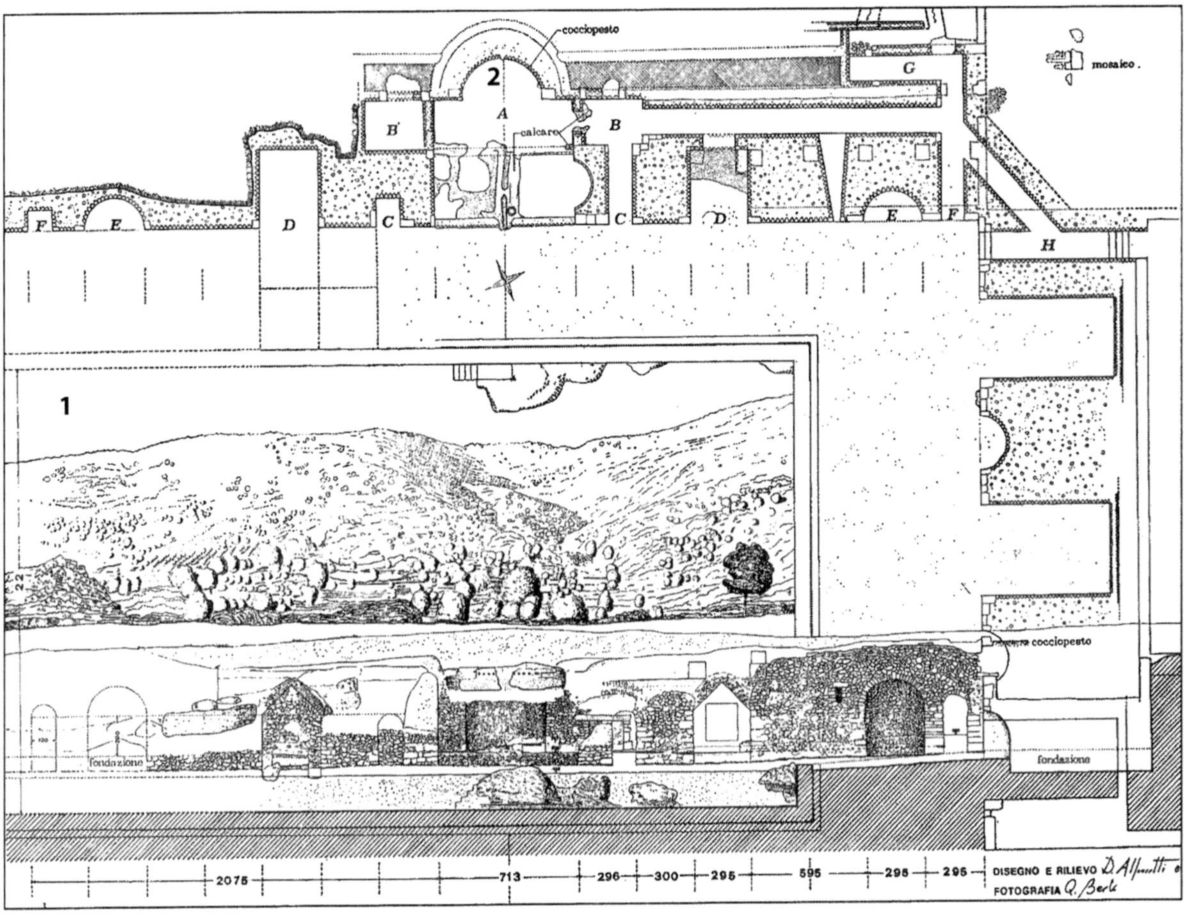

Figure 5. Rieti, *Aquae Cutiliae* (Latium region, Italy). Plan and section of the Roman healing spa with the big pool 1 and the *nymphaeum* 2 (*Termalismo antico* 1999: 209, fig. 107).

The strategic importance of this health resort should be noted: connected to the two consular roads Clodia and Cornelia from the Republican age onward, it experienced, after a prehistoric and republican frequentation, an important monumentalization starting from the Flavian age: not only did Domitian build a sumptuous villa near it, but it is likely that the emperor intervened in the very management of the thermo-mineral center since, among the inscriptions recovered, as many as six mention Nymphs, and in one case these are mentioned as *Numphae Domitianae* (Buonopane and Petraccia 2014; Bassani *forthcoming*).

Subsequently, the site was frequented without interruption until the 4th century AD but was destroyed by the Saracens in the early Medieval period and was soon covered in vegetation. However, the springs continued to be known and used during the Renaissance, so much so that in 1532 a hospice for the sick was erected on behalf of the Hungarian-Germanic College. Between the 18th and 19th centuries, the area was affected by new construction work for a therapeutic plant, which altered part of the ancient remains but also allowed the discovery of some of the buildings from the Roman period. New excavations were made in the 1970s on behalf of the Archaeological Superintendence, but today the area, included in the Bracciano Nature Park, can be visited partially and is in a state of abandon. The cures still practiced in the area between Vicarello and Stigliano are prescribed for breathing ailments, arthritis and rheumatism, including mud treatments.

The northeastern complex (see Figure 7.A) included a cistern 4, two vaulted compartments 5-6 and a building developed axially to the northwest/southeast: this is a big building of large dimensions (c. 40x20m) and with an articulation that seems rather similar to that of the Via Scavi building in Montegrotto Terme and can therefore be ascribed to Type II of the classification of this type of building structures. In room 7 the entrance (c. 16x12m) is recognizable, provided with rectangular exedras (c. 1x0.5m) preserved only on the northern side, perhaps also on the southern side. From here one could enter the interior. The route allowed to reach room 14, the real focus of the building, by crossing two pairs of long rectangular rooms 8-9 and 12-13, similarly the Euganean area, closed to the back by rectangular exedras: from them one could then enter the main

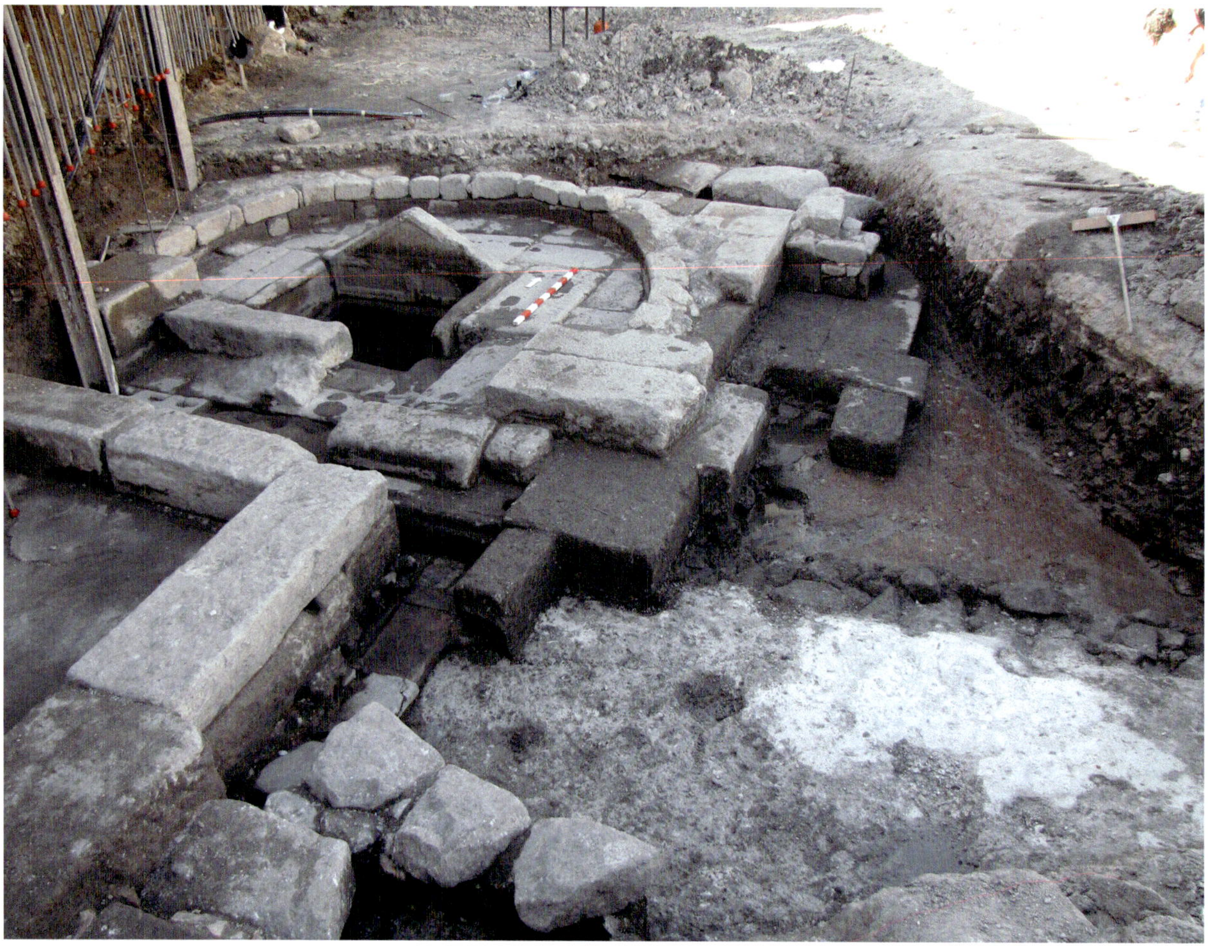

Figure 6. Chaves, *Aquae Flaviae* (Portugal). Photo of the *nymphaeum* in the Roman healing spa (from Carneiro and González Soutelo 2019: 72, fig. 2).

room 14. Furthermore, from entrance 7 two adjoining and specular rooms 10-11 were quadrangular and led to the large mixtilinear hall 14 (9.45x9.2m). The latter was covered by a pavilion vault, and in the center was a rounded cross-shaped fountain, at the sides two rather large apses (c. 6m diam.: Figure 7.B). Finally, at the bottom of the building was a rectangular room 15 introduced by an arch/window, beyond which was a large, deep *nymphaeum* with two brick basins (4.5x1.5m) at the bottom and a marble ladder for water features at the upper level. The ladder was surmounted by the Pentelic marble statue of Apollo (preserved height 1.21m; total height c. 2.10/2.20m), which, constantly washed by the thermo-mineral waters, has reached us in a rather corroded state, and already restored in ancient times. The last rooms served as hallways (16) and service rooms to reach one of the two treatment areas.

During the excavations, marble slab coverings were found for both walls and floors, forming, at least in room 14, geometric floral motifs worked in *opus sectile*; for the walls of the *nymphaeum*, however, mosaic tiles with blue and gold glass paste encrusted with shells and stuccoes were used to recreate the shimmering typical of caves inside springs.

At Vicarello, water was present both in the pool of the central hall 14 and in the *nymphaeum* 15 dominated by the cult statue of Apollo, just as in the supposed *nymphaeum* of Montegrotto, water was probably emphasized both in the large circular pool A of hall 6 and in room 9, should the hypothesis advanced above be correct. In both cases, therefore, the architecture of these building types features as common traits not only the articulation of the complex in alternating rectangular, apsidal and mixtilinear rooms, but also the centrality of spring water (which was under the patronage of Apollo in Vicarello), named in 7 inscriptions, and of the Nymphs. However, we know from recovered materials that other deities were also worshipped here, including Asclepius, Silvanus, Priapus and Pan.

The *nymphaeum* was located at one of the two springs of the health resort, since at the second, which was probably one of the main, the actual health resort sector arose, positioned to the west beyond the stream

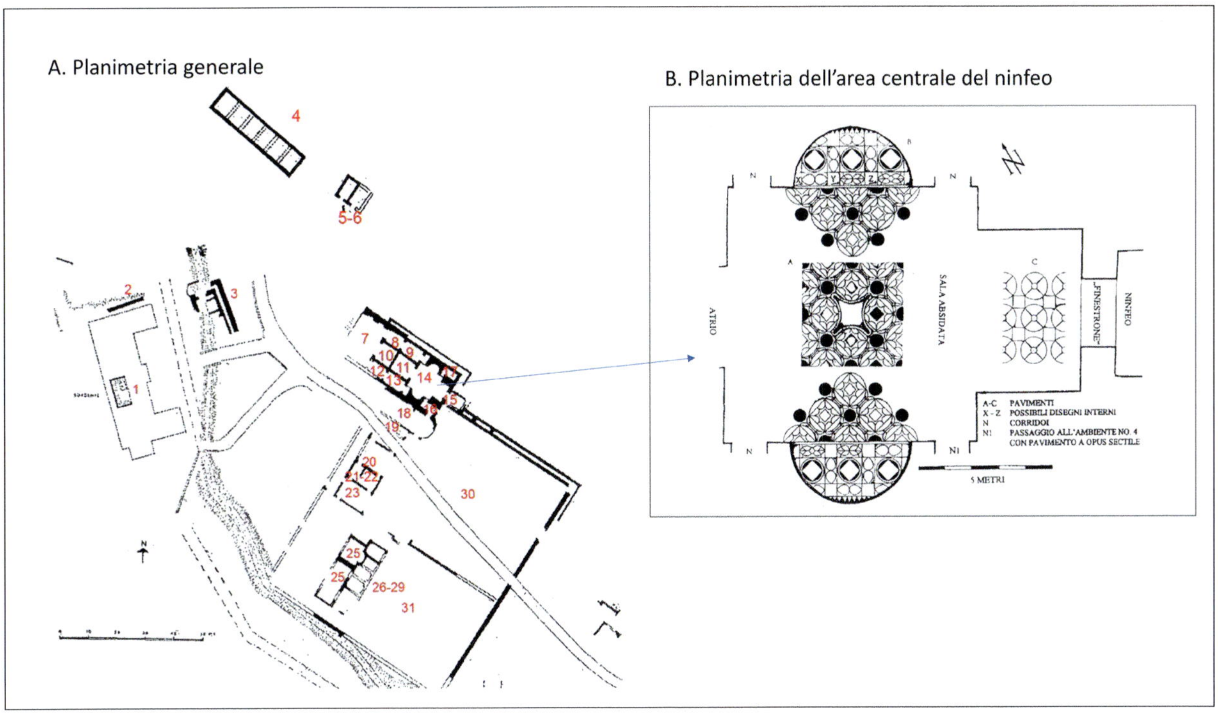

Figure 7. Vicarello-Bracciano, *Aquae Apollinares Novae* (Latium region, Italy). A: Plan of the Roman healing spa; B: plan of the central part of the *nymphaeum* 14 (from Bassani 2022: 115, fig. 16).

(see Figure 7.A, no. 1), where the 18th-19th century establishment later rose. Thus, the *nymphaeum* was close to one of the main springs and to what must have been another sector connected to the cycle of cures and rest provided in this therapeutic station: it is the core extending towards the south-east, which was about 90x75m wide enclosed by a fence. In addition, there were two large, uncovered areas within it used as gardens and/or gymnasia (but remember that we have no definite evidence of gymnastic practices within gymnasiums at healing stations, not least on account of the fatigue involved in thermo-mineral therapies).

To conclude this paragraph, it is important to mention a second case of sacred space corresponding to the Type II of *nymphaea*, that was served by thermal water. I am referring to the sacred complex of Baños de Fortuna in the Murcia region, Spain, that shows similarities both with the polylobate building in Montegrotto Terme and Vicarello (Matilla Séiquer 2006; Matilla Séiquer 2017) (Figure 8). The structure was strictly connected to another sacred thermal place named the Cueva Negra and in the 1st century AD they were used as shrines. In particular, Baños de Fortuna corresponds to a quadrangular structure with some rooms in the entrance area, that were exploited for thermal purposes only in the late phase, because at the beginning they did not present water pipes. Moving inside, the central space was occupied by a rectangular basin with a few steps into which mineral water flowed, coming from the bottom of the building, excavated on that side in the rock: here a semicircular *nymphaeum* flanked by two minor rectangular rooms occupied the main visual axis. Some altars re-used in the modern age building testify the votive activity to the deities worshipped here in relation to the mineral waters.

The building has been interpreted as a shrine as well as a spa for the presence of the pool, accessible by some steps; but in my opinion aspects of worship must have outweighed therapeutic ones: it is hard to imagine that in the structure there could have been at the same time sick people immersing themselves in the rectangular pool and pilgrims and worshippers paying devotion to the spring water, that gushed out at the bottom in the *nymphaeum*. Then, the rectangular pool could be reserved for ceremonial activities and not for curing purposes. In fact, as numerous examples in the Roman Empire show (Bassani, Fusco and Bolder-Boos 2019, *passim*, with bibliography), healing waters in their monumentalized sacred spaces were not meant to be contaminated by the promiscuity of secular use for cures: in the thermal-mineral contexts the healing treatments were assured in specific buildings with pools and rooms, while shrines and sacred springs often monumentalized thanks to basins and *nymphaea* were separated from the profane cures and were worshipped by pilgrims with ex-votos and prayers.

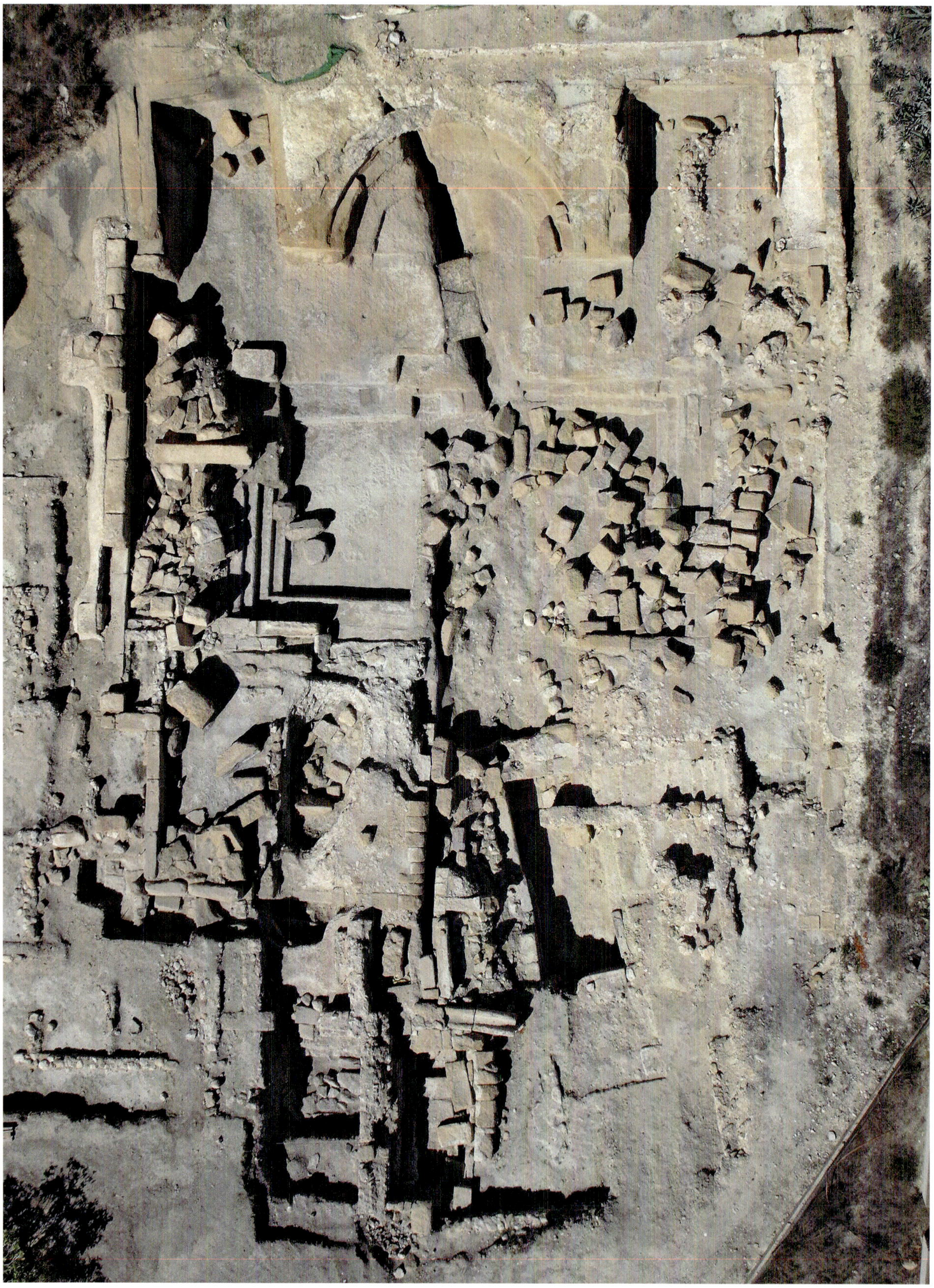

Figure 8. Baños de Fortuna (Murcia region, Spain). Zenith photo of the thermal shrine/bathing with the semicircular *nymphaeum* (from Matilla Séiquer 2017: 146, fig. 16).

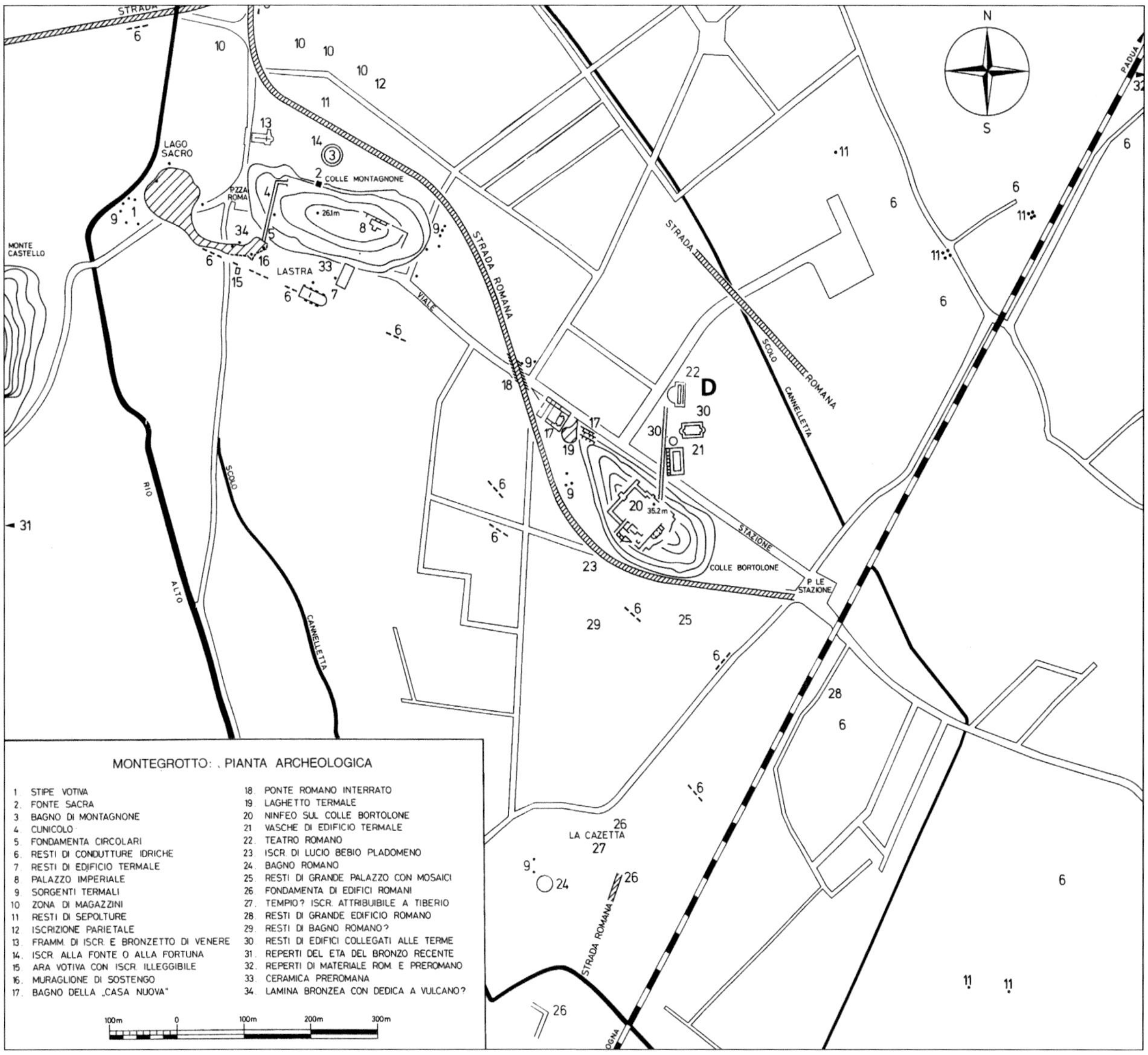

Figure 9. Montegrotto Terme (Veneto region, Italy). Topographical map with all the archaeological remains: the polylobate building is indicated with the letter D within the healing spa of Via Scavi (pools at no. 30 and 21, small theatre at no. 22). It seems to be oriented towards the Roman road found near the area (from Lazzaro 1981: 159, fig. 5).

Food for thought

i would like to conclude this article by pointing out how the comparative analysis between the supposed *nymphaeum* of Via Scavi and the other cases of *nymphaea* examined has allowed to find common and recurring elements on which it is worth focusing our attention.

Indeed, if we consider the Via Scavi building at Montegrotto Terme and the *nymphaeum* at Vicarello, the similarities of the internal articulation of the two buildings are really striking: both provided for multilinear halls accessible symmetrically from one side and from the other with respect to the central hall, provided with a fountain, and both at Montegrotto and at Vicarello the presence of service compartments is documented, to separate or join the *nymphaea* from other sectors of the health resorts. Moreover, the presence of a central pool in the main hall and the existence of an almost processional pathway that passes alongside it in the direction of the inner rooms (which in Vicarello coincide with the actual *nymphaeum* of Apollo) emphasize in both cases the ceremonial experience, prevalent over the bathing one, which indeed seems to be lacking here altogether. In fact, in all the *nymphaea* examined, both Type I and Type II, the water always came from the springs and it seems to be the real protagonist of the different installations, whether small, medium or large: in the contexts considered, the monumentalizing of the springs involved the creation of a room equipped with a fountain/well or real buildings in their own right, with pools and waterfalls in which no curative use was envisaged. Indeed, compared to bathing pools, the *nymphaea* always seem to be clearly separated: this, in my opinion and according to many scholars,[3] was to avoid a promiscuity between pure water and water contaminated by human use. The water in the *nymphaea* was in fact dedicated to the deities who patronized it, while the water used in pools and therapeutic facilities was in any case 'profaned' by its use for the sick. In this sense, Pliny the Younger's famous letter dedicated to the description of the springs of the Clitumnus appears very significant (Plin. *epist.* 8, 8, 2-6; Bassani 2012: 405-406): there the writer specifies that the part destined for the god and other deities was clearly separated by a bridge from that used by men, precisely because in the former the water was uncontaminated, while in the latter it was profaned by use, even if just bathing.

This consideration allows us to underline a further fact, namely that perhaps the separation between the *balnea* facilities and the halls/buildings used for *nymphaea* could also be ascribed to managerial needs: thermo-mineral resorts were visited not only by sick people, but also by pilgrims and travelers, who could pay homage to the deities of the miraculous springs without necessarily carrying out therapy. So, it might have been preferable to provide differentiated routes within the healing complexes, allowing people to reach the sacred springs without mixing with those who had diseases, often highly contagious such as those of a dermatological nature.

In this sense it is worth pointing out that the supposed *nymphaeum* of Montegrotto Terme was oriented eastwards and thus was close to the road of which several sections were discovered in the 20th century near the railway station: in turn it must have been a detour from the major road that from *Patavium* reached the *Aquae Patavinae* and from there continued southward, probably connecting to Via Annia and other consular roads leading to Rome (Figure 9). This could mean that at Montegrotto a traveler could reach the places of worship by following an independent route and deviating from the main road. By offering such an option, those who operated the facility could still obtain an economic return even from a simple pilgrim: if one was not willing to spend money to stop at the healing settlements for several days, one could in any case purchase an ex voto from dealers near the *nymphaeum* and other shrines, such as the *emporium* that existed in the present location of Montirone, near Abano Terme, where vases and *rhytà* were sold (Lavizzari Pedrazzini 1995).

Thus, we can perhaps state that only the continuation of the investigation will allow to confirm or refute the hypothesis advanced here regarding the recognition of the so-called polylobate building of Montegrotto Terme as a *nymphaeum*. Certainly, an analysis on *nymphaea* and places of worship at the thermo-mineral springs intended as destinations of both curative and votive pilgrimage may offer new data for studies on thermalism in Roman times. Observing the structural and material evidence in ancient healing centers with a dynamic perspective, as might have been that of travelers and pilgrims, will perhaps allow us to grasp significant and peculiar aspects of the *aquae* and their customers.

[3] Among which see Abed Ben Kheder *et al.* 2011.

Bibliography

Abed Ben Kheder, A., J. Scheid, H. Broise, and C. Balmelle 2011. Le sanctuaire de source de Jebel Oust (Tunisie). *Les Nouvelles de l'archéologie* 124 : 10-14. (https://journals.openedition.org/nda/1404?lang=en).

Alvino, G. and T. Leggio, 2006. Acque e culti salutari in Sabina, in L. Gasperini (ed) *Usus veneratioque fontium. Fruizione e culto delle acque salutari nell'Italia romana*: 17-53. Tivoli: Tipigraf.

Bassani, M. 2012. La schedatura dei contesti cultuali presso sorgenti termominerali. Osservazioni preliminari su aspetti strutturali e materiali, in M. Bassani, M. Bressan and F. Ghedini (eds) *Aquae Patavinae. Montegrotto e il termalismo in Italia: aggiornamenti e nuove prospettive di valorizzazione*, Atti del Convegno (Padova, 14-15 giugno 2011): 391-410. Padova: Padova University Press.

Bassani, M. 2014. Per una carta distributiva degli spazi sacri alle fonti curative, in M. Annibaletto, M. Bassani and F. Ghedini (eds) *Cura, preghiera e benessere. Le stazioni curative nell'Italia romana*: 161-188. Padova: Padova University Press.

Bassani, M. 2022. L'edificio polilobato in Via Scavi a Montegrotto Terme. Ipotesi per una sua interpretazione. *Rivista di Archeologia* XLVI: 101-123.

Bassani, M. *forthcoming.* Ninfei alle sorgenti termominerali: alcune riflessioni sui casi nel Lazio e in altre regioni, in A. Russo, R. Alteri, A. De Cristofaro (eds) '*Né spelunca o caverna è fra gli sassi*'. *Ninfei antichi e moderni a Roma e nel Lazio. Archeologia e fortuna di uno spazio polisemico*, Atti del Convegno Internazionale (Roma, 13-15 dicembre 2023), Rome: L'Erma di Bretswchneider.

Bassani, M. and M.E. De Venanzi 2024. Hotel Montecarlo nearby the archaeological area of Via Scavi in Montegrotto Terme. Archival sources. *La Rivista di Engramma*, 214:

Bassani, M., M. Bressan and F. Ghedini (eds) 2011. Aquae Patavinae. *Il termalismo antico nel comprensorio euganeo e in Italia*, Atti del I Convegno Nazionale (Padova, 14-15 giugno 2011). Padova: Padova University Press.

Bassani, M., M. Bressan and F. Ghedini, (eds) 2012. Aquae Patavinae. *Montegrotto e il termalismo in Italia:*

aggiornamenti e nuove prospettive di valorizzazione, Atti del II Convegno Nazionale (Padova, 14-15 giugno 2011). Padova: Padova University Press.

Bassani, M., M. Bolder-Boos and U. Fusco 2019 (eds). *Rethinking the Concept of 'Healing Settlements': Water, Cults, Constructions and Contexts in the Ancient World.* Oxford: Archeopress.

Bassani, M., Ch. Destro, F. Ghedini, M.T. Privitera and P. Zanovello 2021. *Montegrotto Terme. Museo del termalismo antico e del territorio. Guida*, Padova: Padova University Press.

Buonopane, A. and M.F. Petraccia, 2014. Termalismo e divinità, in M. Annibaletto, M. Bassani and F. Ghedini (eds) *Cura, preghiera e benessere. Le stazioni curative termominerali nell'Italia romana*: 217-245. Padova: Padova University Press,

Carneiro, S. and S. González Soutelo 2019. Healing by Water: Therapy and Religion in the Roman Spas of the Iberian Peninsula, in M. Bassani, M. Bolder-Boos and U. Fusco 2019 (eds) *Rethinking the Concept of 'Healing Settlements': Water, Cults, Constructions and Contexts in the Ancient World*: 61-79. Oxford: Archeopress.

Colini, A.M. 1979. *Vicarello, la sorgente termale nel tempo.* Roma: Centenari.

Cordiano, G. 2003. Domiziano, Columella e la stipe di Vicarello. Ricerche sugli *Iunii* e sui possedimenti imperiali nella zona del lago di Bracciano in età neroniano-flavia. *Annali della facoltà di lettere e filosofia, Università di Siena* XXIV: 91-116.

Cordiano, G. 2011. *Vicus Aurelii* (Vicarello). La dimora dell'imperatore Domiziano presso le *Aquae Apollinares* Sabatine, la sua articolazione e sorte nel tempo, in S. Accardo (ed) *Sabatia Stagna*: insediamenti perilacustri ad Anguillara e dintorni in età romana: 19-80. Pisa: ETS.

Ghedini, F., P. Zanovello, M. Bassani, C. Destro, M.T. Privitera and M. Bressan 2015. La Villa di Via Neroniana a Montegrotto Terme (Padova): conoscenza e valorizzazione. *Amoenitas* IV: 11-40.

Gros, P. 2011. *L'architecture romaine du début du 3 siècle av. J.-C. à la fin du Haut Empire, I. Les monuments publics.* Paris : Picard.

Lavagne, H. 1988. Operosa antra. *Recherches sur la grotte à Rome de Sylla à Hadrien.* Rome: École française de Rome.

Lavizzari Pedrazzini, M.P. 1995. Il deposito del Montirone (Abano). *Quaderni di Archeologia del Veneto* 11: 109-166.

Lazzaro, L. 1981. Fons Aponi. *Abano e Montegrotto nell'Antichità.* Abano Terme: Francisci.

Matilla Séiquer, G. 2006. La recuperación de los balnearios durante el Bajo Imperio, in *Espacio y tiempo en la percepción de la Antigüedad Tardía: homenaje al profesor Antonino González Blanco. Antigüedad y Cristianismo* XXIII: 159-184.

Matilla Séiquer, G. 2017. El balneario de Fortuna. Visión de conjunto tras la última campaña de excavaciones, in G. Matilla Séiquer and S. González Soutelo (eds) *Termalismo antiguo en Hispania. Un análisis del tejido balneario en época romana y tardorromana en la península ibérica, Anejos de Archivo Español de Arqueología* LXXVIII: 131-170.

Mingazzini, P. 1955. Le grotte di Matermania e dell'Arsenale a Capri – Excursus sui cosiddetti ninfei. *Archeologia Classica* VII: 156-163.

Neuerburg, N. 1965. *L'architettura delle fontane e dei ninfei nell'Italia antica*, Napoli: G. Macchiaroli.

Potter, T.W. 1989. *Una stipe votiva da Ponte di Nona.* Roma: De Luca.

Quilici, L. 1974. *Regio I. Collatia, Formae Italiae X.* Roma: De Luca.

Sensi, L. 2006. Culto delle acque nel territorio di Tuderte, in L. Gasperini (ed) Usus veneratioque fontium. *Fruizione e culto delle acque salutari nell'Italia romana*: 321-353. Tivoli: Tipigraf.

Settis, S. 1973. 'Esedra' e 'ninfeo' nella terminologia architettonica del mondo romano. Dall'età repubblicana alla tarda antichità. *Aufstieg und Niedergang der Römische Welt* I, 4: 661-740.

Termalismo antico e moderno nel Lazio 1999. Regione Lazio, Assessorato Sviluppo Economico ed Attività Produttive, Roma: Quasar.

Tosi, G. 1987. Padova e la zona termale euganea, in *Il Veneto nell'età romana*, vol. II: 157-193. Verona: Banca Popolare di Verona.

Aquae Helveticae Becomes Baden (Switzerland). From the Roman *Vicus* to the Medieval Town

Andrea SCHAER
Independent researcher
andrea.schaer@archaeokontor.ch

Abstract: In my contribution, I will discuss the spatial relationship of ancient healing spas and territory. Taking Baden in Switzerland, the ancient *Aquae Helveticae*, as an example, I would like to discuss the question of the relationship between the baths and settlement areas in the Roman period and subsequent epochs. In doing so, I will ask which influences were decisive for the development of the spa settlement in the different periods.

Keywords: *Baden (Switzerland), healing baths, roman settlement, medieval town*

The site

Baden in the Swiss canton of Aargau lies 25km north of Zurich in the valley of the Limmat river (Figure 1). Here, where the Limmat, one of the three major rivers of the Swiss plateau, cuts through the foothills of the Jura mountains in a so-called Klus (a transverse valley), the most mineralised thermal springs in Switzerland rise in a riverbend, the so-called 'Limmatknie' (knee). Currently, 18 thermal springs are still in use, delivering between 700,000 and 1,100,000 litres of the 47°C hot, highly sulphureous water every day. All springs are at approximately the same temperature; the chemistry of the water is dominated by sodium, calcium, chloride, sulphate and hydrogen sulfide (Na-Ca-Cl-SO4-H2S) (Burger 2011: 96).

In the 21st century, Baden is a lively small town which is currently rediscovering and revitalising its tradition and heritage as a spa town. In recent years, after a long phase of neglect and decline, a renewal and urban upgrading of the spa area has taken place. Its centrepiece is the new thermal baths designed by Swiss architect Mario Botta (Figure 2).

In the run-up to the construction work of the new bathing facilities, extensive archaeological excavations and architectural investigations were carried out (Figure 3). These assessments not only provided new insights into the Roman healing baths, which form the core of Baden's bathing tradition, but they also shed new light on the medieval and modern baths.[1] The new findings make it possible to discuss a wide variety of questions and aspects that go beyond the consideration of bathing operations.

The roman *Aquae Helveticae*

The beginnings of the use of Baden's thermal springs date back to Roman times. The spa town of *Aquae Helveticae,* as Baden was called in Roman times, was located in the *civitas of* the *Helvetii* and from 90 AD, in the province of Germania Superior.

Within the road network of Roman Switzerland, *Aquae Helveticae* lay at the crossroads of the main road that connected the most important settlements of the Swiss Plateau with the Alpine pass routes and the roads leading north towards the Rhine and to the Danube.

The area of the thermal springs was probably already frequented in pre-Roman times by the people living in the area, although there are no traces of settlements in the immediate vicinity of the spring.

In the 2nd and 3rd decades AD, the troops stationed in the nearby legionary fortress of *Vindonissa* (today Windisch/Canton Aargau) built the first bathing facilities at the thermal springs. At about the same time as the thermal baths, a settlement was built on the plateau above the spring area and on the opposite bank of the river, as a bridge spanned the Limmat. The settlement had the status of a *vicus* (Schaer 2015: 20-26). The amenities of the baths and the people from near and far staying here also made *Aquae* a popular stopover and trading place.

In the turmoil of the Year of the Four Emperors in 69 AD, the settlement was destroyed by the troops of the 21st Legion stationed in nearby *Vindonissa* (Schucany 1998; Schucany 2015). The Roman historian Tacitus describes the pillaging of the bathing resort (which he does not mention by name) (Tacitus *Hist.* 67, I). Whether the

[1] The publication of the results of the most important excavations 2009-2018 is currently in preparation: Schaer 2024 and Schaer *et al.* in process. Preliminary reports (some with outdated research) can be found in Schaer 2010a, Schaer 2010b; Schaer 2015 and Schaer 2018 (all of them with further references). A more popular account of the history of the Baden is provided in Schaer 2022.

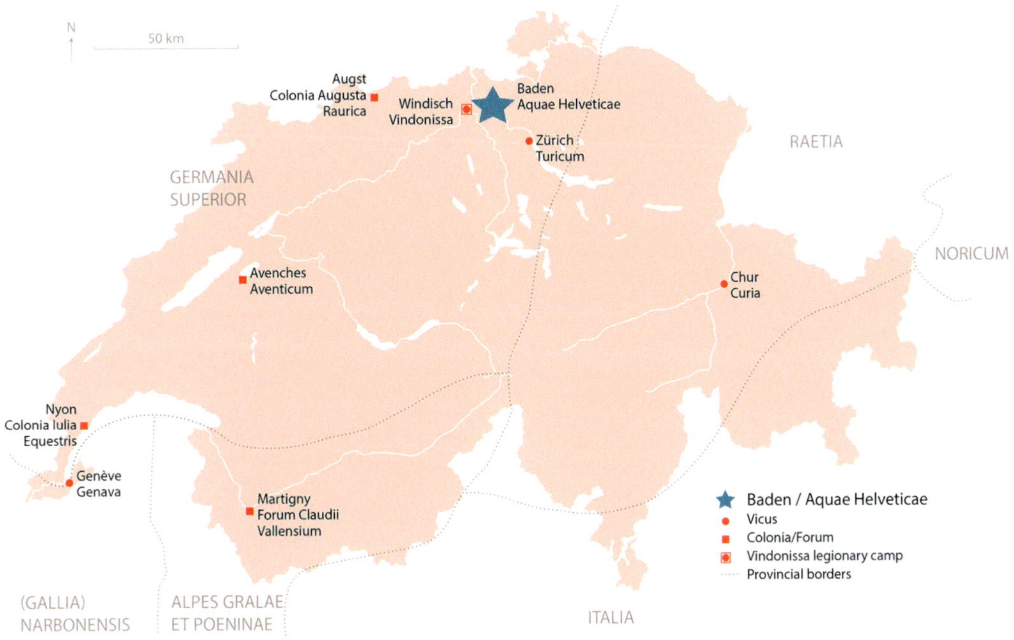

Figure 1. Baden's location in Switzerland. Graphic: Stadtgeschichte Baden/ikonaut/Andrea Schaer.

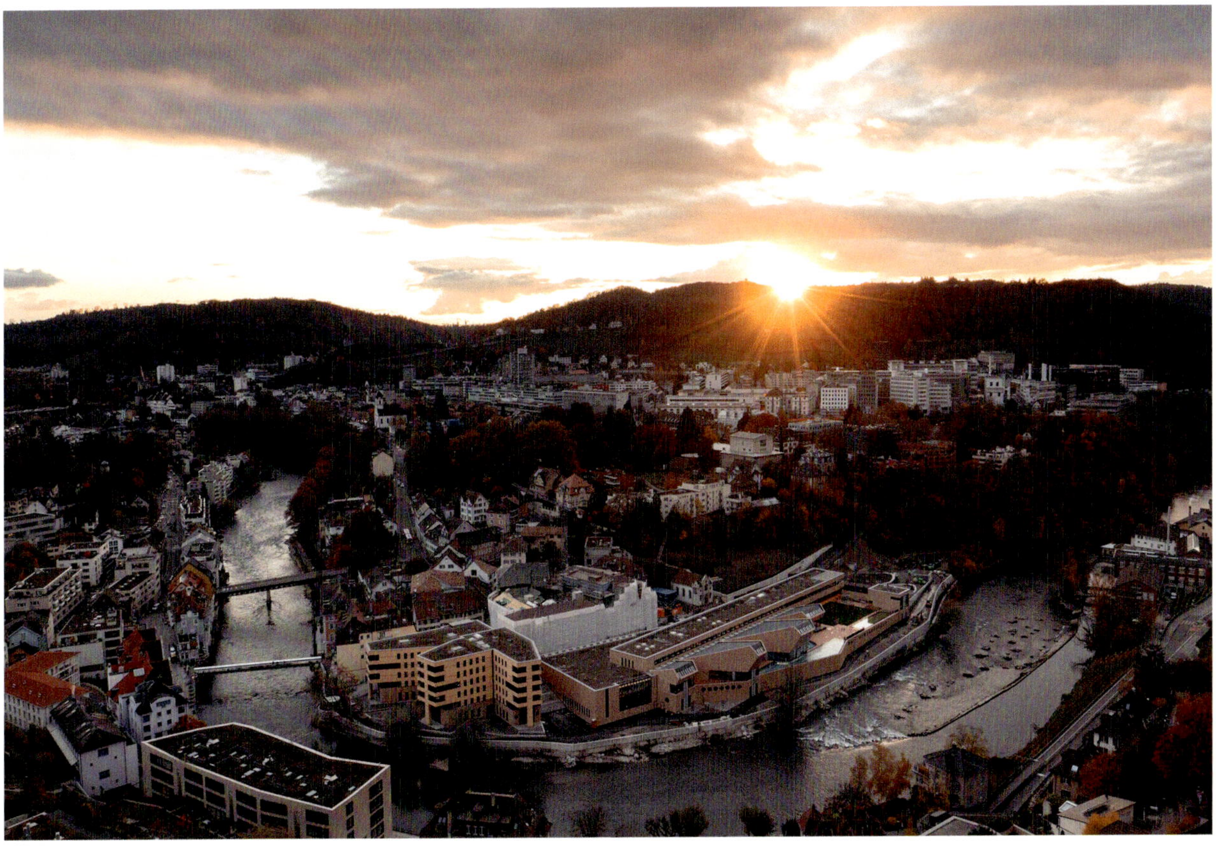

Figure 2. Baden in Aargau in autumn 2022. In the foreground, located directly in the river bend, the new buildings in the spa area. In the background, the old town of Baden. © Switzerland Tourism.

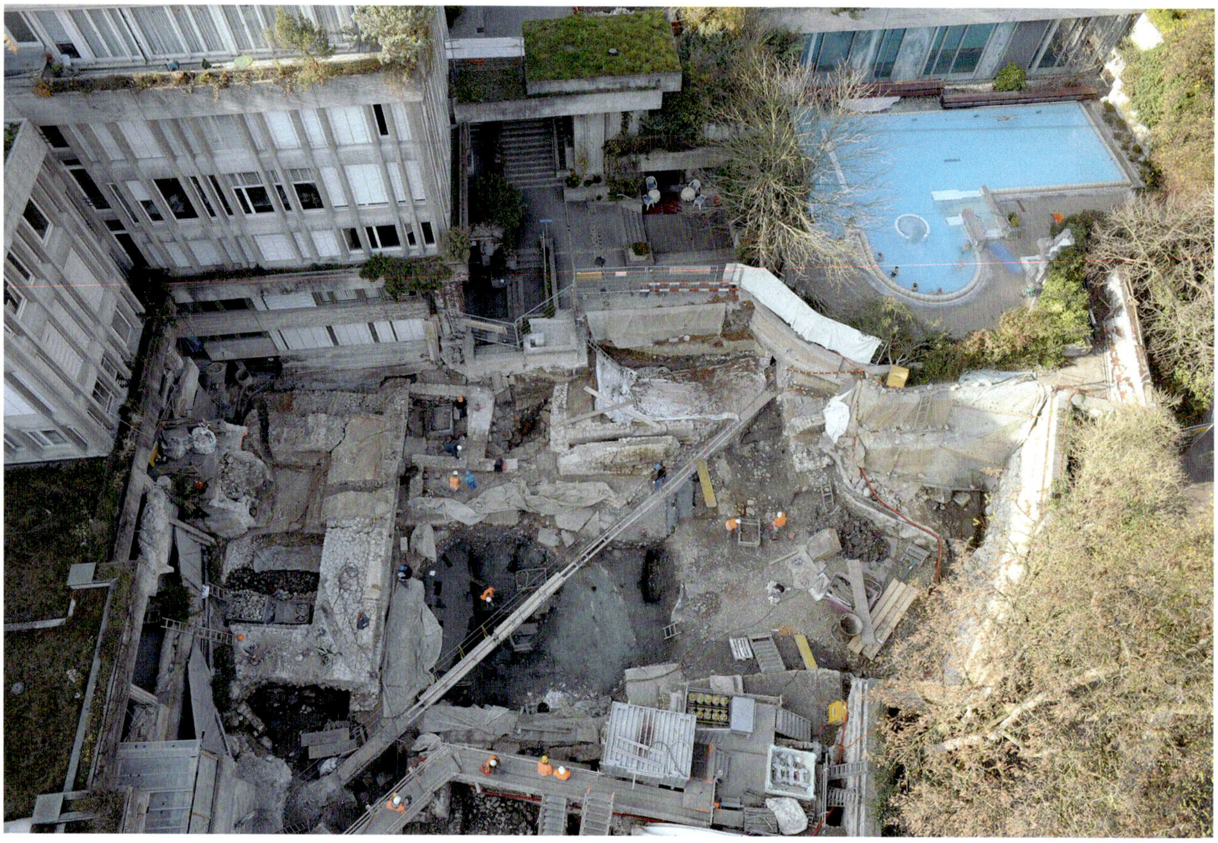

Figure 3. 2000 years of bathing history in Baden. Excavation of the Roman thermae, while the old brutalist public thermal bath is still use in 2011. © Photograph Archaeological Service Aargau/Samuel Mühleisen.

baths were also affected by the destruction has not yet been conclusively determined. This event is not only remarkable as it is the first written mention of Baden e.g. *Aquae* as a spa town. Rather, it also seems to show that the destruction of the obviously quite popular spa town resort was regarded as particularly reprehensible. The destruction of *Aquae* was not accidental. The popular bathing resort was deliberately burnt down, perhaps in order to punish the Helvetian elites who took sides with another emperor than the army did (Schucany 2015: 53–54).

The healing baths in the 2nd century

As in other spa towns, a large-scale redesigning and a monumentalisation of the bathing facilities can be observed in *Aquae Helveticae* around the turn of the first century and in the first decades of the 2nd century AD. Around the middle of the 2nd century, the baths comprised at least five (archaeologically identifiable) large and at least 12 small pools or individual tubs with a total water surface of over 800sqm.[2] Various indications point to the existence of at least three further large basins (Figure 4).

A sacred precinct was located near Baden's main spring, called the (Great and Small) Hot Stone. Here, in 2020, fragments of altars were discovered during excavations. One of them bears an inscription to the divine waters and nymphs (Frei-Stolba *et al.* 2022: 5–9). Further sacred precincts and sanctuaries are to be assumed. Accommodations for the bathers (*hospitalia*) and possibly also a kind of hospital (*valetudinarium*) were located to the west of the baths and sanctuaries (Schaer 2015: 17-21) (Figure 5).

On the location and extent of the Roman settlement

While the bathing area with the corresponding sacred facilities and the thermal baths was built directly at the springs in the fluvial terrace of the Limmat, the residential and commercial settlement was located about 20 metres above on a wide plateau. The riverbank opposite the baths in what is now the village of Ennetbaden was also built over (Wyss and Wälchli 2010; Schaer 2015: 27).

The local topography resulted in a clear spatial separation between the baths area, which had strong

[2] By way of comparison, the water surface of the pools at the new Badener thermae by architect Mario Botta covers approx. 840 square meters.

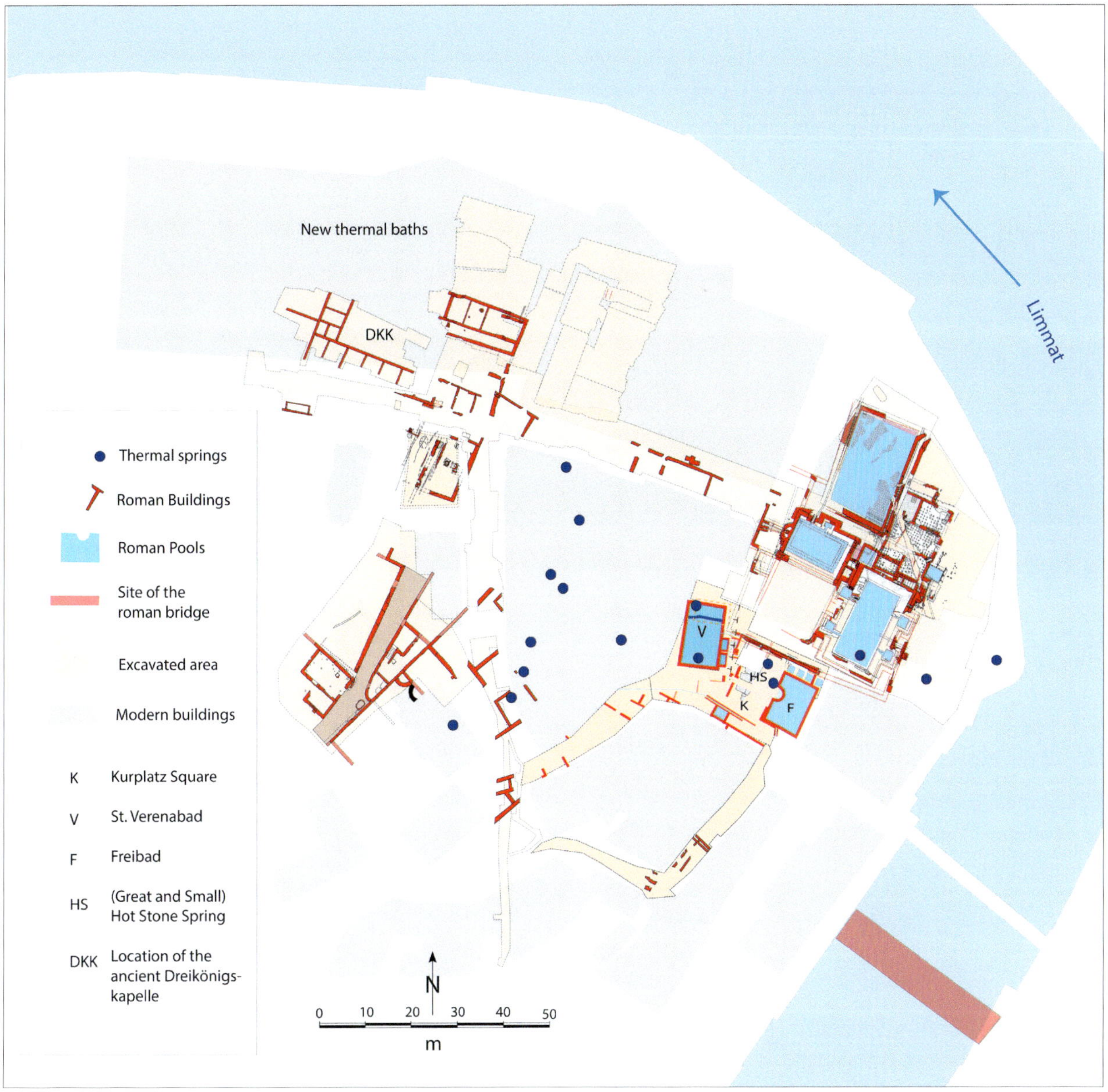

Figure 4. Plan of the roman healing baths in the 2nd century AD. Research status March 2023. © Graphic Archaeological Service Aargau/Rolf Glauser, Markus Fricker; Andrea Schaer.

sacred connotations, and the other part of the settlement which was used mainly for residential and commercial activities.

The settlement extended along two main axes. One ran from the west (*Vindonissa*) to the baths and towards the bridge over the Limmat. The second one ran southwards from the settlement centre towards the southern narrow of the Badener Klus and further on in the direction of *Turicum* (modern-day Zürich). The finds from the settlement as well as finds on the right bank of the Limmat in Ennetbaden indicate that some of the buildings were richly furnished and that wealthy households lived there. Perhaps some of the buildings also served, at least during the bathing season, as accommodation for bathers.

The shape and the perimeter of the settlement can be grasped to some extent through excavations. Graves were found along the arterial roads on both sides of the Limmat (Figure 6). Their location helps us also to reconstruct the approximate extent of the settlement of the later 1st to 3rd century (Figure 7).

As early as the 3rd century, the first buildings in the area of the residential settlement were abandoned. The foundations of a massive fortification wall near the ridge above the baths indicate at least an attempt to fortify

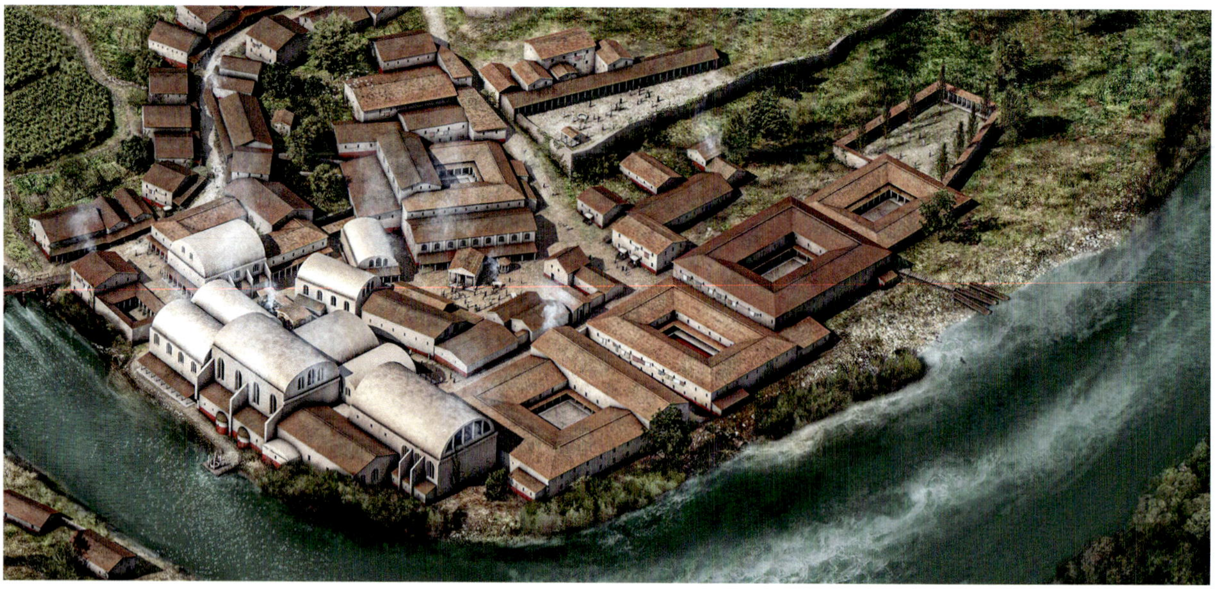

Figure 5. Reconstruction of the healing baths of *Aquae Helveticae* around the middle of the 2nd century. The large bathing pools are located in the buildings with the barrel vaults. State of research 2022. © Historisches Museum Baden/Infostelen Bädergeschichte/Graphic: ikonaut.

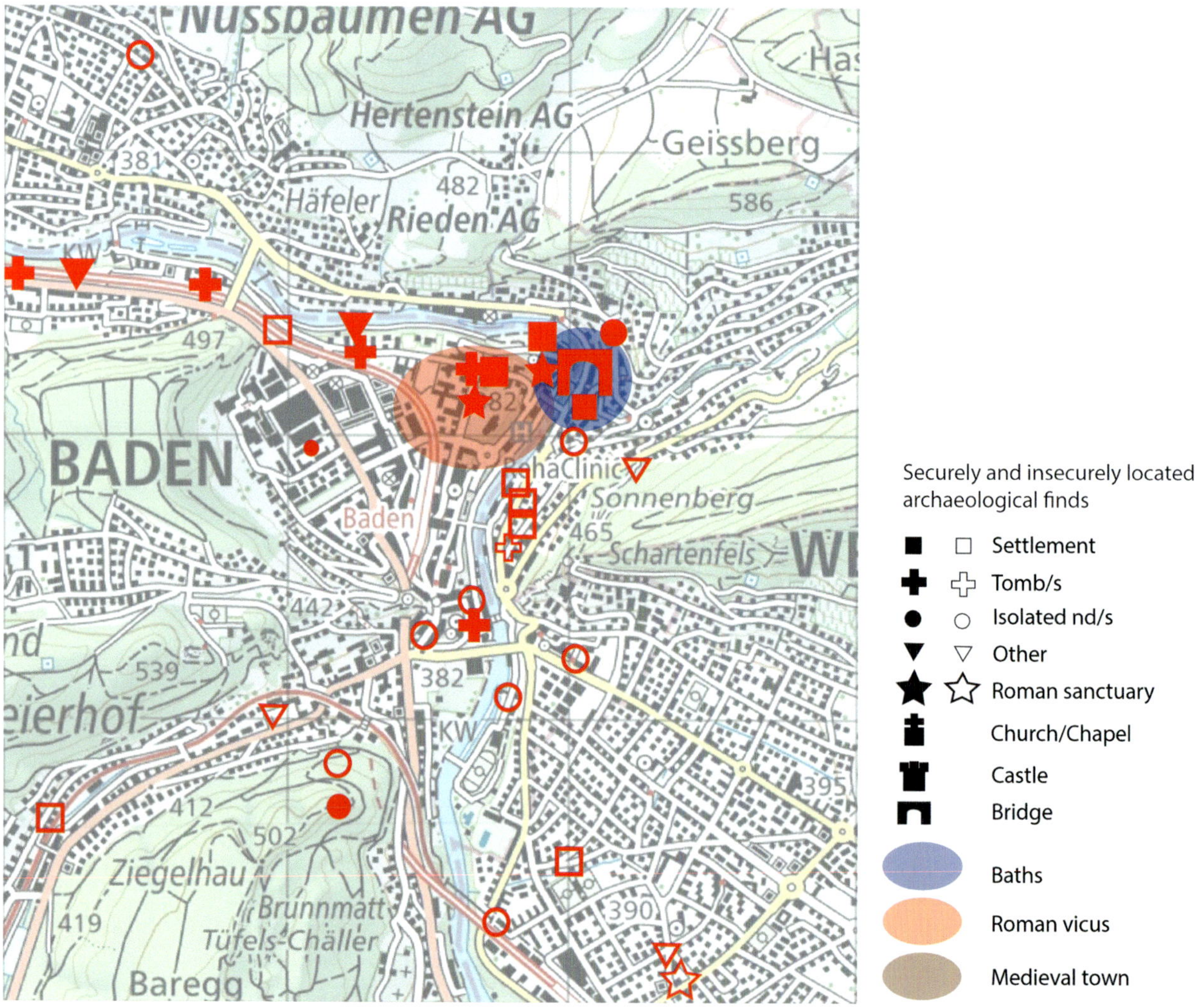

Figure 6. Roman sites in the Badener Klus area. State of research as of March 2023. ©Swisstopo; Graphic Andrea Schaer.

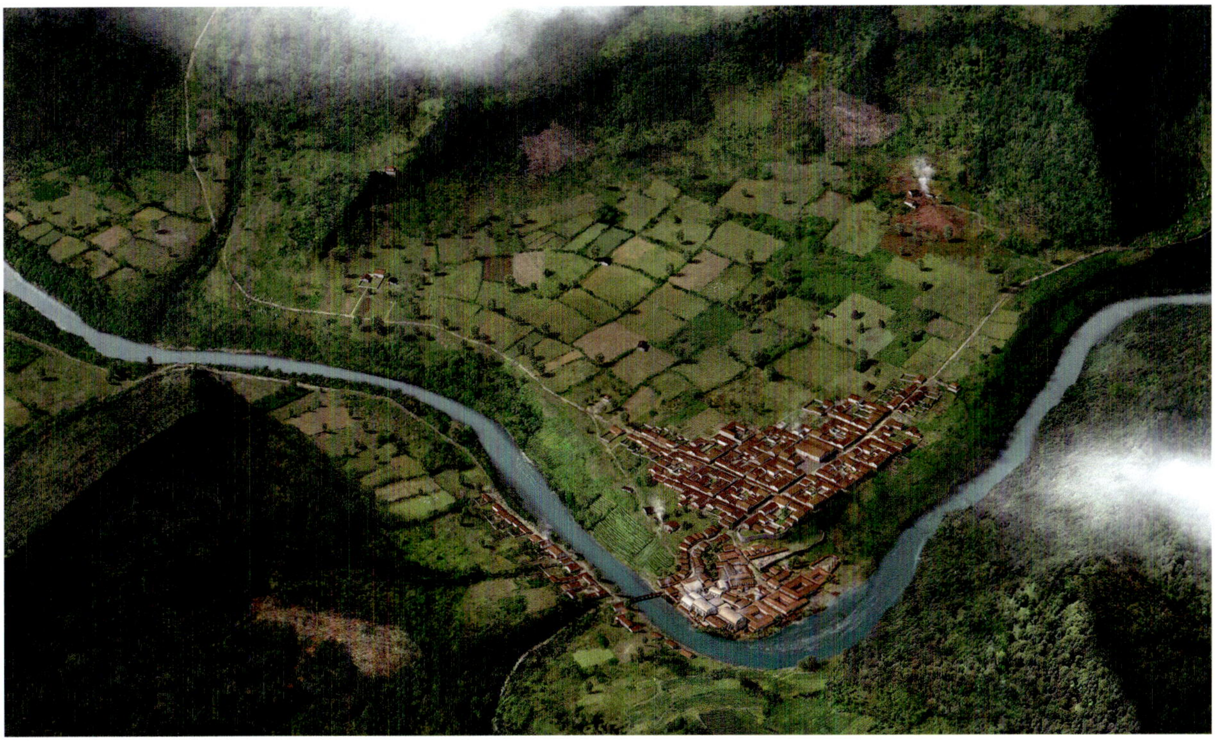

Figure 7. Reconstruction of the Roman settlement and the thermal baths of *Aquae Helveticae*. The image shows how the town may have looked around the middle of the 2nd century. © Historisches Museum Baden/Infostelen Bädergeschichte/Graphic: ikonaut

the baths and a small part of the nearby settlement. The section of wall excavated in 1973, which also contained spolia including a sculpture of Mercury, has remained isolated to this day. Whether the construction was ever completed is still unclear. A late antique fortification of the baths, protecting not only massive buildings but also the location where the Limmat was bridged seems the most plausible possibility. Especially since the baths were probably the most important economic pillar of *Aquae*, their operation therefore had to be secured.

A coin of Valentinian II (dating after 370 AD) as well as the coins from the source of the Great Hot Stone (final coins: Aes of Honorius, 395-402/408 AD) attest that the baths were still being used up until the end of the 4th century AD (Stapfer 2013; Doppler 2007: 113).

The construction work mentioned above and the final coins from the Great Hot Stone, are the last remains of the dense archaeological record of the Baden baths and the settlement of *Aquae Helveticae* before it breaks off.

For the following centuries, there are no viable archaeological or historical sources.

Evidence of activities in the baths in the early middle ages

Graves from the 7th to 9th centuries in the area south of the newly developing settlement as well as in the Small Baths in Ennetbaden, but also two burials in the area of the Large Baths attest to the presence of people in the Baden Klus in the Early Middle Ages (Schaer 2015: 36; Meier 2015: 94) (Figure 8). It cannot be ruled out that the two burials in the Great Baths are possibly connected with the baths themselves. Remarkably, the bones of both burials show traces of illnesses for which a bathing stay at the local sulphur springs would have been a tried and tested means of relief.

A new settlement emerges

In the 8th and 9th centuries, a manor house (*curtis*), with a memorial building, is built about one kilometre south of the spa area at the narrow point at the southern entrance to the Badener Klus. A small settlement begins to develop around this *curtis*. In the late 8th or early 9th century, a Carolingian Hall church of considerable size is built (Sennhauser 2008: 444-448; Meier 2015: 94).

Around 1030, the settlement first appears in written records under the name '*ze badun*' (Old High German for 'at the baths') (Maurer 2008: 413). At that time, the baths were once again the identifying feature of the village and henceforth gave it its emblematic name.

Expansion of the baths in the 11th century

Extensive building work was also carried out in the Great Baths in the 11th or at the beginning of the

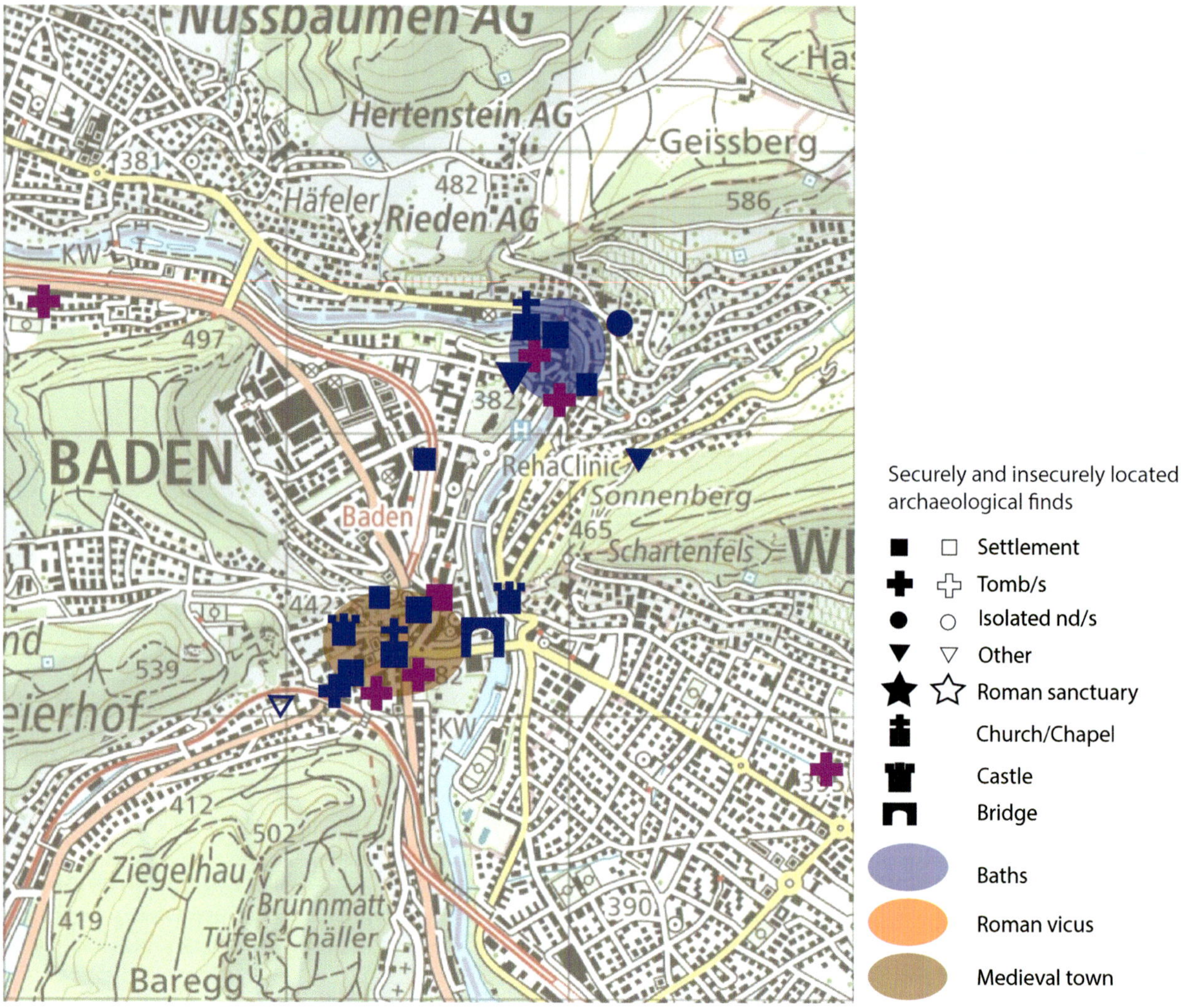

Figure 8. Early medieval and medieval sites in the Badener Klus. ©Swisstopo; Graphic Andrea Schaer.

12th century, indicating an expansion of the bathing facilities and accommodation. Repairs were made to the St. Verenabad, originally a Roman pool that continued to be used up until 1844 (Schaer 2021). In the central area of the baths, various springs were recaptured. Large communal pools were built near the springs, which were probably soon covered with pavilion-like bathhouses (Schaer 2015: 39, 42; Schaer 2018: 200-202). A new stately bathing inn was built on the western edge of the baths, where accommodation had stood in Roman times, and a Romanesque church, the Chapel of the Epiphany (Dreikönigskapelle), was constructed next to it (Sennhauser 2008: 371-373). The new church was almost the same size as the large Carolingian hall church in the settlement (Sennhauser 2008: 457). On the one hand, the unusual dimensions of the Epiphany Chapel seem to indicate that the baths were popular and therefore a church of sufficient size had to be built. However, it may also reflect a special significance of the baths as royal fiscal property and for the chapel as a possible royal foundation (Sennhauser 2008: 457; Maurer 2008: 413-416; Meier 2015: 94).

In any case, the construction work described can only be interpreted as initiated by landlordship and be part of the expansion of an already existing and obviously popular bathing establishment.

The double settlement

From the Early Middle Ages onwards, there were two settlement cores in the Badener Klus: the baths and the new settlement and future town (Figure 9). In between lay the undeveloped area of the former Roman *vicus*.

Why the new settlement core developed at the southern entrance to the Klus and not, like the Roman *vicus*, in the vicinity of the baths, can only be conjectured. Various possible reasons - which may overlap in reality - are to be discussed.

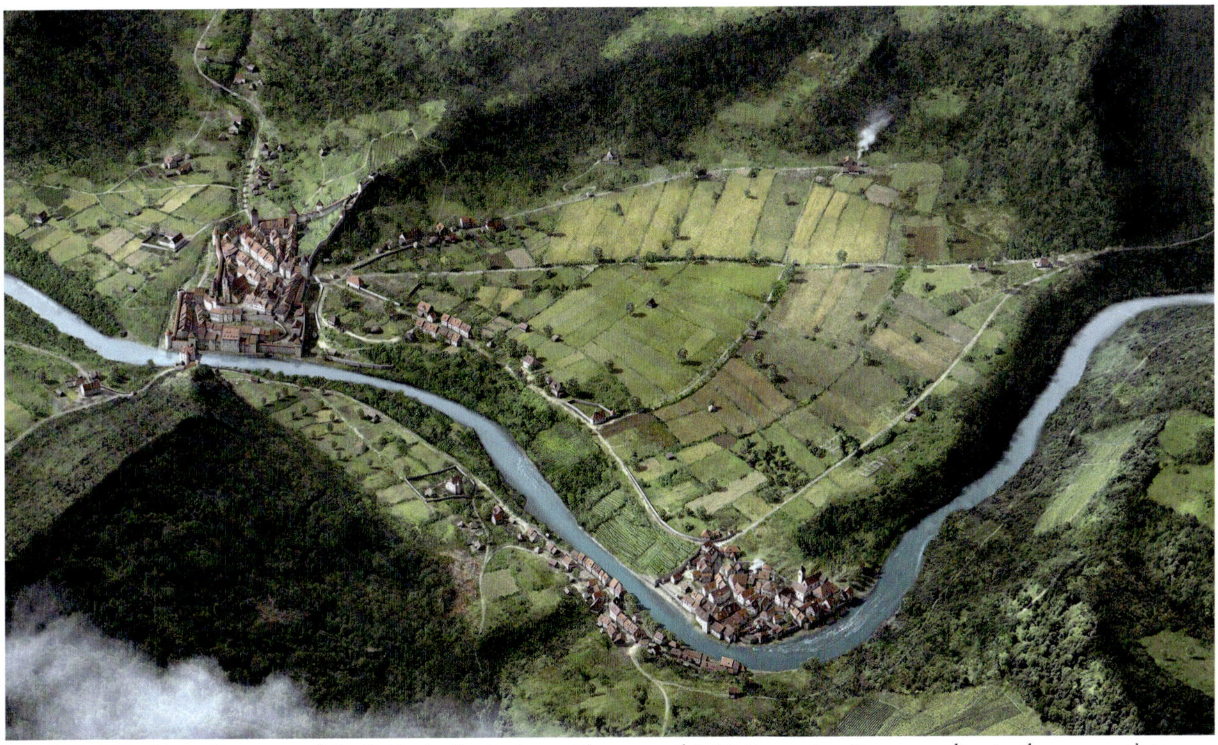

Figure 9. The settlement and the baths in the Badener Klus around 1600. Reconstruction according to the copperplate engraving by Matthäus Merian 1620-1640, incorporating the results of research up to 2015. © Stadtgeschichte Baden/Graphic: ikonaut/Bildebene Joe Rohrer

First of all, the defensively and strategically favourable location of the new settlement at the southern entrance to the Baden Klus should be mentioned. Here, the ridges of the Schlossberg on the left side of the Limmat and the Schartenfels on the right side of the Limmat provide a natural bottleneck that was easy to defend. From the 11th century onwards, the narrows were additionally fortified with the construction of Castle Stein (Frey and Meier 1999). Furthermore, the narrow passage lent itself to the construction of a bridge; such a bridge has been known since the 13th century (Sennhauser 2008: 446; Meier 2015: 96).

The new settlement controlled the access to the Baden Klus and the traffic routes in the Limmat valley and towards the west into the neighbouring Reuss valley. In the politically unstable environment of the early and high Middle Ages with changing spheres of influence and landlordships, this meant a clear advantage over the location of the Roman *vicus* inside the Klus.

It is also conceivable that other factors contributed to the emergence of a second settlement core. For example, existing claims under land law could have played a role in the choice of the new settlement site. However, there are no records of this.

In antiquity, raw materials, which included thermal water, were imperial (fiscal) property (Guérin-Beauvois 2015: 312–318). The early medieval rulers, who saw themselves as the legal successors of the Roman emperors, took over these regalia and fiscal rights. It can therefore be assumed that the thermal springs in Baden, and with them existing bathing facilities and accommodation at the springs, were royal fiscal property in the early Middle Ages and further on until the 13th and 14th centuries. The springs and baths were then administered by the local governors: from the 9th century the Counts of Nellenburg who remarkably also had possessions far from their homelands at Baden-Baden (Germany) (Steiner 2008: 409–411). Later, these rights were passed on to the Counts of Lenzburg and Kyburg, and finally from 1258 to the Dukes of Habsburg (the future kings and later emperors) (Maurer 2008: 416f; Steiner 2008: 408-411; Meier 2015: 94-96). The bathing inns and guesthouses as well as the thermal springs stayed royal i.e. manorial property until the 14th century and were given in fief to the innkeepers (Schaer 2015: 42). As royal fiscal property, the baths possibly had a different legal status than the new settlement. Whether this special status could have contributed to the emergence of two - at least in a spatial sense distinctly separated - settlement areas must remain a hypothesis.

The shifting of the settlement nucleus in the Baden Klus and the emergence of a double settlement - baths and town - in the Middle Ages is an essential characteristic of the spa town of Baden.

While the location of the residential settlement is determined by external factors such as the political and strategic situation and economic considerations, the baths are naturally linked to the thermal springs. Thus, the baths and the residential settlement are subject to different development dynamics.

Translation: Author and Dr Andrew Lawrence, Institute of Archaeological Sciences, University of Berne

Bibliography

Burger, H. 2011. Die Thermalwässer und Mineralwässer im Kanton Aargau und seiner näheren Umgebung. *Mitteilungen der aargauischen naturforschenden Gesellschaft* 37: 91-112.

Doppler, H. W. 2007. Die Münzfunde aus der Quelle «grosser heisser Stein» in Baden AG. *Schweizerische Numismatische Rundschau* 86: 91–116.

Frei-Stolba, R., B. Hartmann, M. Flück, D. Wälchli and J. Baerlocher 2022. Aargauer Neuentdeckungen: Badener Nymphen, Würenlinger Töpfereien und ein Amphitheater. *Archäologie Schweiz as.* 45.2012.3: 4-15.

Frey, P. and B. Meier 1999. Neue Erkenntnisse zur Baugeschichte der Niederen Feste. *Badener Neujahrsblätter* 74: 152–159.

Guérin-Beauvois, M. 2015. *Le Thermalisme Romain en Italie. Aspects sociaux et culturels aux deux premiers siècles de l'Empire.* Rome: École Française de Rome.

Maurer, H. 2008. Vergleichende und Ergänzende Beobachtungen zum hochmittelalterlichen Baden, in H.R. Sennhauser (ed) *Ausgrabungen in Stadtkirche und Dreikönigskapelle Baden 1967/1968. Kirchen und Siedlungsgeschichte von der Frühzeit bis ins späte Mittelalter:* 413–422. Zurich: vdf.

Meier, B. 2015. Baden in der Eidgenossenschaft: Auf den Bühnen der Politik, in F. Furter, B. Meier, A. Schaer and R. Wiederkehr *Stadtgeschichte Baden*: 148–186. Baden: Hier und Jetzt.

Schaer, A. 2010a. Das Dornröschen. Eine archäologische Bestandesaufnahme im Badener Bäderquartier, in Ch. Ebnöther and R. Schatzmann (eds) *Oleum non perdidit. Festschrift für Stefanie Martin-Kilcher zu ihrem 65. Geburtstag* (Antiqua 47): 45–57. Basel: Archäologie Schweiz.

Schaer, A. 2010b (mit einem Beitrag von M. Botta). Mit der Vergangenheit in die Zukunft. 2000 Jahre Bäderkultur in Baden. *Archäologie schweiz as.* 33.2010.1: 24–31.

Schaer, A. 2015. Die Bäder: 2000 Jahre europäische Badekultur, in F. Furter, B. Meier, A. Schaer and R. Wiederkehr *Stadtgeschichte Baden*: 8–91. Baden: Hier und Jetzt.

Schaer, A. 2018. Baden AG – vom Wildbad zum Kurort, in Archäologie Schweiz, Arbeitsgemeinschaft für die Archäologie des Mittelalters und der Neuzeit und Schweizersicher Burgenverein (eds) *Die Schweiz von 1350 bis 1850 im Spiegel archäologischer Quellen. Akten des Kolloquiums Bern 25.-26. Januar 2018*: 197–206. Basel: Archäologie Schweiz.

Schaer, A. 2021. Baden AG, Kurplatz (B.020.2). *Jahrbuch Archäologie Schweiz* 104: 172–173.

Schaer, A. 2022. *Willkommen im Garten Eden. Die Bäder von Baden.* Zürich: Hier und Jetzt.

Schaer, A. 2024. *Ubi aqua – ibi bene. Die Bäder von Baden im Aargau im Licht der archäologischen Untersuchungen 2009-2022. Vol 1 Grundlagen, Forschungs- und Überlieferungsgeschichte von den Anfängen bis 2022* (Veröffentlichungen der Gesellschaft Pro Vindonissa XXXIX/I). Brugg: Gesellschaft Pro Vindonissa.

Schaer, A., R. Stapfer and J. Baerlocher, in process. *Ubi aqua – ibi bene. Die Bäder von Baden im Aargau im Licht der archäologischen Untersuchungen 2009-2022. Vol 2: Auswertung der Grabungen 2009-2012 und 2018 und Chronologie von der Römerzeit bis ins 20. Jahrhundert* (Veröffentlichungen der Gesellschaft Pro Vindonissa XXXIX/II). Brugg: Gesellschaft Pro Vindonissa.

Schucany, C. 1998. Die Brandschichten von Baden/ Aquae Helveticae. Bemerkungen zur Datierung. *Jahrbuch der Schweizerischen Gesellschaft für Ur- und Frühgeschichte* 81: 250–254.

Schucany, C. 2015. Die Helvetier und das Jahr 69 n. Chr. *Jahresbericht der Gesellschaft Pro Vindonissa*: 53–58.

Sennhauser, H. R. (ed) 2008. *Ausgrabungen in Stadtkirche und Dreikönigskapelle Baden 1967/1968. Kirchen und Siedlungsgeschichte von der Frühzeit bis ins späte Mittelalter.* Zurich: vdf.

Stapfer, R. 2013. Baden AG, Bäderquartier, «Limmatknie» (B.010.1). *Jahrbuch Archäologie Schweiz* 96: 192–193.

Steiner, H. 2008. Auf der Suche nach den frühmittelalterlichen Erbauern der Kirche von Baden in H. R. Sennhauser (ed) *Ausgrabungen in Stadtkirche und Dreikönigskapelle Baden 1967/1968. Kirchen und Siedlungsgeschichte von der Frühzeit bis ins späte Mittelalter*: 403–412. Zurich: vdf)

Tacitus, Publius Cornelius. *Historiae.* Transcription used by H. Vretska (ed) 2009. P. Cornelius Tacitus, *Historien.* Latin/German. Stuttgart: Reclam.

Wyss, S. and D. Wälchli 2010. Neues aus Aquae Helveticae. Das rechte Limmatufer. *Badener Neujahrsblätter 85*: 138–151.

Repositioning a Spa in Space and Time: The Bagneres-de-Bigorre Spa (Hautes-Pyrénées, France)

Laurent COSTA

Research Engineer at the French National Centre for Scientific Research (CNRS) – PhD, The Huma-num Paris Time Machine (PTM) Consortium MSH Mondes, 21, allée de l'Université, 92023 Nanterre Cedex.
laurent.costa@cnrs.fr

Richard SABATIER

Government-accredited Architect (DPLG), Chairman of the Observatory for Archaeology and Heritage in Haute-Bigorre (OAPHB), 6, rue Gambetta, 65200 Bagnères-de-Bigorre.
oaphb65.gmail.com

Abstract: From 2016 to 2020, the archaeological survey of an ancient underground collecting tank in the spa district of Bagnères-de-Bigorre in the Hautes-Pyrénées (France) updated the narrative surrounding the extraordinary history of this site, thanks to the input of new technologies and participatory science.

Directly established on the spring that supplies its thermal mineral waters, Bagnères-de-Bigorre developed its spa activities long before the advent of the spa industry during the Second Empire (1850). An ancient bathing area discovered in 1823 bears witness to this development, as do the municipal archives. From the 1660s-1670s onwards, local civil society began to develop the town's balneotherapy industry, establishing close links with the private residences of the Bourbon monarchy and the great Academies.

The research we are carrying out shows that this balneotherapy industry is also closely linked to the irrigated pastoral production systems that structure the local mountain environment. From the mountain pastures to the spa town and beyond, via the terroirs, the barns, the villages and the fields, a veritable 'water supply edifice' irrigates the crops and serves the homes of local residents and associated structures.

In Bagnères-de-Bigorre, in the early 2000s, the abandonment of the old gravity-fed catchments in favour of the extraction of thermal waters through the use of deep boreholes completed a cycle of some fifty years during which the distribution of water had been radically redesigned and rebuilt for reasons of efficiency and hygiene. Through this process, the waters once present were literally erased from the urban landscape, although they have been maintained higher up in the mountains.

Together, the Observatory for Archaeology and Heritage in Haute-Bigorre (OAPHB) in partnership with UMR *Archeologies & Sciences de l'Antiquite* (ArScAn) and the French Club Alpin of Bagnères-de-Bigorre, are running participatory GIS workshops. Via cross-generational knowledge sharing, vector map representations of the water systems giving structure to the landscapes of the local valleys have been developed, while the skills needed to manage them by gravity have brought together a number of local associations. Going back to the sources, again and together, thus offers possibilities.

Keywords: *spas, thermal cures and balneotherapy, water systems, geohistorical GIS, collaborative sciences.*

Introduction

Like many European spa towns, the Roman origins of Bagnères-de-Bigorre were alleged at a very early point in the historical record. From the turn of the 17th century, publicity given to the discovery of scattered objects, including two votive altars, attested to a Roman presence in the area. With these few material facts fuelling the imagination, antiquarians have extrapolated a history for this spa town dating back to Roman antiquity (Jazé-Charvolin 2016; Carribon 1999). A short while later, during the construction of the municipal thermal baths in the 1820s, the partial uncovering of an ancient bathing area provided spectacular evidence that the hot springs had indeed been used since Antiquity. In the 2000s, with the epigraphy of a votive altar having proved authentic, the town's major new spa complex was named *Aquensis*, thus reiterating this extrapolation of historical context.

From 2016 to 2020, the archaeological survey of an ancient collecting tank in Bagnères-de-Bigorre[1] gave new impetus to this issue by raising the question of how these springs and this system were integrated into the urban fabric over the long term. The study of this hot water collecting tank, and then the extension of this approach to include the cold surface water irrigation systems, channels and ditches, has driven our team to consider the Grands Thermes area of Bagnères-de-Bigorre as one single integrated unit with its vast forest and pastoral thermal park opening out onto mid-mountain ranges. The aim was to shift the perspective and observe all the gravity-fed water supply systems

[1] Works described in *Cahiers Archéologie en Haute-Bigorre* [Notebooks on Archaeology in the Haute-Bigorre region]: Notebook 1 (2015-2016): An ancient canal in Bagnères-de-Bigorre; Notebook 2 (2017-2018) Water systems and balneotherapy; Notebook 3 (2019-2021). Sharing our natural waters. Media library of the Community of Municipalities of Haute-Bigorre.

taking in and releasing natural waters *in situ*, in order to create a new research subject that would enable us to assess the resilience of these systems over the long term. Because of the water supply complex that gives it its structure, Bagnères-de-Bigorre – a spa and then a spa town – forms part of the layering of irrigated landscapes in the Haut-Adour Valley, which is in itself a vast water supply edifice made up of water catchments, streams, channels, ditches, basins, fountains, baths, etc., but also of people who have developed practices and know-how, and of the biotopes and biocenoses associated with them. These run-off waters make the Haut-Adour a place with a history and longevity that is due as much to its natural aspects as to the social elements they create, by catalysing cooperative projects ranging from transition to tourism to pastoral micro-farms (Letang and Knauf 2022; Bouneau 2005).

Such a return to our roots raises a number of questions of substance and form that this article sets out to address. Whether it be in the spa town, proposing to free thermal mineral springs from the now useless straitjacket of their catchments, or in pastoral units that inhabitants are seeking to re-establish with the support of farmers, the aim here is to apply an approach based on research and action[2] and to establish a knowledge development project based on a contributory and participative dynamic. Here, archaeology, as an integral part of a digital humanities approach, is no longer simply a means of gathering information before destroying landscapes, but becomes rather a means of achieving synergy for the redeployment of possible transformations, possible points of ecological resilience, possible economic development and, above all, a shared knowledge of the terrain (Lamothe 2021).

Hydrogeological context of thermal mineral waters

Bagnères-de-Bigorre is a spa town that has its origins in a very limited hydrogeological complex in which rainwater collected at the summit of a small mountain massif adjoining the town (Mont Bédat) emerges hot at the base of its slopes and through the alluvial soil on which urban settlements have developed. At a distance of fifteen hundred metres, a second resurgence point is located away from the centre, deep in the park in the Salut Valley. (Figure 1)

This circulation of water takes place through a system of syncline folds made up of Jurassic and Cretaceous limestone. After conveying the captured rainfall very deep into the earth, this system returns those waters at a temperature of between 50°C and 30°C, loaded with calcium sulfate principles that they have collected by dissolving Triassic gypsum and anhydrite (Nartet and Soule 1986) during their underground journey. This hydrogeological system corresponds to the spa town's rural setting. The slopes of the Monné, Tucou and Bédat peaks combine to form a small basin that feeds the Aygo Tebio ('*warm water*') stream, which rises deep in a nearby valley.[3] At the mouth of this valley, its thalweg widens and joins the Adour after running parallel to the river for 8 kilometres. Resulting from a vauclusian-type spring, the stream sometimes swells after heavy rainfall to the point where it begins a second resurgence. The town centre and its spa district were flooded to a height of 1.50m during the 100-year flood. A recent flood in July 2023 is a perfect illustration of this type of event.[4] The hot springs bubble up from the diaclastic rocks of the foothills and through the alluvial deposits on which the town centre and its spa district have developed. Although the epicentre of the hot springs (50°C) and the baths have been closely linked since at least Antiquity[5], it was not until the early medieval Renaissance that the town was established and developed directly around its thermal mineral resources and the infrastructure it inherited. (Figure 2)

Historical and societal context of a spa town

From the diaclases overlooking the town or through the alluvial deposits on which it is built, the technical methods used to capture the hot waters have shaped the long history of this spa and then spa town, which has been developing since ancient times, well before the advent of the spa industry. To collect water through the limestone, horizontal tunnels had to be dug to reach the main source of a spring and bring the water by gravity to a bath or fountain. These water catchments, located in the Reine district above and behind the main thermal bath complex (Grands Thermes), were mainly used by religious and consular institutions. Drawing water from beneath the town and its surroundings through the gravel and peat of the alluvial soil was easier and less costly than digging a tunnel in the rock. These catchments are in the form of either lower-pressure columns or emergence pools. Like a well, the water compressed by the subsoil finds a means of expansion and rises to the surface to feed pools or underground basins.

It is interesting to note that it is at the junction of these two types of catchment – at the point where the water is warmest – that the site of the ancient spa is located,

[2] https://hal.science/hal-01490609

[3] The Aygo Tebio is fed by a small watershed measuring 3.29km2 located upstream of Bagnères-de-Bigorre town centre. Cf. Report presenting the Risk Prevention Plan (RPP), Hautes-Pyrénées Prefecture, March 2010.

[4] https://www.ladepeche.fr/2023/06/04/hautes-pyrenees-les-orages-provoquent-des-inondations-a-aste-et-bagneres-de-bigorre-11240910.php

[5] As demonstrated by the partial discovery of a bathing area in 1823 during the construction of the Grands Thermes thermal bath complex.

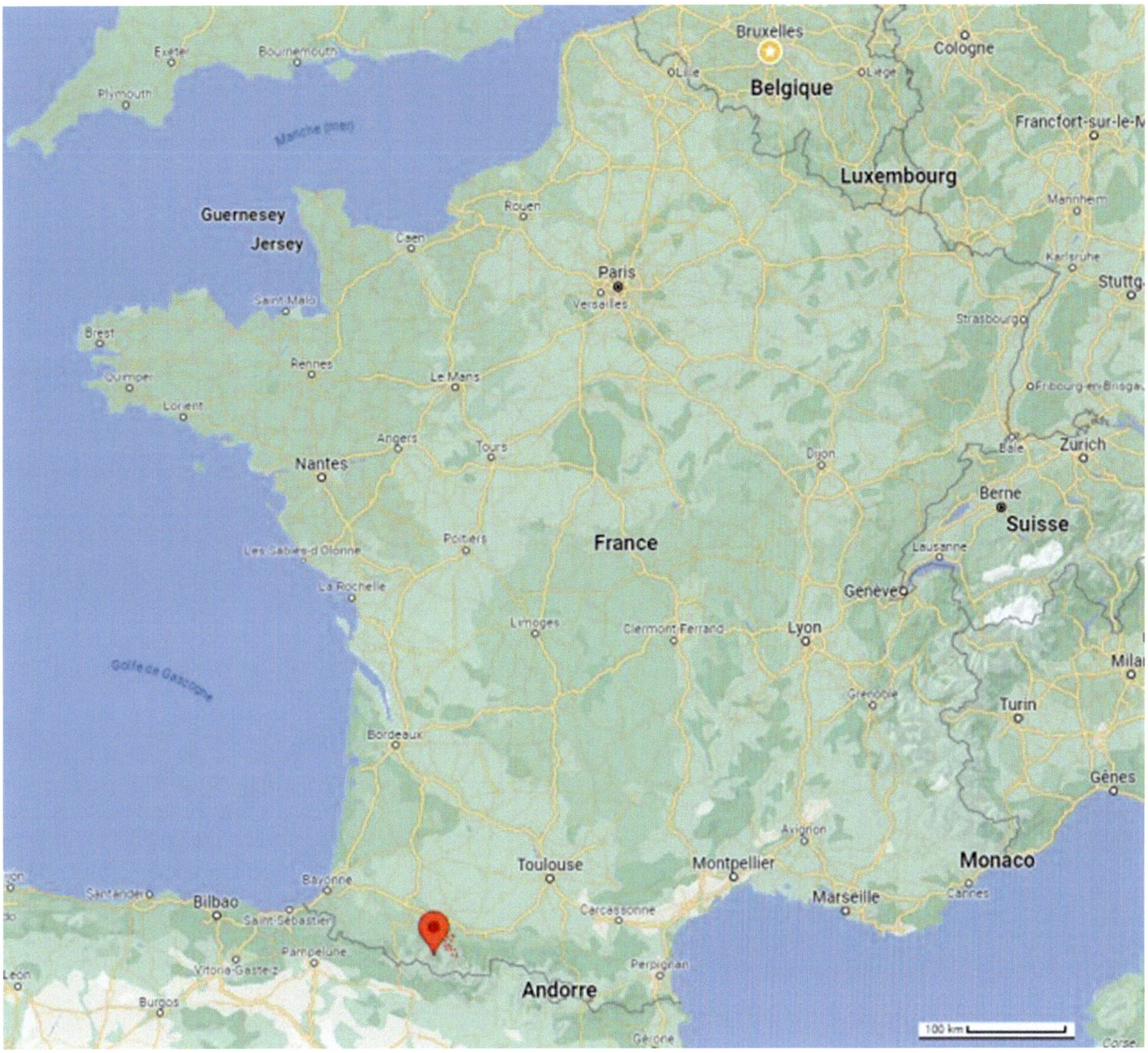

Figure 1. Location of Bagnères-de-Bigorre (France). Google maps. © Google map

as is the Grands Thermes municipal complex today (Figure 3).

A bird's-eye view from 1668[6] shows the baths in the form of rectangular pools in the open air inside and outside the town. The municipal archives have preserved medieval edicts that sought to regulate the use and customs of these pools, which catered for everyone, including domestic animals. As far as we know, from the 16th century onwards, vaulted baths equipped with one or two bathtubs supplemented and then replaced these open-air pools in order to satisfy a desire for modesty and comfort for an urban clientele who came to experience the waters. (Figure 4)

The relative simplicity of catchment through alluvial deposits led to an increase in the number of private establishments. By the end of the 18th century, there were more than thirty. Most were owned by doctors who sought to set themselves apart from the competition by advertising their waters as suitable for curing a particular pathology. One prominent man, whose family has produced several mayors, bought a former public bathhouse and renovated it to increase its capacity. This would become the Bains de Salut. In this same pre-revolutionary period, the consuls asked the engineer from the Public Highways Office of the Pays d'État de Bigorre to design a new bath as a gift for the first-born son of King Louis XVI.[7]

[6] 'Sent to Mr Coignet to present to Monseigneur Colbert, Minister of State', 1668, Vincennes Archives.

[7] The Bain des Pauvres was replaced by the Bain du Dauphin, now known as the Bain du Roi de Rome. This small establishment with two swimming pools was designed by Louis Moisset, an engineer with the Public Highways Office. It was inaugurated in 1781.

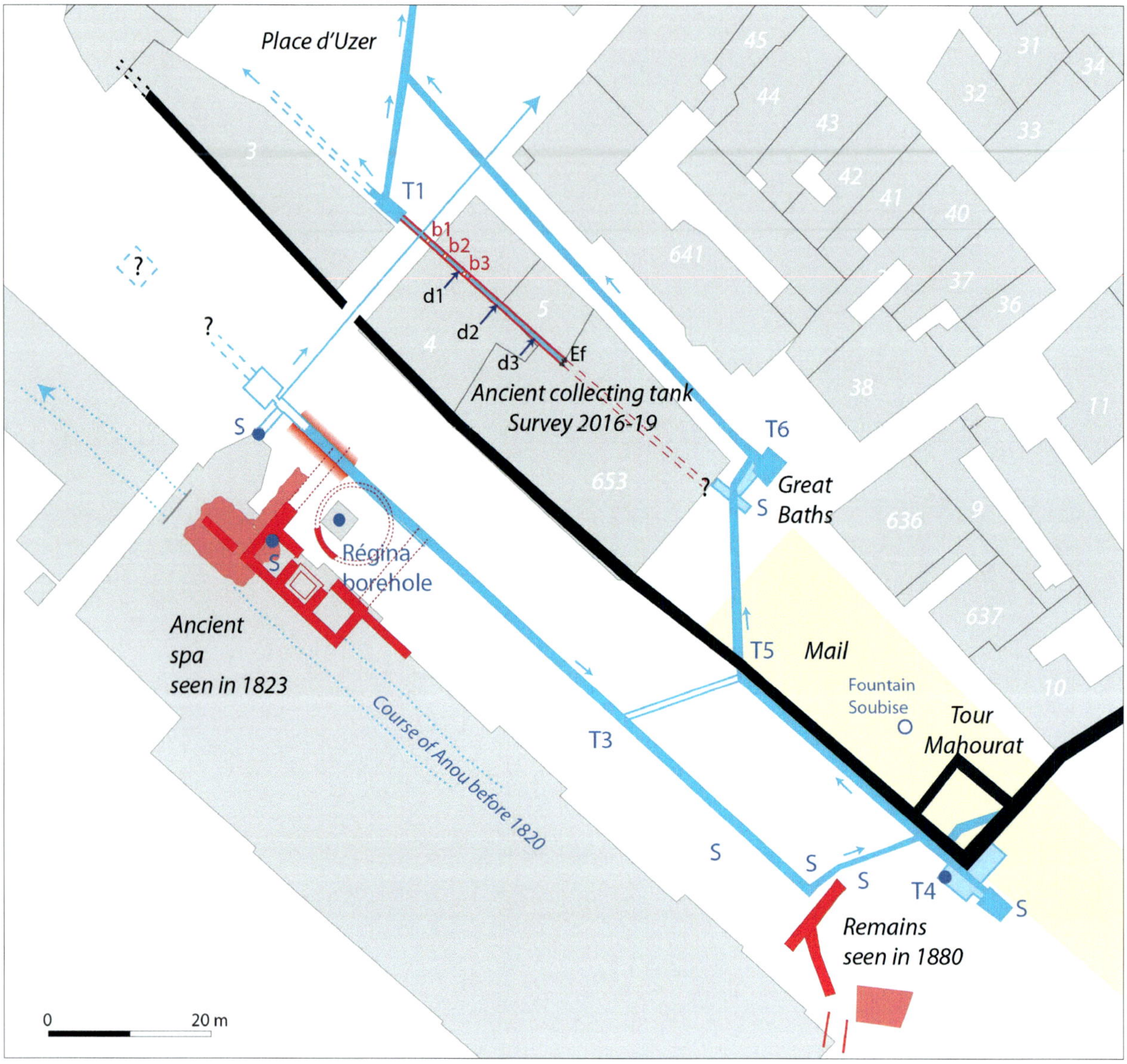

Figure 2. Plan of the ancient baths based on a repositioning of the Milestone outline. © OAPHB 2020

At the dawn of the French Revolution, Bagnères-de-Bigorre was a highly socially structured spa town, attracting a select clientele (Roux 2008-2009). The arrival of Madame de Maintenon and the recovery of the Duc du Maine, whom she accompanied, are described as the inaugural moment in this boom, which would be sustained by the links that figures in local society forged with renowned spa visitors and by the decision to place some of the town's children in service in the private residences of the King and Queen.[8] From the end of the 17th century, people from the area held positions such as private secretary to the King, chambermaid or bodyguard to the Queen. In return, they sent doctors, botanists, geographers, and fountain builders ... and these monarchical influences survived the Revolution. The current Grands Thermes bath complex in Bagnères-de-Bigorre was inaugurated in 1828 by the Duchess of Berry (1798-1870), daughter-in-law of King Charles X.

Designed using a range of industrial arts and applied sciences, this large establishment, bringing together some forty public springs, would eventually mean the disappearance of the private baths that were once the feature of the spa district, and beyond. From this point on, the municipality controlled the hot springs, while the local community continued to welcome and entertain visitors seeking thermal cures in the spa.[9] The

[8] The Cuilhé and Bertholet-Campan families, including Mrs Campan, Dumoret, Dufourc d'Antist, etc.

[9] However, no grand hotel was ever built, despite a last, belated attempt in the period between the World Wars. Hotel capacity continued to be boosted by civil society, which was expanding and renovating its stock, while customers with more modest means found accommodation through rental companies and in a number of religious institutions.

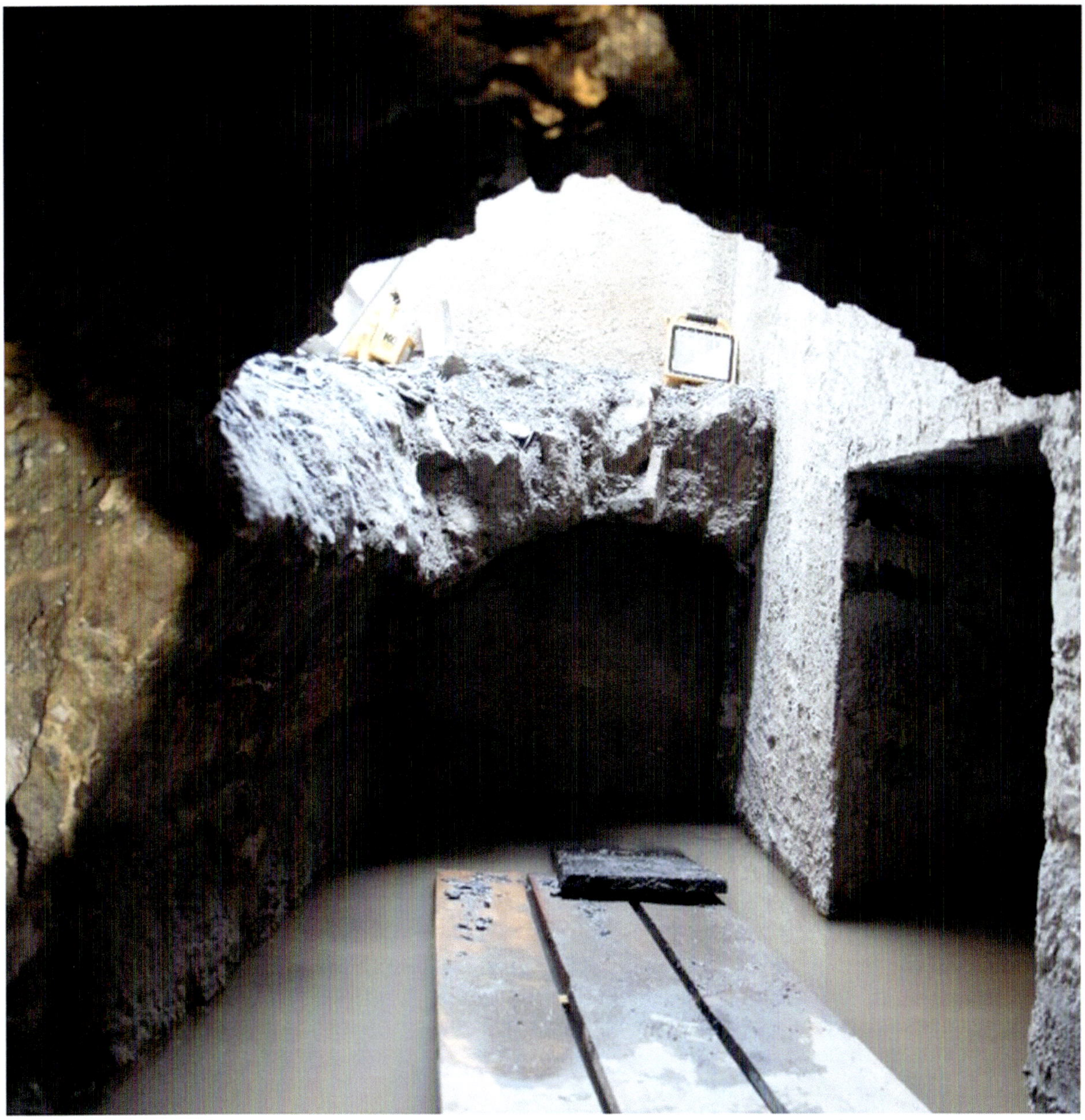

Figure 3. Photo of the ancient collecting tank. © R. Sabatier 2016

first gaming hall was opened in the early years of the 18th century. Arrangements were then made for the development of promenades. Around 1780, the upper reaches of the stream leading to the new Bains de Salut were transformed into a Rousseauist promenade under the name Vallon de Salut, while lines of trees were planted to provide shade for the paths and tracks leading up to the mountain pastures. The development of promenades continued in the 19th century. Guides to the region's health resorts at the time praised the scenery and the rest areas set up near springs and in farms where people drank milk in the cool shade of centuries-old chestnut trees. A ferruginous spring (mineral spring waters containing salts of iron) transformed into a neoclassical bar dedicated to the Duke of Angoulême was also inaugurated in 1828 by his wife. Linked to an avenue on the plain, the development of which combined a new district administrative office, a convent, a grand hotel and villas with surrounding grounds, a new promenade was laid out on Mont Bédat to provide a route to the spa district. These developments are the expression of a romantic approach to natural phenomena, in which the worship of natural springs is a response to a Christian conception of nature and its wonders, although it does not exclude an interest in vernacular

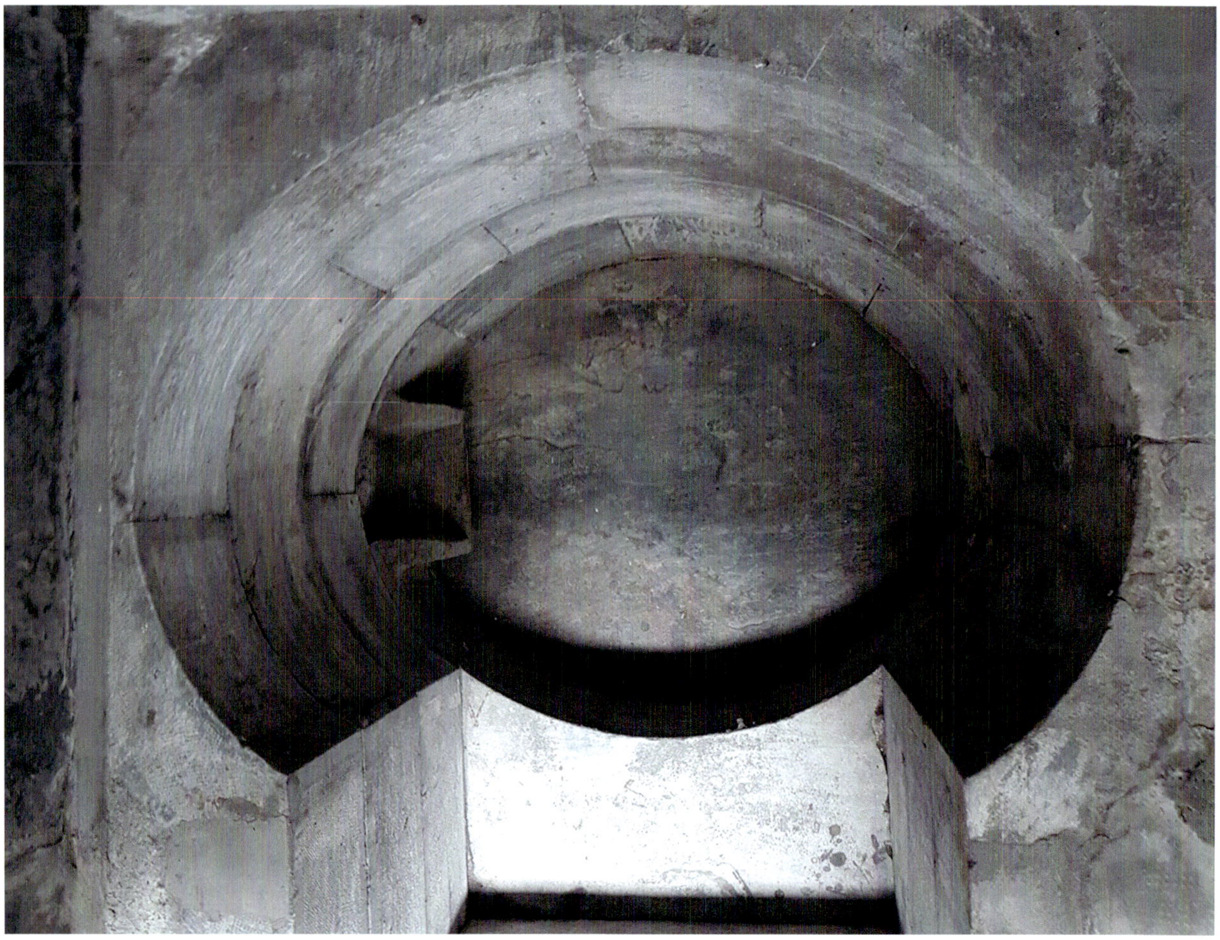

Figure 4. View of one of the ponds to receive service water from small canals in a house. R. Sabatier 2017

practices,[10] which will continue to be threatened by modern changes.[11] (Figures 5a y 5b).

This *cultural and medical* balneotherapy (Scheid *et al.* 2015) would become an industry under the Second Empire.[12] As in Spa in Belgium, these promenades to the springs are the legacy of a time when people did not know exactly what to do with their waters: should you bathe in them, shower in them, drink from them or even inhale their vapours? By this time, the academies of the Age of Enlightenment had undertaken a classification of their curative principles: soda waters, sulphur waters, sulphate waters, etc. But while technical devices were increasingly conditioning the way in which bodies came into contact with the waters, the use of springs was not abandoned. In Bagnères-de-Bigorre, as numerous views and photographs show[13], moorland and summer pastures dominated the small mountains that support the hydrogeological setting of the spa. The Second Empire's Law on the Restoration of Mountain Land[14] (RTM) was the means by which the small massif was

[10] John Scheid, Archaeologist, Teacher at the Institut de France, *Religion, institutions and society in Ancient Rome*. 12 lessons given at the Collège de France (201?-2016).

[11] Bagnères-de-Bigorre, with its poet Philadelphe de Gerde (Claude Duclos, 1871-1952), would be one of the anchor points of the Félibrige movement (focussed on protecting and promoting Occitan language and culture).

[12] It was in this pioneering spa that an industrial concept of balneotherapy was born and developed during the Second Empire. In the 1860s, the town fulfilled the requirements of the new laws regulating spa resorts. The railway station was inaugurated in 1865, and the Grand Casino – equipped with a 'neo-thermal' swimming pool – in 1885 by Monaco's Société des Bains de Mer (SBM), while the Grands Thermes thermal bath complex dating from 1828 was already being updated by hydraulic engineer François de Neufchâteau.

[13] In particular, the watercolour view by Louis-Denis Leleu, Land Registry Officer, preserved in the Hautes-Pyrénées Départemental Archives.

[14] *Restaurer la montagne.* Exhibition catalog, Comissioner Benoît Coutancier, Museon Arlaten, Musée départemental d'ethnographie d'Arles, France. 2004. In France, the 'restoration of mountain land' (RTM) was an operation to stabilise and restore soil on mountain slopes. Because of the specific context and risks involved, it calls on specialised civil engineering, plant engineering and ecological engineering techniques adapted to different environments (steep slopes, cold, temperate, hot or tropical climates). The department of the same name responsible for carrying out these operations was created in the 19th century within the Water and Forestry Service, and still exists at the beginning of the 21st century within the National Forestry Service.

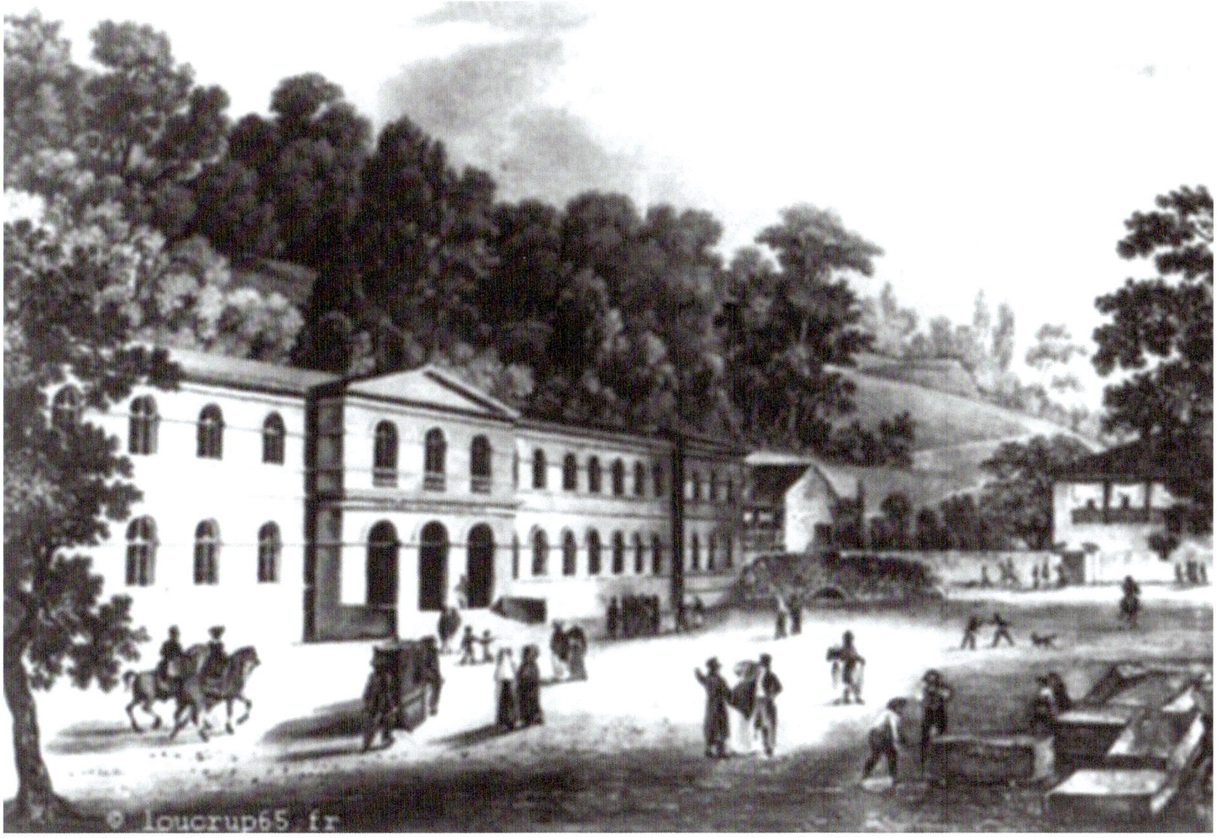

Figure 5a. View of the spa district of Bagnères in the 19th century and today. Here, the main thermal bath complex in 1828, when it was inaugurated. François DANDIRAN, milieu XIXe siècle © Médiathèque Bagnères-de-Bigorre

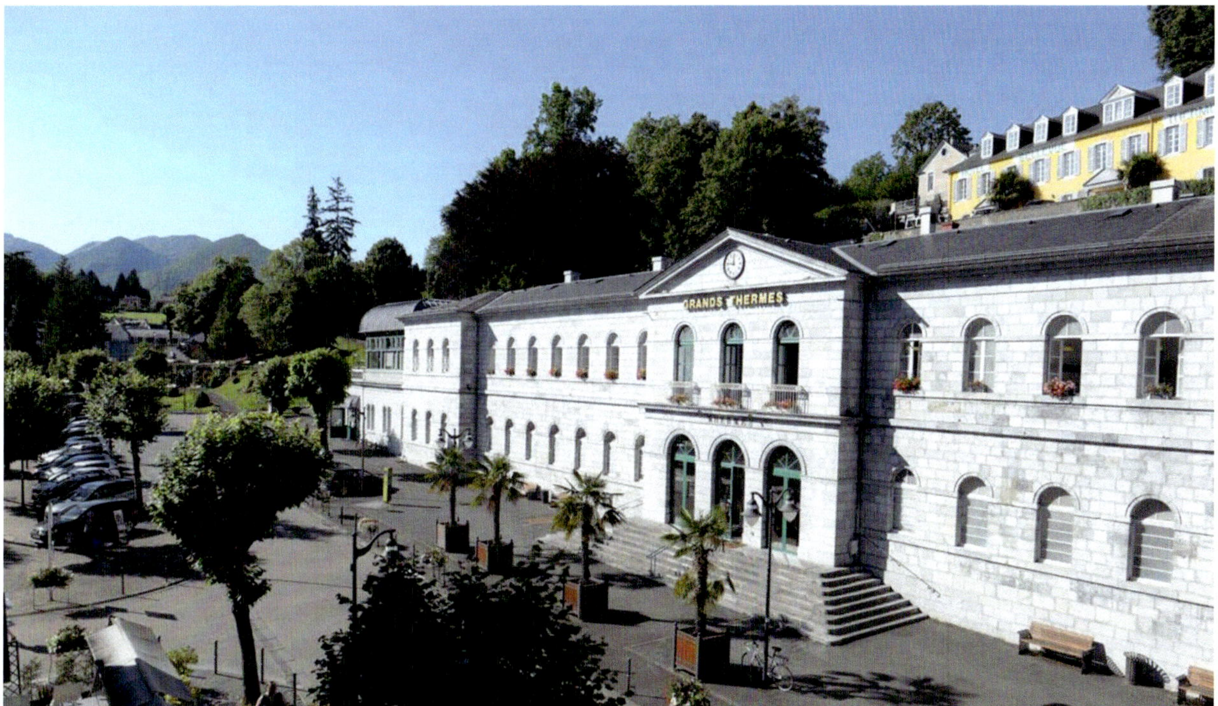

Figure 5b. The main complex in 2023. © R. Sabatier 2020. © R. Sabatier 2020

afforested, and the company Ramond[15] took advantage of this to fund the Association for the Restoration of the Bigorre Mountains. Nurseries were set up by members of the association, supported by the Water and Forestry Service. The summits of Mont Bédat and Mont Olivet are then covered by a mixed wood forest planted with various species of trees. Near a grotto, a discreet Fairy Fountain was created, with an inn next door. And, as the plantings expanded, new paths were created. With the mountains being regenerated through the forest and protection of water resources, the promenade, now understood as a means of oxygenating the body, added the curative action of the air and sun[16] to that of the water. At the time, the company Ramond was in contact with the very pioneers of forest ecology,[17] who were also working on the afforestation of Mont Aigoual, in the Massif Central, where the summit was to be the site of a weather station from 1885. Ten years earlier, Ramond had itself embarked on the construction of a high-altitude weather station, which was to become the Observatoire du Pic du Midi de Bigorre.

In Bagnères-de-Bigorre, from the end of the 17th century onwards, a close relationship was forged between the growth of the spa industry and the development of the natural sciences.

From natural to industrial waters

The last major cholera epidemics in Paris – in 1832 and again in 1854 – provided scientific evidence of a cause-and-effect relationship between water pollution and health. The Imperial Decree of 1853 on the creation of the Compagnie Générale des Eaux was in line with these developments. For spas investing in industrialising their activities, the Law of 14 July 1856 on *the conservation and development of mineral water springs*[18] made their accreditation subject to a number of conditions.

For Bagnères-de-Bigorre, the 1864 Small Channel Plan[19] reflects the need to update water management on a regular basis. While the small service channels and drains in the middle of the streets disappeared, the fountains, gutters in the new pavements and irrigation systems in the English-style parks and gardens increased in number. While losing its medieval appearance, Bagnères-de-Bigorre was to become the 'Venice of the Pyrenees'. Laying underground pipes in the streets to supply spring water fit for drinking and distributing it to forty public fountains cut the underground routes of the small channels running along the streets or passing from block to block to supply private homes with service water. It was therefore necessary to record and represent their underground routes so that the impact of the works could be measured and solutions identified. This precaution on the part of local councillors with regard to the 'water rights'[20] associated with these works is highly expressive of a culture of water and the conditions conducive to its evolution and its revolutions. At the time, water was everyone's business.

As far back as the 16th century, Salluste de Bartas noted the skill of the people of Bagnères in managing both hot and cold waters closely and separately.[21] The abundance of water in this mountainous region and the power of its flow led successive societies to use it to irrigate the land, supply houses with service water, power the mills and clean the streets, while the hot springs were reserved for medical care. These multiple uses were not *the prerogative of the spa town, but of the whole valley*, from the communal summer pastures to the fields on the plain, from the pastoral enclosures in the mid-mountains to the resort and beyond, via the market town and the villages. In the new urban promenades, in the new parks and resort gardens, and in the renovated streets, everyone saw the allegory of the living, sparkling, whispering waters of the mountains.

The new drinking water standards decreed in 1914 and implemented by local authorities between the wars, followed by public health policy from the 1970s onwards, were to revolutionise this water culture and profoundly change the spa atmosphere of the town.

From the silence of a city of water... to an approach based on water supply chains

In the mid-1970s, when you got off the train at the station, you would walk up the avenue and arrive in Bagnères-de-Bigorre on a hot summer's afternoon to gradually become aware of the new silence of this spa town.

[15] This learned society was founded in 1865 by: Emilien Frossard (1802-1881), the pastor who re-founded Protestant worship in the Hautes-Pyrénées, Charles Packe (1826-1896), British officer, and Henry Russel-Killough (1834-1909), Irish explorer, who were joined by Farnham Maxwell-Lyte (1828-1906), photographer. Several of these members had previously been among the founders of the London Alpine Club (1853).

[16] This afforestation of the thermal and pastoral promenades of Bagnères-de-Bigorre inspired a project to build a sanatorium and then a mountain hotel, also promoted by Ramond.

[17] Charles Flahault (1852-1935), Botanist, Professor at the Université de Montpellier, and Georges Fabre (1844-1911), Forestry Engineer and Meteorologist.

[18] The Law of 14 July 1856 on the conservation and development of mineral water springs relates to the declaration of public interest and the scope of protection of springs, inspections, and the general operating conditions of spa establishments.

[19] Kept by the town's Technical Services Department, the Small Channel Plan, dated 1864, takes the form of an atlas including a general layout plan and 23 land use plans at a scale of 500. Scanned by the OAPHB, can be accessed online via the Haute-Bigorre GIS (https://oaphb.fr/sig/).

[20] Water rights are perpetual rights attached to the water intake and not to the structure conveying the water to that point. As such, these works are covered by perpetual water rights for a specific use and are therefore exempt from any authorisation or renewal procedure (Wikipedia).

[21] *'And although there is little space between his flow, as cold as ice, and the pain-relieving bath, he holds back his nature, and will not in the slightest mix his cold with his fire'*, Salluste de Bartas (1544-1590) *Les Œuvres poétiques*, volume 1, page 248, about Bagnères-de-Bigorre.

Some fifty years on, the final year projects of two architecture students (Dedieu and Vertallier 2015), whose aim was to set up a participatory workshop open to local residents as part of their degrees, revealed the residents' recurring nostalgia in relation to the loss of this close lin#k between waters and town. At the same time as this study, the rediscovery of an ancient collecting tank under the spa district resulted in an inventory survey of this underground structure.[22] This survey enabled the establishment of a research team, which was first created as a branch of the company Ramond in 2017 and then became independent in 2018 in the form of the Observatory for Archaeology and Heritage in Haute-Bigorre (OAPHB)[23].

In 2015, a 'Natural Waters' workshop was set up with the local authority to bring together stakeholders and experts to discuss this issue. It was followed by a second in 2016. These two sessions provided an insight into the current state of thermal mineral management at the resort[24], and more specifically the abandonment of the old gravity-fed catchments in favour of the installation of deep boreholes to secure the use of hot water. Like in other spa towns, such as Bath in England's Somerset, the town centre of Bagnères-de-Bigorre, including its spa district, was built and developed in direct contact with the resurgence of thermal mineral waters. These deep boreholes make it possible to control piezometric disruptions linked to the risk of interference with the underlying water table during the final phase of the ascent of hot water. Indeed, the current urban layout, which has evolved since the Middle Ages, is characterised by the absence of cellars, apart from the old semi-buried private baths. This situation is particularly indicative of the activity of the hydrogeological substrate.

At the beginning of the 2000s,[25] in accordance with the requirements imposed by the Ministry of Health, Bagnères-de-Bigorre drilled two deep wells to replace the gravity-fed catchments that had previously supplied the town. The consequence of this advance was a modification in the monitoring of these waters, which now circulate under pressure from the hydrogeological subsoil to the various points where they are used. However, the fact that the old water catchments were no longer in use did not mean that they were obsolete, since they remained direct monitoring points for the thermal mineral aquifer. At the end of the drilling work, Antéa Group submitted a memorandum to the town emphasising this new state of neglect of the springs owned by the municipality[26] and pointing out two areas requiring vigilance[27], while at the same time a major spa was being added to the town's treatment establishments[28]:

- To ensure that '*currently neglected springs are brought into and maintained in compliance with (...) the conditions necessary for safeguarding the quality of thermal mineral water ...*'.
- To maintain '*these flows at defined, fixed levels to ensure that a balance is maintained between the pressure of the thermal water and that of the other aquifers, a guarantee of safety for the protection of the quality of the resource*'.

For our observatory, this question of the neglect of the springs was a key issue at the time of its creation. The hydrogeologists' recommendations sought to protect the town from the loss of corporate memory inevitably associated with this upheaval in the management of its thermal mineral resource. The staff assigned to maintenance and surveillance now had to refocus their tasks on the contingencies of the new water supply installation storing and transporting hot water under pressure, which is now more prone to bacteriological development.[29] Although rare in the case of spa resorts in France[30], this risk of outbreak is nevertheless feared because of its catastrophic impact on the reputation of spa resorts.

But this visible loss of a corporate memory[31] relating to the extensive overhaul of water management was not

[22] https://oaphb.fr/wp-content/uploads/2021/01/Prospection-Inventaire-Bagne%CC%80res-de-Bigorre-2016-Drac-Occitanie.pdf

[23] https://oaphb.fr/

[24] The first two sessions of this workshop were held in 2015 and 2016, bringing together the Fountains Department of the Château de Versailles National Estate and the companies Antéa Group and Eiffage.

[25] According to the Ministry of Health and Prevention: '*The water used for therapeutic purposes in a spa must be natural mineral water (...) It is defined by its original purity and is distinguished from other waters by the nature and stability of the essential physical and chemical elements it contains (minerals, trace elements). Since the 2000s, strict microbiological requirements have been laid down by regulations, relating to the resource and to the points of utilisation in the spa establishment (Decree of 19 June 2000 amending the Decree of 14 October 1937, as amended, relating to the monitoring of mineral water springs)*' In: *Eaux thermales, eaux minérales naturelles utilisées à des fins thérapeutiques dans un établissement thermal* [*Thermal waters: natural mineral waters used for therapeutic purposes in a thermal spa*] (website updated in January 2021).

[26] *Protection de la ressource hydrothermale / Etat de délaissement des sources minérales du patrimoine communal [Protection of hydrothermal resources / State of neglect of municipal mineral springs]*, Antéa Group / Town of Bagnères-de-Bigorre, July 2002. This memorandum is based in part on the description of water catchments provided by BRGM under the title 'Département des Hautes-Pyrénées / Stations thermales et sources thermo-minérales' (Departement of Hautes-Pyrénées / Thermal spas and mineral springs) by Marie Nartet and Jean-Christophe Soulé, Ministry of Industrial Redeployment and Foreign Trade, December 1985.

[27] Ibidem, page 20.

[28] Since the early 2000s, the deep boreholes have supplied the main municipal Grands Thermes thermal baths complex, the Thermes de la Reine private spa (bought by the town in 2020), the Aquensis spa and the Functional Rehabilitation Centre at Bagnères-de-Bigorre Hospital (which terminated its contract with Semetherm in 2019).

[29] Decree of 22 October 2013 on health monitoring and surveillance analyses of packaged waters and natural mineral waters used for therapeutic purposes in a spa establishment or distributed in public refreshment areas.

[30] In France, only 1% of spas are affected by such a situation.

[31] Corporate memory, or organisational memory, refers to all the knowledge and know-how within an organisation taken as a whole: managers and employees, whether this relates to a region, a company, an association, etc.

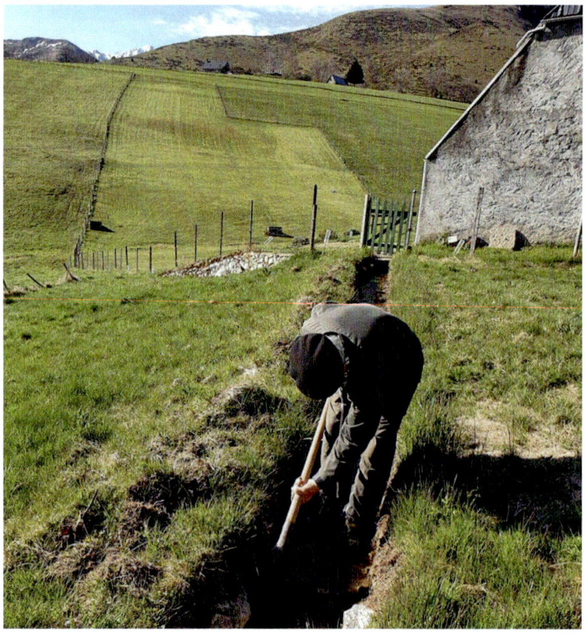

Figure 6. View of the valley and irrigation channels in the mid-mountain region. Photo by R. Sabatier 2021

confined to thermal mineral waters. It also affected all the water supplies that once brought life to the 'Venice of the Pyrenees', inherited from the embellishments designed by the Public Highways and Mines engineers of the Second Empire. The recent neglect of the springs and their catchments was compounded by the removal of water gutters on pavements and the drying up of fountains and ditches along promenades, parks and gardens in the town. Although mountain water remained free, this decline in the urban spa landscape was partly due[32] to the delegation of the drinking water service to private companies from the 19th century onwards, and then to the fact that its distribution and potability became chargeable during the 20th century. In addition to the disappearance of natural water run-off in the fountains, pools and gutters of the spa district, we had to add the fact that we had forgotten about the flooding of the Aygo Tebio. Today, the discontinuation of maintenance of the cofferdams protecting the thresholds of the houses here demonstrates the lack of transmission of local knowledge between old and new occupants. This is the most worrying as these thresholds have lost some of their height as a result of the roadway being raised to bring it into line with the Disability Law. With neither pavements nor gutters, the urban fabric of the town centre means that the ground floors of houses and businesses are now more exposed to the hazards of flooding, making it all the more important to update our knowledge of natural gravity-fed water systems. Could what the engineers of the Second Empire achieved to improve the resort, based on the gravitational principle of the natural path of a drop of water, not be applied differently today? This has led us to focus our work not only on learning about a heritage that has been forgotten, but also on the dynamics of the landscapes of a valley where the many water-based systems – whether dormant or active – are still generating know-how and projects that seek to appreciate the water that falls from the sky or bubbles up from the depths of the rocks and to manage this resource economically in order to irrigate the valley once again through its many small streams (Figure 6).

The resilience of the living waters of the Haut-Adour

We observed that further up the valley, local associations had been working for some time to take over from local authority workers in the upkeep of mid-mountain pastures, maintaining an infrastructure and the associated know-how. While the archaeological survey undertaken in 2016 enabled us to gain a better understanding of the complexity of the water supply substratum providing the structure for the town of Bagnères-de-Bigorre[33], from 2019 our work would extend to the gravity-fed water supply systems of channels and ditches irrigating the land and mountain pastures of the Haut-Adour. This extension of our studies enabled us to see that the old irrigation systems for the mountain pastures and meadows also established the structure of the town of Bagnères-de-Bigorre, its districts, its promenades, its vast thermal park, etc.

With this in mind, in 2021 our team brought together a small team of residents for a consultation to discuss the current situation of the springs in that thermal park. From this first formal exchange, it emerged that because it accommodated the catchment field for the hydrogeological cycle of the thermal mineral waters, this large thermal park was directly involved in the spa town's thermal cure economy. This economy cannot be reduced solely to the efficiency of the mechanical extraction system installed some twenty years ago in the spa town. The natural waters, grasslands and woods that make up the resort's vast thermal landscape are essential to its redeployment in the light of our current climate and, above all, to the fact that the inhabitants of these areas play an active part in this overall system. In Bagnères-de-Bigorre, the environment of the springs in the town and in the thermal park is now in decline, with car parks now even being installed at some

[32] The other cause of this subsidence is the withdrawal of the pastoral production system historically associated with the resort's large thermal park.

[33] Archaeological survey carried out as part of the Observatory for Archaeology and Heritage in Haute-Bigorre, initially within Ramond and then from November 2018 as part of an association under the Law of 1901 (OAPHB) in order to meet the development and management expectations of the Collective Research Programme *Water Systems and Balneotherapy in Occitania* (2018/2020). Refer to the association's website: https://oaphb.fr/Qui sommes-nous.

resurgence points. This is why we felt it was necessary to set up a laboratory of springs with the following three objectives:

- Describing the water systems of the spa town and its vast park as corollaries to those of the pastoral valley;
- Acknowledging the importance of springs as both societal and ecosystem locations;
- Proposing to local residents that they once again become partners in the protection and maintenance of this tangible and intangible heritage.[34]

Since we can no longer claim that the upkeep and development of our habitats can be ensured by delegating services alone, we need to come together at a spring, to share our knowledge and the associated vicissitudes, so as to anchor our scientific and societal questions in the reality of the local landscape's economy. We knew that, in the common sense, a spring is a place where water emerges naturally from the ground after an underground journey, and that journey will dictate its quality: potable, mineral, thermal or even unfit for consumption. In a spa resort such as Bagnères-de-Bigorre, most of the springs have been collected and channelled into reservoirs, fountains, pools and baths, as well as gutters and sometimes drinking troughs. The small Spring Laboratory team therefore decided to begin its work at the Fontaine des Fées fountain in the Bédat woods near the town, in an attempt to appreciate the site *in situ* and thus explore this past in a different way. We worked together at this spring, watching, measuring, surveying, smelling, listening, naming the things seen, showing them to others, discussing them and listening to each other in this way ... and by hearing each other, building a new narrative. The team was lucky enough to include a number of young professionals: a landscape architect, an archaeologist, an archivist, an artist in residence, a visual artist and a historian ... Along the way, despite their professional commitments, each of them – based on his or her individual skillset – took the time to go and draw up a survey or a sketch, take photos, grab maps, write, and glean some archive information.

A programme of weekly meetings and session reports was then put in place. Following the ten meetings held between April and October 2021[35], it emerged that all the springs contributing to the context of the listed site of Mont Bédat and Vallon de Salut had been updated by the Regional Environment Office in 2007[36], and above all those new perspectives had been identified with the development of participatory workshops based on a new tool: the Haute-Bigorre Geographical Information System (GIS)[37]. This tool was developed as part of a partnership between the OAPHB and the Huma-num Paris Time Machine (PTM) Consortium[38]. The various participatory workshops we organised involved both a group of secondary school students[39] and members of five local associations[40], both active and retired, all of whom are working to maintain the mid-mountain landscape.

This initiative is part of an open science and participatory science approach in which digital humanities are the preferred medium for building and sharing knowledge. The workshops are structured around:

[34] The concept of 'intangible heritage' emerged at the end of the 1980s and deals with traditional cultures. In this case, this relates to the usages and know-how associated with the gravity-fed management of natural waters.

[35] A report on this first 2021 session of the Spring Laboratory can be found in Notebook 3, *Archéologie en Haute-Bigorre* (Archaeology in the Haute Bigorre region), published by the OAPHB in the chapter 'Des eaux naturelles, des herbages, des bois' – *En héritage, le grand parc thermal de Bagnères-de-Bigorre* (Natural waters, grasslands and woods' – A legacy, Bagnères-de-Bigorre's vast thermal park) p. 143 to 190 (https://oaphb.fr/publications/).

[36] The Mont Bédat and Vallon de Salut site was listed in 2007 by the Regional Environment Office (DREAL) with the aim of 'raising awareness of the picturesque and historic character for which this site is renowned, particularly in the history of Pyrenean thermal baths'. Its 244-hectare perimeter overlaps the catchment area of the thermal mineral resource.

[37] The Haute-Bigorre GIS was set up in 2020 as part of a CNRS programme to develop research infrastructures. Run jointly by the OAPHB and the Huma-num Paris Time Machine (PTM) Consortium, with the support of the Geomatics team for the Département of Hautes-Pyrénées – which has provided access to the databases of the National Institute for Geographical and Forestry Information (IGN) – this geographical information system contextualises the data acquired by the OAPHB's research by comparing it, using geolocation, with a series of maps and plans, drawings and photos, both old and new, documenting the Haut-Adour Valley. This geohistorical GIS can be accessed in a modulated way. A public version is available on the OAPHB website. Like Google Maps, the Haute-Bigorre GIS gives you access to maps that allow you to find your way around in everyday life and to travel back in time: you can currently see the town of Bagnères-de-Bigorre in 1771 (Plan Terrier, a property map with agricultural use illustrated), in 1791 (topographical plan), in 1810 (Napoleonic land register), and in 1864 (Small Channel Plan) for the time ...

[38] The Huma-Num Paris Time Machine Consortium has become the Time Machine Projects (https://paris-timemachine.huma-num.fr/) and is a consortium funded by the CNRS Huma-Num research infrastructure. It is managed by the UMR 7041 ArScAn (http://www.arscan.fr/). Members of these two workshops can access the Haute-Bigorre GIS using a personalised code giving them expert access. The work in progress can be consulted on the OAPHB website under the GIS heading (https://oaphb.fr/sig/) and on the website of La Fabrique Numérique du Passé (https://www.fabriquenumeriquedupasse.fr/pages/homepage/?flg=fr) where the *Bagnères-de-Bigorre, historical milestones* tab gives access to the set of data already georeferenced.

[39] This group is made up of eight students from the Lycée Victor-Duruy in Bagnères-de-Bigorre, accompanied by two of their teachers, one of whom is the Academic Contact for Digital Technology for the Académie de Toulouse.

[40] In addition to the eight students from the Lycée Victor-Duruy in Bagnères-de-Bigorre, the other participants are members of the associations for Pierre des Esclozes (https://www.campan.fr/vivre-a-campan/associations/patrimoine/pierre-des-esclozes/), Rigoles de Gaye (https://www.campan.fr/vivre-a-campan/associations/patrimoine/les-rigoles-de-gaye/), Sentiers de Campan (https://www.campan.fr/vivre-a-campan/associations/patrimoine/les-sentiers-de-campan/) the Grange Foraine barn site located in the Lesponne valley in Bagnères-de-Bigorre (https://grangeforaine.com/contact/) and the French Club Alpin of Bagnères-de-Bigorre (https://www.caf-bagneres-bigorre.com/).

- Small channels underlying the town centre of Bagnères-de-Bigorre, based on a land register atlas prepared in 1864 for the installation of forty public fountains;
- Mid-range mountain irrigation systems which, until the inter-war period, supported the valley's pastoral production system based on intensive grassland farming.

The idea was to take two very different levels of the valley landscape as a starting point, to work with local people to highlight the gravitational water supply systems that take water from rivers at their source, through channels and ditches, and carry it to the land, the villages and the town, before returning it to its natural course.

From a formal point of view, we then supervised two teams based respectively on the work of two students supervised in Haute-Bigorre by the OAPHB[41] to carry out two workshops:

- The GIS workshop on 'Irrigation in mid-mountain areas', which brings together a dozen active members from six associations, is working on the seasonal pastoral habitat of the Haut-Adour region, linking the mountain pastures to the grasslands via irrigation channels and ditches. In the light of the detailed studies (Buisan 2001-2012) carried out on the *courtaous*[42], the team intends to develop a topographical description of this extensive pastoral system. For the time being, the aim is to define and test methods for recording and describing both the routes of the channels and all the associated structures. At the end of the first sessions, there were already numerous potential projects: reactivating a pastoral unit using gullies that have now been abandoned, continuing to maintain the irrigation of a residential area, rebuilding shepherds' huts, re-opening paths, etc. All of these projects have the potential to contribute to the revival of local pastoral production and to the transition of the tourism offering.
- The 'Small Channels' workshop, which began in 2022 and will be continued in 2023, is currently enabling teams of secondary school students from the Lycée Victor-Duruy to learn about GIS while at the same time learning how to read under-used historical documentation (old maps). For two hours a week from October to February, with field trips and video-conferences, the students are accompanied by a team of history and mathematics teachers from the school, two members of the OAPHB, a member of the Time Machine Projects consortium, an architect and a divisional engineer. During the first session, which started at the beginning of September, a presentation of the 1864 Small Channel Plan was made in the offices of the town's Technical Services Department. This was followed by two excursions during which the pupils were able to meet local residents and a garden historian from the Versailles Fountains Department. They then set about digitising all the water supply chains represented in the Small Channel Plan to create a database that can be used in current digital systems. This cross-disciplinary and interconnected approach to education, which is highly compatible with the expectations of this generation, is proving to be very promising. In particular, it makes it possible to combine an appreciation of the local environment and its history with current issues in the subject areas in which secondary school pupils are learning the fundamentals. A second session is planned for 2023, and this will add other aspects to the database.

This cross-generational, cross-social, cross-neighbourhood and cross-terroir approach to the valley is in some ways an expression of the resilience of the landscape (Robert 2021). Far from expressing a defensive or protective reaction against the inevitable erosion of time, these perspectives represent a move towards possible transformations, possible *ecological resilience* (Robert 2021). Indeed, for the new generations, it is no longer a question of conserving and safeguarding, but of doing, acting and undertaking. (Figure 7)

Age of service water supply to private homes in town

The complete survey of the town's water supply structure in 1864 provides an initial overview of the unique systems specific to each of the four districts making up the walled town as seen by Louis de Froidour in the 17th century (circa 1625-1685). This late meeting point – for which we have no assurance as to its completeness – brought together four districts, each represented by two consuls sitting as a college under the authority of the Count of Bigorre (Sabatier 2015). According to historiographical tradition, it was the Bourg-vieux and Bourg-neuf areas that served as the original basis for the foundation of the contemporary

[41] In 2021, a geomatics student worked on the Bagnères-de-Bigorre 1864 Small Channel Plan as part of his placement. In 2020, an architecture student studied the water supply chains in the Haut-Adour mid-range mountains as part of her final qualification.

[42] In the Haut-Adour region, a *courtaou*, or *courtaú*, generally refers to a more or less large group of pastoral enclosures used for rearing cattle in summer pastures. Each of these enclosures generally includes a hut and a yard with a lean-to and a stable. Cooled by a spring or stream, a *leyté*, a stone shelter for storing milk from milking, was associated with each courtaou.

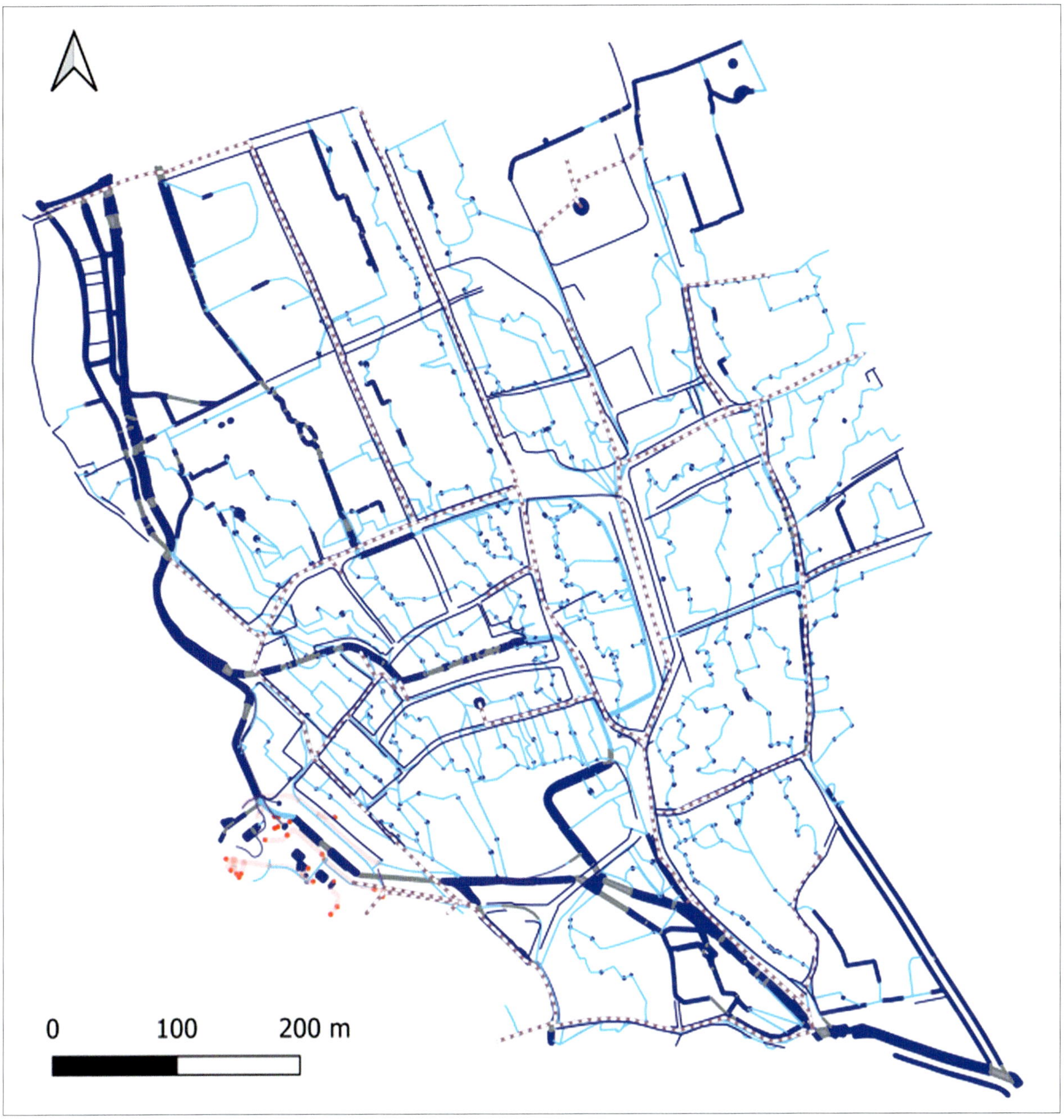

Figure 7. View of the Small Channel Plan after vectorisation. By OAPHB / ArScAn 2023

town by the Comte de Bigorre (11th/12th century), followed by the two adjoining suburbs: *Caouteres*[43] and *La Hount*[44]. (Figure 8)

These four neighbourhoods are clearly distinguishable by their plot structure and the water systems that run through them. You can see the regular layout of the old and new towns, for which the 'padlock'[45] shape is characteristic of the foundations laid in the time of the Count. Those of the two suburbs are more irregular, and one incorporates a first market place. In the absence of an in-depth morphological analysis, the layout of the boundaries remains approximate. What is quite clearly visible, however, are the large surface

[43] Caouteres, steam rooms in Gascon, according to Jean-François Lenail, archivist-paleographer, former Director of the Hautes-Pyrénées Départemental Archives. This district, formed at the gates of the old town, led to the hot springs and steam baths.

[44] La Hount, Gascon for 'fountain', named after a large drinking water fountain in this suburb.

[45] In the foothills of the Pyrenees, the foundations of the market towns resulting from the first medieval revival (10th/11th century) are characterised by a street serving deep strips of land on either side. At each end of the street is a gate. The market is located outside the town. The advent of the 'bastide' movement (13th/14th century) integrated commercial functions at the heart of urban planning.

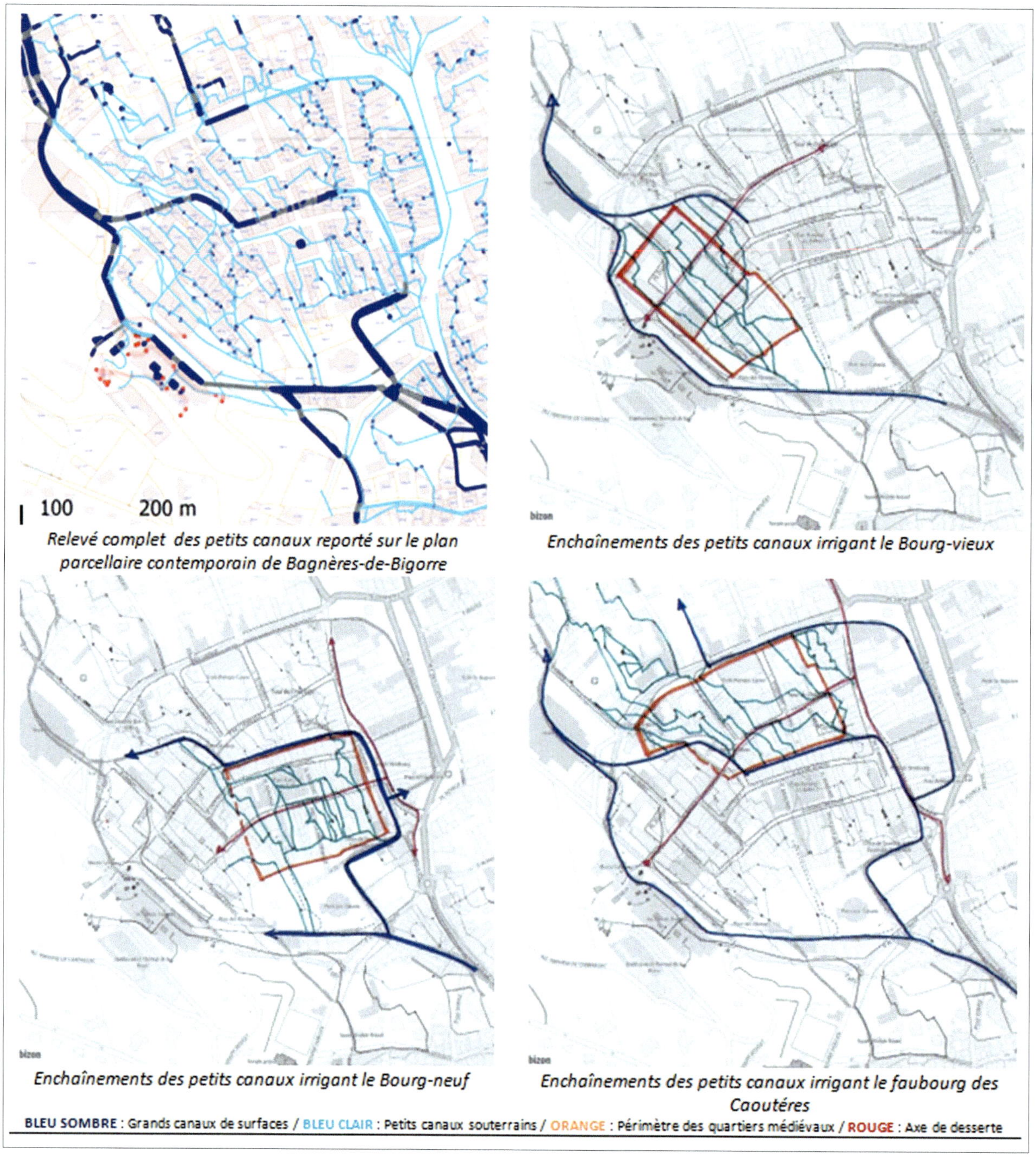

Figure 8. The organisation of three of the four districts of Bagnères-de-Bigorre. © OAPHB / ArScAn 2023

milling channels that clearly outline the shape of the town and its surrounding walls. This reading leads us to wonder about the rampart, which was paid for by the consuls and was completed very late (if at all), and about the layout of the channels, which seems to us to be earlier. Indeed, the shape of these channels (narrow and shallow) makes them unsuitable for use as moats, and they are also easy to walk through, but they are perfectly suitable for supplying mills and houses with service water.

We have then spoken on numerous occasions about water supply sequences, as the small channels do not – strictly speaking – form a network in the strict sense of the term, but rather successive sequences running from a water intake on an upstream channel to an outlet. Reading the database, we can therefore see the assemblies and probable phases in which these sequences of underground channels, troughs and manholes are formed, arranged organically or planned so as to serve the blocks of a single district. The most regular, orthonormal groups correspond to the first two planned districts. The water system links serving the blocks of the two suburbs are more random in form, as if developed piecemeal in an attempt to avoid the obstacle of a rampart, which can then be guessed at. The result is a water distribution system based on gravity, either in the form of a bundle or a comb cutting more or less perpendicularly through the service axis of each of the districts. The water supply network connected to the plots is also distinct from the road network. It was not until the installation in 1864 of the first network, in the strict sense, to supply the forty public fountains that the water distribution route and the public roads became one and the same.

The structure of the series of small channels serving the old town is particularly noteworthy as it is laid out as a whole parallel to the axis of the large ancient collecting tank that we surveyed. This straight ancient collecting tank, which has proportions identical to those of the Gard aqueduct, has its current water course at around three and a half metres below the current surface of the town, namely at paleosol level. It runs for around three hundred metres parallel to the course of the Aygo Tebio, irrigating a thalweg with hot springs on which ancient baths have been built. The small channels in the old town, on the other hand, are located at minus eighty centimetres, and thus at the level presumed to be the ground in the medieval period. However, their routes follow the general direction of the stream rectified by the collecting tank built by the ancient engineers.

Conclusion: Working together to develop tools for interpreting the shapes of the town and the shapes of water

In addition to their social dimension, these workshops have produced (and will continue to produce) original data that can be used to identify the key features of the town's landscape. As demonstrated by the way in which plots of land and roads were laid out, the layout of the small channels that ran beneath the town until the 1970s reveals how this *spa town*[46], which developed its baths in Antiquity and then at the end of the Middle Ages, and became a spa resort in the 19th century, had inherited a culture of sharing water, with the shape of the town and the shape of the water intertwined. To this we must add rights and duties, which in this case are one and the same. In fact, what this work reveals is that it is not about the register of land ownership, or about the register of publicly owned land, but about the necessary building of solidarity between residents, block by block, district by district, market towns and suburbs, and about the gradual construction of an urban fabric over the long term.

In this case, the use of digital tools to build interactive workshops has made it possible to vectorise the various water system objects and integrate a number of old sources into an accessible application that anyone can use today. In these historical sources, which give us a glimpse of the successive states of the land, these particular water system objects – the small channels – which can be identified on the fine scale of the plot of land and are described in detail in the 1864 Small Channel Plan, have helped to provide a unique image of all the surface milling channels, small underground channels distributing service or household water to private containers, roadside gutters, catchments and supply points for thermal mineral waters, including reservoirs and basins, as well as an initial pipe-based supply network for forty drinking water fountains.

This document describes the culture of hydraulic engineers and surveyors in 19th-century France, enabling us to capture the very peak of the spa town's beautification and a status inherited from the construction of these water supply systems. This idea of the omnipresence of water in the urban and agropastoral landscape of Bagnères-de-Bigorre disappeared from the 1970s onwards because of the need to comply with health standards and to make way for the car and property developments that restricted areas for water expansion in the town. The consequences of this disappearance are now being assessed in terms of their impact on the resort's thermal environment and its resilience in the face of climate hazards, which are all the more sensitive given that part of Bagnères-de-Bigorre town centre lies directly in the Vaucluse floodplain of the Aygo Tebio stream, and the town is directly exposed to climate hazards that are now set to increase in frequency and volume. In this case, the proposal put forward in this article clearly falls within the field of digital humanities and makes it possible to reactivate a memory for shared engagement that carried this thermal landscape, at once urban and natural. This is a memory which is currently perhaps not lost but at least reduced to a single technical approach, one that misinterprets the medical and cultural scope of balneotherapy. So how can we consolidate, or even retie, this thread?

The archaeological surveying of an ancient collecting tank, part of an underground water supply to the thermal district, combined with the study of surface irrigation systems, channels and ditches, led the team to make these hydraulic systems used to take in and then release natural water locally its subject of research. It is at the point of delivery of water from a spring – a

[46] *Vicus aquensis*, spa town, name attributed to the ancient town of Bagnères when it appeared engraved on an ancient votive stone. *Vicus aquensis* is not its name, but the generic designation of an administrative category of territorial management at the time, on a par with civitas aquensis, Aachen in Westphalia.

fountain, a bath, a shower – just as it is at the point of delivery of water taken from a river – a meadow, a pond, a basin, a street – that complex heritage and environmental objects are now anchored, nourished and deployed in search of a future: a former private spa, an urban promenade dominated by the car, a park leading to abandoned farms and mountain pastures, and so on.

In Bagnères-de-Bigorre, although the natural spring and river waters continue to replenish the old, abandoned water catchments, percolate through the soil and sometimes flood the thermal district, they are constrained by the accumulation of successive occupations of the thermal mineral site. In the Place des Thermes, the stratigraphy overlying the paleosol of the Aygo Tebio thalweg is estimated at around 3.50 metres. As a counterpoint, the resilience of the natural waters observed in the mid-mountain pastures of the Haut-Adour Valley questions a form of balneotherapy where post-war medicalisation has not prevented rampant discrediting, a situation that still weighs heavily on resorts that have nevertheless regularly improved their facilities and invested in climate control systems and then in *thermoludisme* (the use of the properties and benefits of thermal water to rest, restore vitality and well-being)[47]. Its considerable archaeological and hydrogeological potential, as well as its accessibility to the public within the framework of the thermal park, offer the opportunity to experiment with the capacities of thermal mineral springs to reconstitute biotopes and biocenoses. To this end, an in-depth survey is under way to gain a better understanding of the interface between the old concrete catchments, now no longer in use, and the rocky facies of the resurgences they cover. In conjunction with a number of official bodies, the aim will be to propose a process of reconstruction and deconstruction that could help to release some of these emergences.

Secondary school students are beginning to understand the significance of open waters, which, from the very beginnings of agriculture and animal husbandry, have generated one of the earliest forms of law. These are forms that have continued to evolve since the development of their driving forces, from mills to the industrialisation of all our activities, and in particular the balneotherapy industry. The members of several associations, working together and with support, are already collaborating on projects to record and map the fine networks of streams, channels and gullies that make up the headwaters of the Haut-Adour watershed. Returning to our roots, once again and together, is the right place to start.

[47] While the 1947 Ordinance recognises spa treatments as therapeutic, and subject from that point to reimbursement by the social security system, spa literature, dictionaries and other encyclopedias show that the Academies, still waiting for tangible proof, continue to use the conditional to qualify the therapeutic capacities of thermal waters. Today, according to the Ministry of Solidarity and Health, '*a spa is an establishment that uses water from one or more legally authorised mineral springs, or sludge and gases derived therefrom, on site or by direct supply, for the internal or external treatment of spa visitors*'. Public Health Code, Article R. 1322-52, 2021.

Bibliography

Bouneau, Chr. 2005. *La mise en valeur de l'équipement thermal pyrénéen du Second Empire à la crise des années trente: l'hygiénisme au service d'une nouvelle économie montagnarde*. Presses universitaires de Perpignan, 305-325. Licence OpenEdition Books. https://www-cairn-info.inshs.bib.cnrs.fr/revue-internationale-d-intelligence-economique-2022-2-page-43.htm

Buisan, G. 2001-2012. *Des cabanes et des hommes: Vie pastorale et cabanes de pâtres dans les Pyrénées, La vie montagnarde* (2011) and *Hier en Vallée de Campan* (2012), CAIRN.

Carribon, C. 1999. Un panorama de l'histoire du thermalisme en France: A. Authier and P. Duvernois 1997. *Patrimoine et traditions du thermalisme*, Toulouse, Edit. Privat. In Annales du Midi: revue archéologique, historique et philologique de la France méridionale, vol. 111, n°226, 1999. By D. Porté (ed) *Saint-Sernin de Toulouse à la fin du Moyen Age. Des reliques et des hommes*, 272-274.

Dedieu, L. and A. Vertallier 2015. *Réinventer ensemble un territoire. Une ville du Haut-Adour, Hautes-Pyrénées.* End-of-studies project at the Ecole Nationale Supérieure d'Architecture (Ensa) de Versailles under the guidance of Richard Sabatier, Government-accredited architect (DPLG), DEA EHESS, teacher and researcher; February 2015 session; presentation brochure, Documentation and Information Centre (CDI), Ensa Versailles. https://oaphb.fr/wp-content/uploads/2020/12/Re-inventer-ensemble-un-territoire-EnsaV-2015-BD.pdf

Jazé-Charvolin, M.R. 2016. *Les stations thermales: de l'abandon à la renaissance. Une brève histoire du thermalisme en France depuis l'Antiquité, In situ* [Online], 24 | 2014, online since 11 August 2016, accessed on 14 September 2023. DOI: https://doi.org/10.4000/insitu.11123

Lamothe, M. 2021. *Lectures patrimoniales du thermalisme: quand le patrimoine culturel immatériel et le patrimoine architectural et paysager se nourrissent réciproquement*, Les Cahiers de Framespa [Online], 38 | 2021, available online since 25 October 2021, accessed on 13 September 2023. URL: http://journals.openedition.org/framespa/11943; DOI: https://doi.org/10.4000/framespa.11943.

Letang, P. and A. Knauf 2022. L'implantation d'un complexe thermal comme facteur d'attractivité : rôle et enjeux de l'intelligence territoriale, *Revue internationale d'intelligence économique* 14, n°2, 43-61.

Nartet, M. and J-C. Soule 1986. *Département of Hautes-Pyrénées / Thermal spas and mineral springs*, Geological and Mining Research Office (1986), Ministry of Industrial Redeployment and Foreign Trade.

Robert, S. 2021. *La Résilience: persistance et changement dans les formes du paysage*, Interdisciplinarity, Sciences and Humanities Collection, ISTE éditions.

Roux, L. 2008-2009. *Le thermalisme européen au XVIIIe siècle: Etude comparative de quelques villes d'eaux, France, Angleterre, Belgique, Suisse, Italie, Allemagne.* Master 2 Humanities and Social Sciences thesis. Specialism: History of international cultural relations and exchanges. Université Pierre Mendès-France. Grenoble.

Sabatier, R. 2015. *Un édifice dans son paysage*, Newsletter of the company Ramond.

Scheid, J., M. Nicaud, D. Boisseuil and J. Coste (eds) 2015. *Le Thermalisme: Approches historiques et archéologiques d'un phénomène culturel et médical*, Paris. CNRS.

Space and Place around the Sacred Pool of Bagno Grande at San Casciano Dei Bagni (Toscany, Italy)

Jacopo TABOLLI
Dipartimento di Studi Umanistici, Università per Stranieri di Siena
jacopo.tabolli@unistrasi.it

Emanuele MARIOTTI
Dipartimento di Studi Umanistici, Università per Stranieri di Siena
emanuele.mariotti@unistrasi.it

Abstract: This paper presents the discovery of an intact Etruscan and Roman votive deposit within a sacred hot pool at Bagno Grande, San Casciano dei Bagni (province of Siena, Italy). This sanctuary was in use at least from the beginning of the 3rd century BCE to the end of the 4th century CE. 25 litres of hot water (42 degrees Celsius) still flow into the sacred pool of the sanctuary every second.

A series of ritual closing actions took place throughout these centuries at an institutional level, thus preserving into the hot mud the stratification of the votive deposit. Almost 7000 coins, hundreds of votive carved woods, and over 20 bronze statues and statuettes have been found. This is one of the largest votive deposits ever found in the Mediterranean and certainly the largest within a thermo-mineral spring.

Due to the possibility of investigating the stratigraphy of the deposit, the interdisciplinary team working in the excavation is expanding our understanding of the complexity of a votive context.

This paper investigates both this complexity and the potential of the Bagno Grande sanctuary in order to decode the system of ritual and cult actions that took place diachronically around and within the sacred pool. The paper is also focused on the multicultural and polylingual elements that characterized the transition between the Etruscans and the Romans, and how these elements were 'cast' into the mud within the sacred pool.

Keywords: Sanctuary, thermal and mineral-medicinal waters, Etruscan and Roman votive deposit

Bagno Grande and its sanctuary

In the vast majority of publications on the archaeology of thermo-mineral sites, and especially in those focused on ancient spas, the assumption that Romans constituted the origin of communal use of bathing into hot water often occurs. Although the scale of the Roman phenomenon is certainly without precedents, looking at the evidence in Italy, and especially taking into account the archaeological record associated to thermo-mineral springs, it should stressed that in many cases Romans consistently selected sites that were already in use in pre-Roman times.[1] Moving beyond the traditional narratives and aiming at decolonizing the archaeology ancient spas, the excavation at the thermo-mineral sanctuary of Bagno Grande at San Casciano dei Bagni (Siena, Italy) is bringing to light a sacred site that from the late 4th century BCE to the beginning of the 5th century CE had at its core a hot spring (Mariotti and Tabolli 2021; Mariotti, Salvi and Tabolli 2023; Osanna and Tabolli 2023). From this spring, located to the north of the sanctuary, still flow nowadays 25 litres of hot water at 39.5/41 degrees Celsius per second. This site was abandoned a once again in use probably since the fifteenth century without interruption. After an earthquake that occurred in 1575, the Medici from Florence promoted the construction around pools of a small portico that was built on top of the ruins of the Etruscan and Roman sanctuary, and especially overlaps the northern half of the Roman temple built around a sacred pool. While this late Renaissance portico has undergone stages of abandonment in 1700s and 1800s, the pools still function as open-air public bath for the local community (Fotini, Ledda and Morelli 2023) (Figure 1).

The Romanization of the territory of the Etruscan city-state of *Clevsi*/*Clusium*/Chiusi, where San Casciano dei Bagni was located in antiquity, was a long process, beginning in the 3rd century BCE and reaching 89 BCE where the entire area received Roman citizenship (Paolucci 1988a; Paolucci 1988b; most recently Carpentiero and Felici 2021). This economic and political gradual meting process between Etruscan and Roman ruling of the area occurred at a time in which the sanctuary of Bagno Grande was already in use. San Casciano and its Bagno Grande marked the southernmost border of the city-state of Chiusi, located along the ancient road that from Chiusi reached the seaside and the city-state of Vulci (Tabolli 2021). For whoever was coming from the sea into the inland city-

[1] On pre-Roman thermo-mineral sites, where evidence of communal practices have been identified, see Tabolli 2023c, with bibliography.

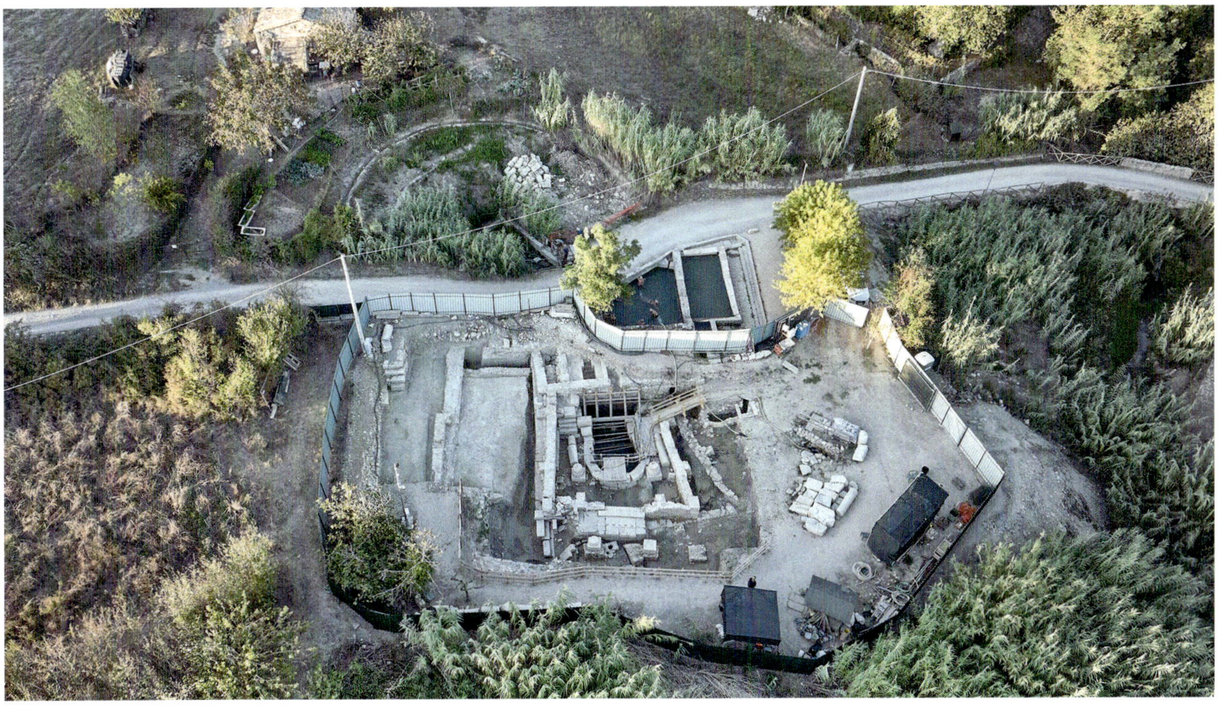

Figure 1. Aerial photo of Bagno Grande, from the south (photo by Gabriele Forti, copyright: Comune di San Casciano dei Bagni and SABAP-SI).

state, the location of this thermo-mineral shrine – as well as the others for which we have little structural evidence, such as Doccia della Testa[2] – would be the ideal access point. At the same, this site time functioned for the mother town as a 'business card' to display its power and at the same time to safely allow for a place of interregional trades.

The ongoing excavation revealed the presence of a pre-Roman pool made of travertine blocks (most probably built before the 3rd century BCE), probably with an oval shape, located at the center of a semi rectangular space, 10m large, oriented towards the south-southeast. Due to the preliminary results of the excavation, it is still early to define this place as an 'enclosure' or already a 'temple' with at its core the thermo-mineral water collected into a pool. This site underwent a dramatic transformation at the beginning of the 1st century CE when the earlier pool was partially dismantled while a new and elongate pool was built on top of it and now inside what appears to have been a tetrastyle temple[3]. This time of entire reconstruction occurred together with the ritual deposition into the dismantled pool of over thirty-five large bronzes statues and statuettes, depicting devotees or divinities, of three zoomorphic figurines, of over twenty anatomical organs, and of about ten plates embossed with representations of faces and eyes, alongside parts of natural elements, such as tree branches and fruits.[4] All these metal objects prior to the dismantling of the area had to be located somewhere into the shrine, probably along the edges of the earlier pool. These metal and natural donations were accumulated and intentionally placed in a single moment into the ruins of the pool, following an event, which affected, probably in the Tiberian age, the earlier structure. The discovery of a flint arrowhead, probably dating to the Eneolithic period (and reused at the time of the ritual), and of a bronze model of thunderbolt, collected within the layer of tiles that marked the dismantling of the earlier structure and pool may refer to the actual event of the impact of a lightning bolt (Cuda and Mustone 2023; Tabolli 2023b) (Figure 2). According to the Etruscan *ars fulguratoria*, collecting and burying those statues and sacred ornaments hit by a thunderbolt corresponded to the ritual of *fulmen condere* or *fulgur conditum*.[5] (Figure 2). The small model certainly depicts a *fulmen trisulcum*, the most destructive lightning bolt, as Festus recalls.[6] The model, made of cast bronze, in fact it is incomplete, proving that in a moment of the ceremony it was intentionally broken as part of a ritual of expiation. This place buried under tiles and the hot mud became subsequently a bidental (Mercattili 2005). Therefore, in the 1st century CE with the restructuring of the building, in the form

[2] Iozzo 2013; most recently Arbeid 2023 and Mariotti 2023b.
[3] On the tetrastyle temple, see below.

[4] For the preliminary publication of the ex-votos discovered, see Mariotti, Salvi and Tabolli 2023; Osanna and Tabolli 2023.
[5] Tabolli 2023b with references to Pfiffig 1975: 135-138; Mercattili 2005; MacIntosh Turfa 2012: 59-60.
[6] Tabolli 2023d.

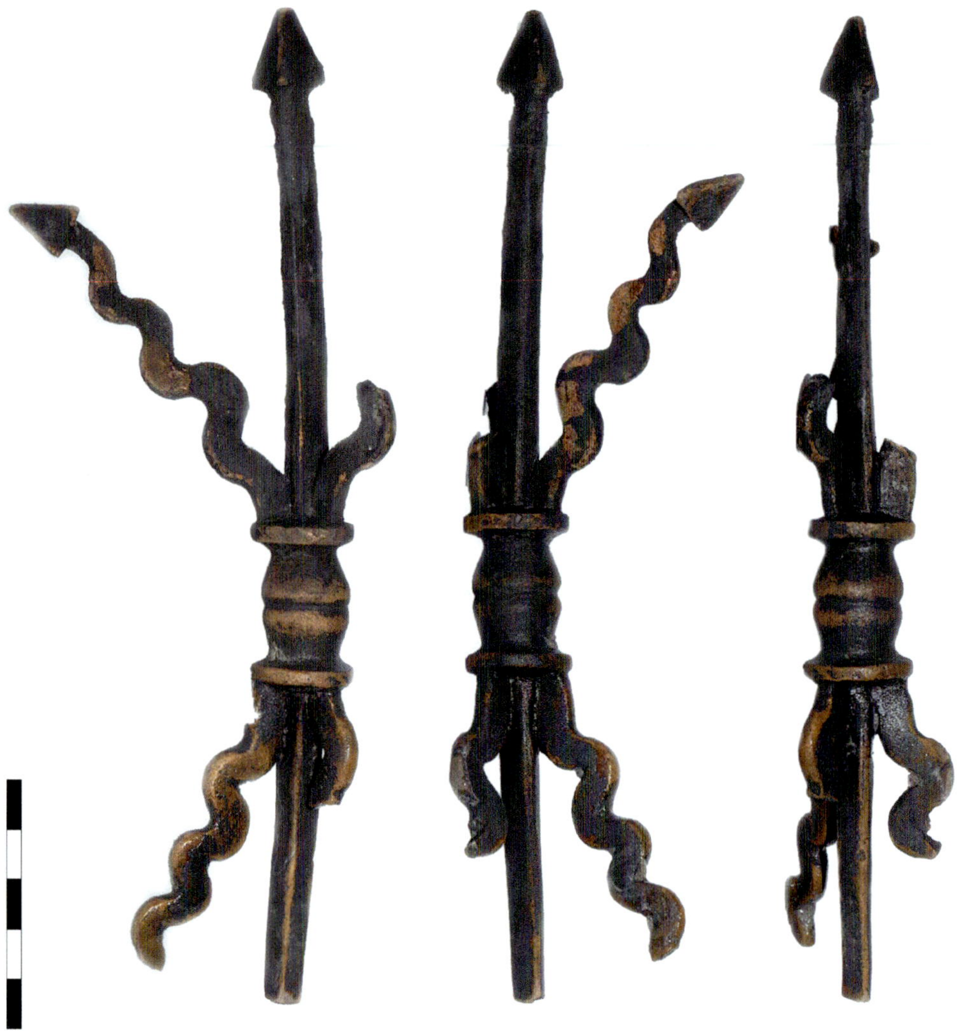

Figure 2. The bronze lightning bolt marking the ritual of *fulgur conditum* (photo by Francesco Marsili, copyright: Comune di San Casciano dei Bagni and SABAP-SI).

of a temple, the pool was enlarged to the south where more than six thousands of bronze coins (Pardini 2023; Pardini and Carbone 2023) were offered between the 1st and the late 4th centuries CE, together with a small number of earlier bronze ex votos that were not buried under the ritual *fulgur conditum*.

A large corpus of inscribed ex votos have been uncovered until now at Bagno Grande, both in Etruscan and in Roman scripts. In Etruscan, the name of a single deity appears in six inscriptions: *Flere Havens*, the deity of the Hot Spring (Maggiani 2023). This female deity is also depicted in one of the bronze statues buried under the *fulgur conditum*. In Roman times, from one goddess to a multitude of deities, *Flere Havens* probably become *Fons Caldus* (masculine in Latin) and, starting from the end of the 2nd century BCE, also Apollo and Fortuna played a significant role in the sanctuary (Gregori 2023). Asclepius and Hygeia are also present in Roman Imperial times, while Isis played a central role in the last two centuries, between the end of the 2nd and the 4th centuries CE (Caracciolo and Tabolli 2021).

The architecture of the shrine

The imperial building shows a succession of various restoration phases, which, however, kept its architecture almost unchanged until the beginning of the 5th century CE, when the complex was orderly decommissioned. At this time, large parts of columns and stone blocks were laid into the sacred pool to hide and to protect its sacred contents (Mariotti and Tabolli 2021, Mariotti, Tabolli and Salvi 2023). As we have seen the building consists of a semi rectangular structure, orientated north to south, with its entrance on the southern side. The northern part of the building is still covered by the portico that was built on top of the Roman ruins after the earthquake of 1575. Thus,

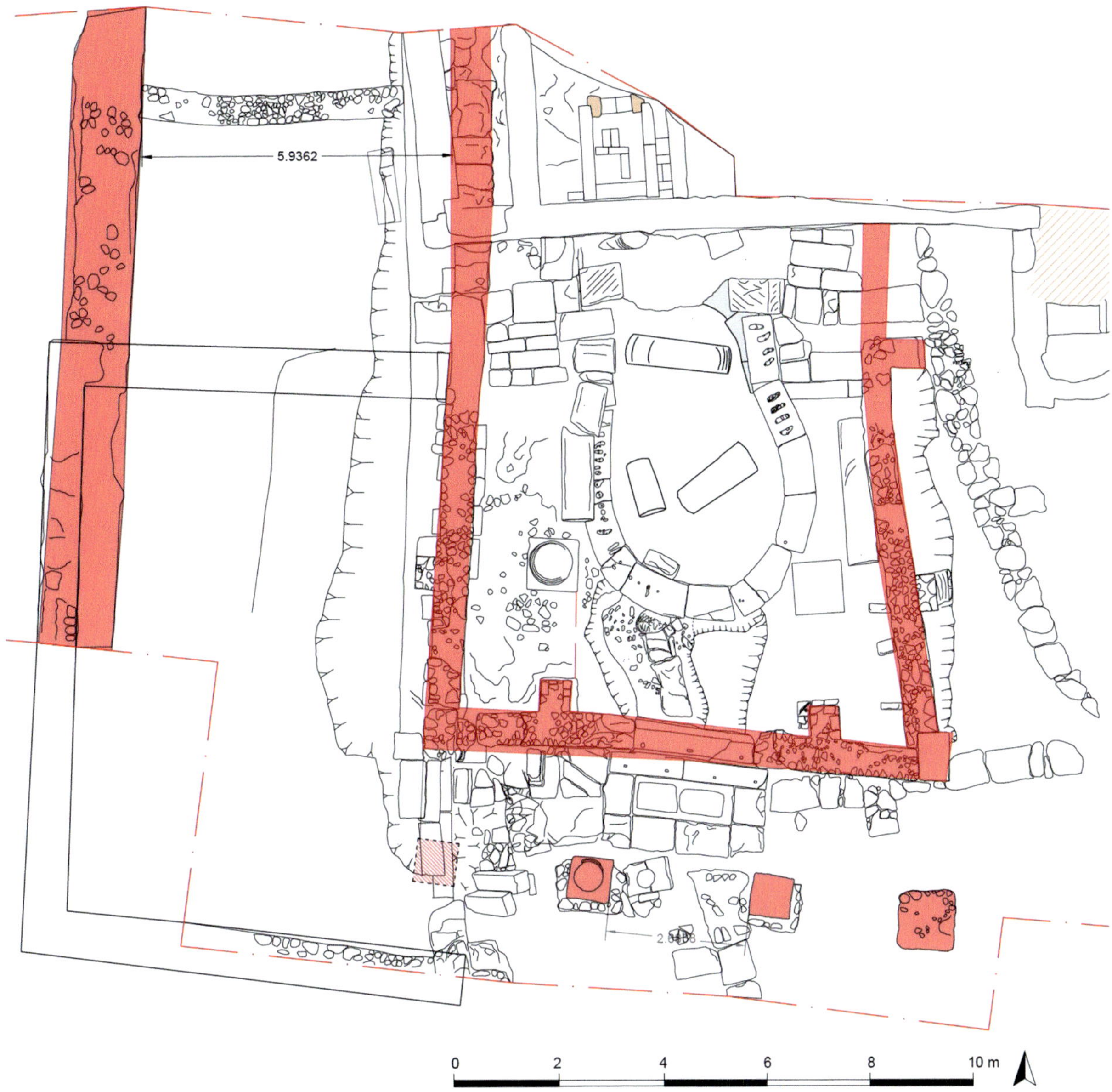

Figure 3. General plan of the site, with the perimeter of the Roman temple highlighted (after Mariotti 2023).

our reconstructions of this part of the temple must be considered hypothetical.

In the southern part of the sacred building, three column bases of the entrance propylaeum have been identified. The two central plinths are preserved, one with an Attic base,[7] while the third base is lost.[8] The distance between the columns is 2.66m, corresponding to 9 Roman feet,[9] while the entire wheelbase corresponds to 3.55m, equal to 12 Roman feet. The third plinth was located at the south-eastern corner of the building, and it is preserved only in its preparation, that was unearthed during the 2023 excavation campaign. A fourth column at the south-western corner probably collapsed between the 3rd and 4th centuries CE and completed the architectural system of the façade of the temple. Therefore, the sacred building must have had a tetrastyle entrance (Mariotti 2023: 34-35) (Figure 3).

Inside the building, the sacred pool occupied a large part of the available space. The sacred pool extends from south to north, with an elongated shape, of probably 30 feet[10] in length. However, geophysical analyses indicate a possible total extension of the

[7] No. 3 in the catalogue of architectural decorations in Camporeale 2021: 180, tab. 2.

[8] No. 4 in the catalogue of architectural decorations in Camporeale 2021: 180, tab. 2.

[9] References are intended to the accepted metric equivalent for the Roman foot (*pes*) of 29.6cm. Hultsch 1882.

[10] If our hypothesis (30 feet) is correct, the length of the pool, whatever the shape of the structures around or above it, would correspond to that of the south front (entrance) of the building.

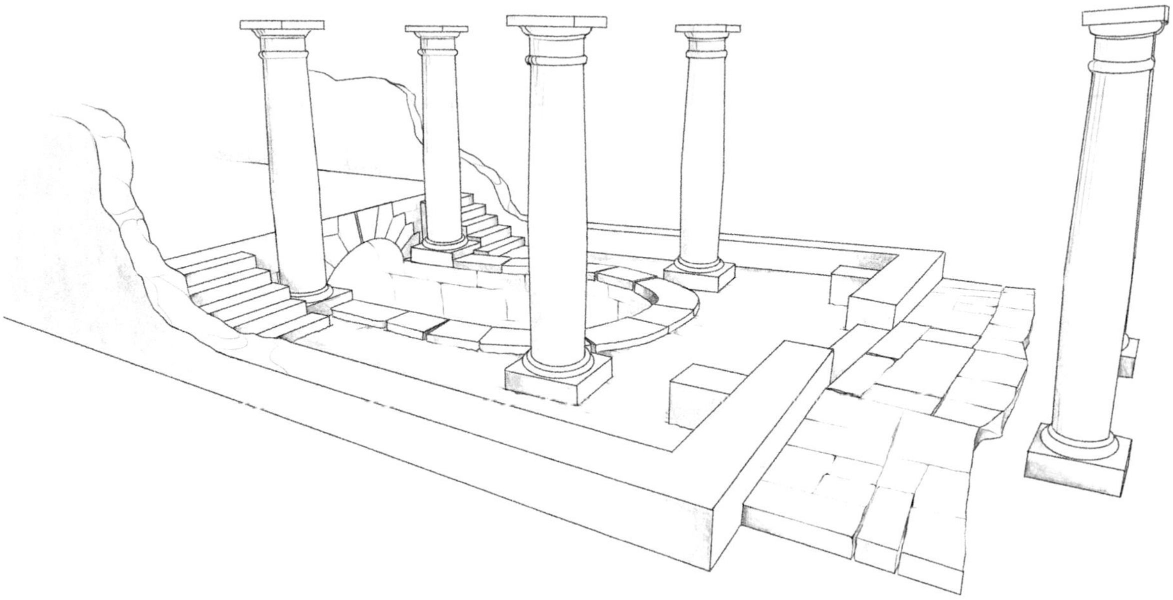

Figure 4. Hypothetical view of the temple (drawing by G. Ghelli and C. Felici, after Mariotti and Carpentiero 2023).

entire sacred building for approximately 50 feet to the north, thus ending close to the modern structures. For what is visible after the end of the 2023 excavation campaign, the pool an apsidal shape on the southern edge, continuing northwards with straight walls, with maximum width of 3.26m, equal to 11 Roman feet for a visible length of 5.32m, equal to 18 Roman feet (Figure 4).

An arch made of travertine squared blocks - 3.80m wide, equal to 13 Roman feet – have been found with some blocks still *in situ,* on both sides. This arch probably marked the separation between the southern part of the building and the northern part, allowing also for the creation of spaces at different elevation. On the west side of the pool, a staircase was located, with at least three steps preserved, having a tread of approximately 30cm each one. On the east side, there must have also been a similar staircase, where only one step is preserved. Here, however, late Renaissance interventions have affected this side of the structure, because of the overlapping presence of the baths that were created around the spring after 1575. The presence of the arch and steps, on both sides of the pool, suggests that the building was elevated in its northern portion towards the spring, thus creating a sort of 'podium' (Figure 5). Collapsed architectural elements within the sacred pool appear to be portions of a 'vaulted' canal of brick and mortar. Although there is no decisive evidence at the current state of research, it cannot be excluded that the northern part of the pool was therefore entirely covered.

The discovery of portions of columns and travertine stonework inside the pool, in addition to those already identified, allows for the reconstruction of the height and number of the Tuscan columns that held the inner structure, aligning on both long sides of the pool.[11] Thirteen travertine parts, already identified in 2020-2021, are related to the decoration of the building,[12] including 4 attic bases, 2 Tuscan capitals, 6 portions of columns and a corbel. In addition, two more column portions were recovered inside the pool during the excavation of 2022, for a total of 8 remaining parts. Considering that the columns inside the building must have reached a height of 15 feet (or 4.44m),[13] a minimum number of four columns - or more likely six - can be identified. Looking from the complete excavation plan and trying to define the original architectural design, the general measurements seem to follow the Roman foot measurements, and in particular, it is possible to notice a recurrence of multiples of 3 foot[14] (Figure 4).

[11] On the problem of roofing in hot *balneas*, see in general Vitr., V, 10. This issue also concerns the general appearance of the building, its inner porch and its roof.

[12] For the catalogue of architectural decorations, see Camporeale 2021: 180, tab. 2.

[13] According to Camporeale, following the Vitruvian proportion (the height of Tuscan column is equal to seven times its lower diameter), it is possible to reconstruct a height of 15 feet, or 4.44m, starting from a diameter of 64.5cm for the inner columns, and 3.50m for the outer columns of the propylaeum (starting from a base diameter of 50cm) (Camporeale 2021: 182).

[14] The width of the façade wall of 8.90m correspond to 30 feet, the width of the pool to 4.45m (15 feet). The total length of the building that can be reconstructed on the basis of resistivity anomalies also seems to be within the range of 45-50m.

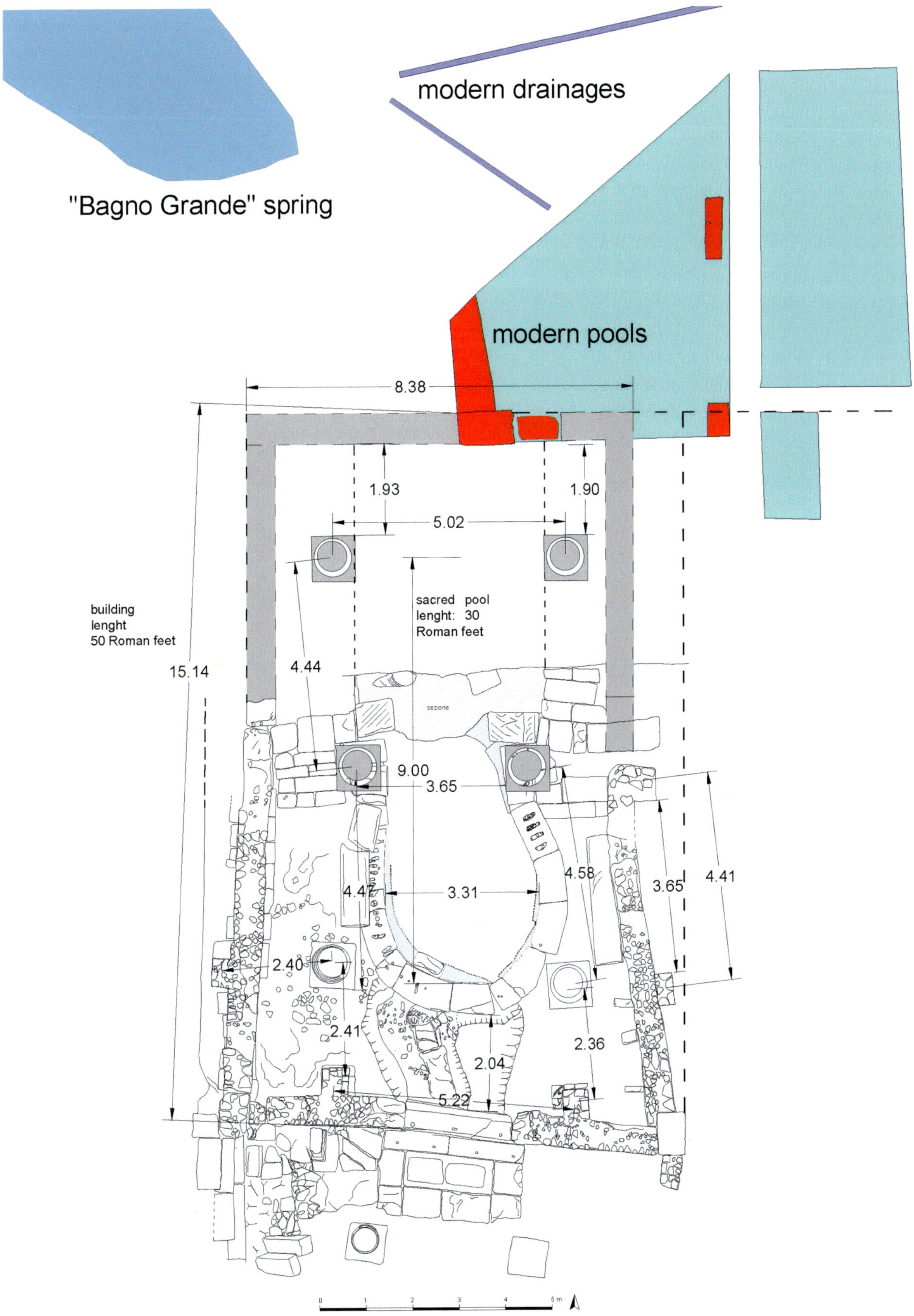

Figure 5. Reconstruction of the ideal measurements in Roman times (after Mariotti 2023).

From a functional point of view, we face a building that, in the early Imperial age, and particularly in the first thirty years of the 1st century CE, must have housed the 'sacred pool' located south to the spring, thus delimiting the sacred space and the healthy waters near the spring. From this point of view, the pool - surmounted by a large supporting arch and flanked by two flights of stairs, which allowed access to an upper level - conferred a 'cave-like conformation' to the structure, which is typical for spring sanctuaries of the pre-Roman and Roman age. This subdivision of spaces could also correspond to a functional and ritual division. The southern part of the sacred pool was open-air, allowing for the sacred water to receive offerings, on top of the earlier *fulmen conditum*. The northern portion at a higher elevation, probably with a podium, had the water flowing into a 'canal' perhaps vaulted and covered. The presence in this norther part of fallen other *ex votos*, such as *arae* and 'donari', as well as *ornamenta*, such as marble statues, suggest that ritual and votive actions were also taking place in this area, although the excavation is still preliminary.[15]

Inside the building, the columns around the sacred pool held the roof. On the southern façade wall, a propylaeum, formed by the above mentioned four columns and probably surmounted by a double-pitched roof, must have given monumentality to the entrance.

Therefore, in an effort to try to identify the original construction project of the building, we realized that perhaps the original idea was never actually put into practice. In other words, it is likely that the masonry emerging from the excavation was not only based on a construction project, that was built from scratch, based on a pre-established module, but also it was the result of subsequent adaptations to pre-existing structures. It is indeed possible to refer the adopted architectural solution to the presence of a monumental (or partially monumental) structure that already existed at an earlier period. The votive offerings from the 3rd-2nd centuries BCE, later deposited at the bottom of the pool at the time of the construction in the Tiberian period, refer to this earlier period (Mariotti, Tabolli and Salvi 2023). In any case, the Bagno Grande sanctuary must have been part of a larger complex with cult buildings, other therapeutic structures, in addition to other possible thermal baths that were open to the public and structures related to the practice of medicine (Mariotti, Salvi and Tabolli 2023).

Are there comparanda for the sanctuary of Bagno Grande?

On the basis of the information gained so far from the excavation, the typological peculiarity of the Etruscan and Roman architecture of Bagno Grande stands out. In fact, no precise comparisons can be identified, but rather general references based on some elements of similarity, in contexts that are sometimes distant, both geographically and chronologically.

The monumentalization of the spring identifies San Casciano as a true 'spring sanctuary' (Gros 2001: 492-495; Scheid 1991; Scheid 2007-2008) with a complex monumental apparatus around the *krene* (the spring). The first construction phase of the sanctuary must have presented the spring in its natural form, with minimal architectural additions,[16] as in the thermal sites of Valchetta near Veio,[17] in Bath (*Aquae Sulis* in England) and Baden (*Aquae Helveticae*) in Switzerland (Yegül 1992). As in the examples of *Aquae Helveticae* or *Augusta Traiana* in Bulgaria, at a second stage often rectangular rooms with large baths occupying almost the entire space of the structure represent the most characteristic element of roman bath sites (Yegül 1992: 111).

A more advanced stage in the development of thermo-mineral spas involves the combination of several naturally heated thermal environments and artificially heated ones, up to the creation of full-fledged thermal spas, such as the examples of Civitavecchia and Bath (Yegül 1992: 111).

In the case of Bagno Grande, the pool located next to the spring accommodates the sacred waters coming from the spring, as it is the case with Bagno di Romagna (Ortalli 2004) (near Forlì-Cesena), which was built on an initial nucleus, dating to the end of the 2nd century CE and then enlarged in the 1st-2nd century CE and used until the 5th century CE. In *Aquae Tauri* in Civitavecchia, at the site of the Ficoncella, the *calidarium* consists of a large pool, entirely carved and modelled in the travertine bedrock, fed by at least three hot water springs that reached it by means of channels, that were also carved in the rock (Yegül 1992: 111-117; Chellini 2002: 88-94).

The explicit process of monumentalization of the spring at Bagno Grande find a good comparison in the Roman sanctuary of Aisillo at Bevagna, in the province of Perugia (Albanesi and Picuti 2009: 133-179). Here, recent excavations, carried out by the Archaeological Superintendency of Umbria between 2002 and 2005,

[15] Travertine altars and denarii were found during the 2023 excavation in the sacred pool, with early imperial inscriptions (under study), and parts of marble statues (possibly an Apollo). These objects were deposited (and even thrown) into the sacred pool when it was closed at the beginning of the 5th century CE.

[16] Yegül 1992: 110. This would represent the first stage of development of thermo-mineral thermal sites.

[17] Better known as the Queen's Baths. Chellini 2002: 81-82; Fusco 2011: 262.

brought to light an area organized around a circular pool and a courtyard with portico, surrounded by various rooms with different functions. In this case, the organization of the spaces and the recovered materials suggest that the structure was in use from the 2nd century BCE and at least until the 3rd century CE. This chronological span is quite similar to the ancient life of Bagno Grande. Other examples of monumental spaces related to sacred springs appear in sites such as Fordongianus in Sardinia, *Aquae Flaviae* in Portugal, or *Aquae Iasae* in Croatia (Bacchus and Serra 1998: 1213-1255; Carneiro 2016: 289-298; Kusan Špalj 2015). They feature organized spaces, porticoes, large paved areas for the reception of visitors, as well as steps to descend into the pool (*piscinae* as *natatio*).

The Bagno Grande differs from all these sites for two reasons: a) at the moment, no structures have been identified that would allow for the descend into the sacred pool, which did not function as a *natatio*, also due to the depth of the pool itself, about 4m[18] (we must imagine removable elements that would allow access for the maintenance of the pool itself); b) the tetrastyle entrance and the podium in the northern part of the building represent a significant difference from the architecture of sites known.

The sanctuary of the Bagno Grande appears to be the core of a large and articulated system, even if it is still largely 'invisible'. Despite the small excavation area - when compared to the ancient extent of the site (of approximately 4 hectares) - the topography of the site is becoming to be increasingly clearer, as demonstrated by the presence of the large wall in mixed work in the western portion of the excavation area: the structure, although identified only for a few meters and with multiple reconstructions, seems to delineate the *tèmenos* of the imperial period. To the north of the spring, on the other hand, there is a concrete building, already surveyed in the 2017 archaeological map (Pocobelli 2021: 121-130) and hypothetically interpreted as a cistern for collecting drinking rainwater.[19] On the adjacent plateau, to the east, geophysical surveys ascertained the presence of other structures (Felici and Morelli 2023: 20-27; Carpentiero and Felici 2021: 131-144). The spring, therefore, and the described sacred complex, were surrounded by structures whose destination is still unknown and that represent one of the future objectives of our research.

[18] There was a channel for the outflow of water located in the southern part of the sacred pool and indicated by the projecting bas-relief of a bull (Mariotti 2023a). The canal, identified by the excavations of 2023, continued outside the sanctuary towards the south-east.

[19] This hypothesis remains to be confirmed: the building, although clearly of Roman date and with external *opus caementicium*, is currently occupied by a shed for farming and therefore is only partially visible.

Bibliography:

Albanesi, M. and M.R. Picuti 2009. Un luogo di culto d'epoca romana all'Aisillo di Bevagna. *Mélanges d'École française de Rome*, Antiquité 121, n°1: 133-179.

Arbeid, B. 2023. Ex-voto dalla stipe di Doccia della Testa, in M. Osanna and J. Tabolli (eds) *Gli dei ritornano. I bronzi di San Casciano*: 66-69. Rome: Treccani.

Bacchus, G. and P.B. Serra 1998. Forum Traiani: il contesto termale e l'indagine archeologica di scavo, in M. Khanoussi, P. Ruggeri, C. Vismara (eds), *L'Africa romana, Atti del XII Convegno di studio (Olbia, 12-15 dicembre 1996)*: 1213-1255. Sassari: Editrice Democratica Sarda.

Bassani, M., M. Bolder-Boss and U. Fusco 2019 (eds). *Rethinking the Concept of 'Healing Settlements': Water, Cults, Constructions and Contexts in the Ancient World*. Padua: Archaeopress.

Camporeale, S. 2021. L'architettura del santuario: materiali da costruzione, tecniche edilizie e decorazioni, in E. Mariotti and J. Tabolli (eds) *Il Santuario Ritrovato. Nuovi Scavi e Ricerche al Bagno Grande di San Casciano dei Bagni*: 171-186. Livorno: Sillabe.

Caracciolo, G. 2021. Prima degli scavi: le iscrizioni pro salute dal Bagno Grande, in E. Mariotti and J. Tabolli (eds) *Il Santuario Ritrovato. Nuovi Scavi e Ricerche al Bagno Grande di San Casciano dei Bagni*: 187-191. Livorno: Sillabe.

Carneiro, S. 2016. The water supply and drainage system of the Roman healing spa of Chaves (Aquae Flaviae), in J.M.F Garrido, A. Formella, J.A.F. Brea, M.G. Gesteira, F.P. Fermín Pérez Losada and V.R. Vázquez (eds) *Termalismo y Calidad de Vida, Libro de Actas del I Congreso Internacional de Agua (Ourense (España), 23-24 de septiembre de 2015)*: 289-298. Ourense: Universidade de Vigo.

Carpentiero, M.G. and C. Felici 2021. Topografia e indagini non invasive nell'area del Bagno Grande: ricostruzione della viabilità storica e del paesaggio antico di età romana, in E. Mariotti and J. Tabolli (eds) *Il Santuario Ritrovato. Nuovi Scavi e Ricerche al Bagno Grande di San Casciano dei Bagni*: 131-144. Livorno: Sillabe.

Chellini, R. 2002. *Salutary and sacred spring waters in Etruria (Italiae Regio VII). Archaeological research and ancient topography*. Oxford: BAR.

Felici, C. and G. Morelli 2023. La geofisica del santuario, in E. Mariotti, J. Tabolli and A. Salvi (eds) 2023. *Il Santuario Ritrovato 2. Dentro la Vasca Sacra. Rapporto Preliminare di Scavo*: 21-28. Livorno: Sillabe.

Fortini, A., M. Ledda and P. Morelli 2023. Senza soluzione di continuità: il Bagno Grande dalla tarda antichità ad oggi, in E. Mariotti, J. Tabolli and A. Salvi (eds) 2023. *Il Santuario Ritrovato 2. Dentro la Vasca Sacra. Rapporto Preliminare di Scavo*: 71-85. Livorno: Sillabe.

Fusco, U. 2011. Archeologia dell'acqua: il sito di Campetti a Veio (Roma), in M. Bassani, M. Bressan and F. Ghedini (eds) Aquae Patavinae. *Il termalismo antico nel comprensorio euganeo e in Italia. Proceedings of the First National Conference (Padua, 21-22 June 2010)*: 261-279. Padua: Padua University Press.

Gregori, G.L. 2023. Le iscrizioni latine su votivi di bronzo: divinità, devoti, formulari, in E. Mariotti, A. Salvi and J. Tabolli (eds) *Il Santuario Ritrovato 2. Dentro la Vasca Sacra. Rapporto Preliminare di Scavo:* 195-204. Livorno: Sillabe.

Gros, P. 2001. *L'architettura romana dal III sec a.C. alla fine dell'alto impero II d.C.* Milano: Longanesi.

Hultsch, F.O. 1882. *Griechische und römische Metrologie.* Berlin: Weidmann.

Iosso, M. 2003 (ed.). *Iacta stips. Il deposito votivo della sorgente di Doccia della Testa a San Casciano dei Bagni,* Florence: Polistampa.

Kušan Špalj, D. 2015. *Aquae Iasae. Nova otkrića iz rimskog razdoblja na području Varaždinskih Toplica. Recent discoveries of Roman remains in the region of Varaždinske Toplice.* Zagreb.

Maggiani A. 2023. Le iscrizioni etrusche su votivi di bronzo. Le divinità e i suoi devoti, in Mariotti, E., Salvi, A. and Tabolli J. (eds) *Il Santuario Ritrovato 2. Dentro la Vasca Sacra. Rapporto Preliminare di Scavo:* 181-193. Livorno: Sillabe.

Mariotti, E. and Tabolli, J. (eds) 2021. *Il Santuario Ritrovato. Nuovi Scavi e Ricerche al Bagno Grande di San Casciano dei Bagni,* Livorno: Sillabe.

Mariotti, E. 2023a. Il Bagno Grande in the 2021 and 2022 excavation campaigns, in E. Mariotti, J. Tabolli and A. Salvi (eds) 2023. *Il Santuario Ritrovato 2. Dentro la Vasca Sacra. Rapporto Preliminare di Scavo*: 29-48. Livorno: Sillabe.

Mariotti, E. 2023b. Afrodite ai Bagni, in M. Osanna and J. Tabolli (eds) *Gli dei ritornano. I bronzi di San Casciano*: 70-71. Rome: Treccani.

Mariotti, E. 2021. Il Santuario Rivelato: gli scavi 2019 e 2020 al Bagno Grande, in E. Mariotti and J. Tabolli (eds) *Il Santuario Ritrovato. Nuovi Scavi e Ricerche al Bagno Grande di San Casciano dei Bagni*: 145-170. Livorno: Sillabe.

Mariotti, E., A. Salvi and J. Tabolli 2023 (eds) *Il Santuario Ritrovato 2. Dentro la Vasca Sacra. Rapporto Preliminare di Scavo.* Livorno: Sillabe.

Ortalli, J. 2004. *Bagno di Romagna nell'antichità. Le terme, l'insediamento, il territorio.* Florence: All'Insegna del Giglio.

Osanna, M. and J. Tabolli 2023 (eds). *Gli dei ritornano. I bronzi di San Casciano.* Rome: Treccani.

Pardini, G. 2023. Le offerte monetali nella vasca. Questioni preliminari e prospettive di ricerca, in E. Mariotti, A. Salvi and J. Tabolli (eds) *Il Santuario Ritrovato 2. Dentro la Vasca Sacra. Rapporto Preliminare di Scavo*: 255-268. Livorno: Sillabe.

Pardini, G. and F. Carbone 2023. I rinvenimenti monetali in M. Osanna and J. Tabolli (eds), *Gli dei ritornano. I bronzi di San Casciano.* 148-155. Rome: Treccani

Paolucci, G. 1988a. *Archeologia in Valdichiana.* Chianciano Terme: Multigrafica editrice.

Paolucci, G. 1988b (ed). *I Romani di Chiusi.* Chianciano Terme: Multigrafica editrice.

Pocobelli, G. F. 2021. Il progetto della Carta Archeologica delle 'Acque', in E. Mariotti and J. Tabolli (eds) *Il Santuario Ritrovato. Nuovi Scavi e Ricerche al Bagno Grande di San Casciano dei Bagni*: 121-130. Livorno Sillabe.

Scheid, J. 1991. Sanctuaires et thermes sous l'Empire *romains*, in *Le thermes romains. Actes de la table ronde de Rome*: 205-216. Rome: École Française.

Scheid, J. 2007-2008. Le culte des eaux et des sources dans le monde romain un sujet problématique, déterminé par la mythologie moderne. *Cours et travaux du Collège de France. Résumés. Annuaire* 108: 621-637.

Tabolli, J. 2021. Ai confini meridionali di Chiusi tra Bronzo Finale e prima età del ferro, in E. Mariotti and J. Tabolli (eds) *Il Santuario Ritrovato. Nuovi Scavi e Ricerche al Bagno Grande di San Casciano dei Bagni*: 33-39. Livorno Sillabe.

Tabolli, J. 2023a. Dentro la vasca sacra, in E. Mariotti, A. Salvi and J. Tabolli (eds) *Il Santuario Ritrovato 2. Dentro la Vasca Sacra. Rapporto Preliminare di Scavo*: 101-116. Livorno: Sillabe.

Tabolli, J. 2023b. Tra divinazione e medicina termale, in E. Mariotti, A. Salvi and J. Tabolli (eds) *Il Santuario Ritrovato 2. Dentro la Vasca Sacra. Rapporto Preliminare di Scavo*: 235-247. Livorno: Sillabe.

Tabolli, J. 2023c. The Etruscan and Roman thermo-mineral sanctuary of Bagno Grande at San Casciano dei Bagni (Siena): aims and perspectives 'behind-the-scenes' of the ongoing multidisciplinary research project. *Folder* 556: 1-23.

Tabolli, J. 2023d. Il fulmine in bronzo e la punta di freccia in selce, in M. Osanna and J. Tabolli (eds) *Gli dei ritornano. I bronzi di San Casciano*: 80-81. Rome: Treccani.

Yegül, F. 1992. *Baths and bathing in Classical antiquity.* New York: Mit Pr.

Transformation of Residential Architecture into Private and Public Baths in Late Antique Baiae

Gioconda DI LUCA
Università degli Studi di Roma 'Tor Vergata'
latericium@hotmail.com

Abstract: The setting of Late Antique Baiae (Bacoli, Naples), its architectural transformation and the subsequent changes in everyday life included one important peculiarity that could be considered almost a rule. This was the process of extensive re-arrangement of private houses into private or public *balnea*, attested in numerous examples across the site.

An obviously lucrative business of providing bathing services, accompanied by a number of other social amenities, proliferated across the place quite significantly during the 3th and 4th centuries, and also became the backbone for the establishment of bathing facilities of Late Antique *episcopia*. Processes of transformation of residential into bathing architecture resulted in some quite ingenious solutions.

Considering the outstanding number of cases of these transformative processes in Baiae, I have chosen the most illustrative ones, belonging to similar contexts and sharing the same ideas of creating representative spaces which would cultivate and promote Roman bathing culture.

Thus, these processes will be represented and discussed through some case-studies: *balnea* arranged in private houses using natural hot sulphurous jets, and then balnea in private contexts heated by fire, and bath complexes built *ex novo* by rearranging a previous building or creating new ones.

All the examples, in their architectural planning, purpose and use, testify to changes in local needs during the Late Antique centuries and also demonstrate innovative and interesting improvisations in the process of transformation of residential architecture into places of leisure, body care, healing spa and entertainment across the region, as the contemporary writers say.

Keywords: baths, healing spa, Baiae, Late Antiquity

The setting of Late Antique Baiae, in the Phlegraean Fields, its architectural transformation and the subsequent changes in everyday life included one important peculiarity that could be considered almost a rule. This was the process of extensive re-arrangement of private houses into private or public *balnea*, attested in numerous examples across the site (Figure 1).

An obviously lucrative business of providing bath services, accompanied by different social amenities, proliferated across the place quite significantly during the 3rd and 4th centuries, and also became the backbone for a likely future establishment of bathing facilities of *episcopia*. Processes of transformation of residential into bathing architecture resulted in some quite ingenious solutions.

Most of these transformations were due primarily to changes in social make up of the users of Baiae. The site was always frequented for its thermo-mineral sources, making it an attractive place, also because it was not too far from Rome (Medri 2018; Di Luca 2020; Miniero *et al.* 2022: 325-327). But in Late Antiquity, we are far from the magnificence of the Julio-Claudian age, when the imperial court frequented the *sinus Baianus*. In fact, between the end of the 1st century AD and the Severan age, we witness a phenomenon of abandonment by the capital's upper class and their progressive but inexorable replacement by the local middle class who took full advantage of the lack of interest in Baiae (Di Luca 2020; Miniero *et al.* 2022: 333-334). In Late Antiquity, however, the senatorial elite returned: Baiae was now part of a strategic circuit because of the nearby port of Miseno, one of the main infrastructures supplying Romw. In this dynamic, the small wellness centre with its thermo-mineral waters and still active sulphurous steam is proposed as a functional location for those involved in the arrival of goods in *Misenum*, attracting the new Roman ruling class in Late Antiquity (Figure 2). This situation is familiar to us since the same happens in Ostia due to its relationship with Porto in the same period. But Baiae also offered well-being for body and mind and a landscape.

Considering the outstanding number of cases of these transformative processes in Baiae, I have chosen the most illustrative ones, belonging to similar contexts, and sharing the same ideas of creating representative spaces which would cultivate and promote Roman bathing culture.

Thus, these processes will be represented and discussed through some case studies, divided into three groups:

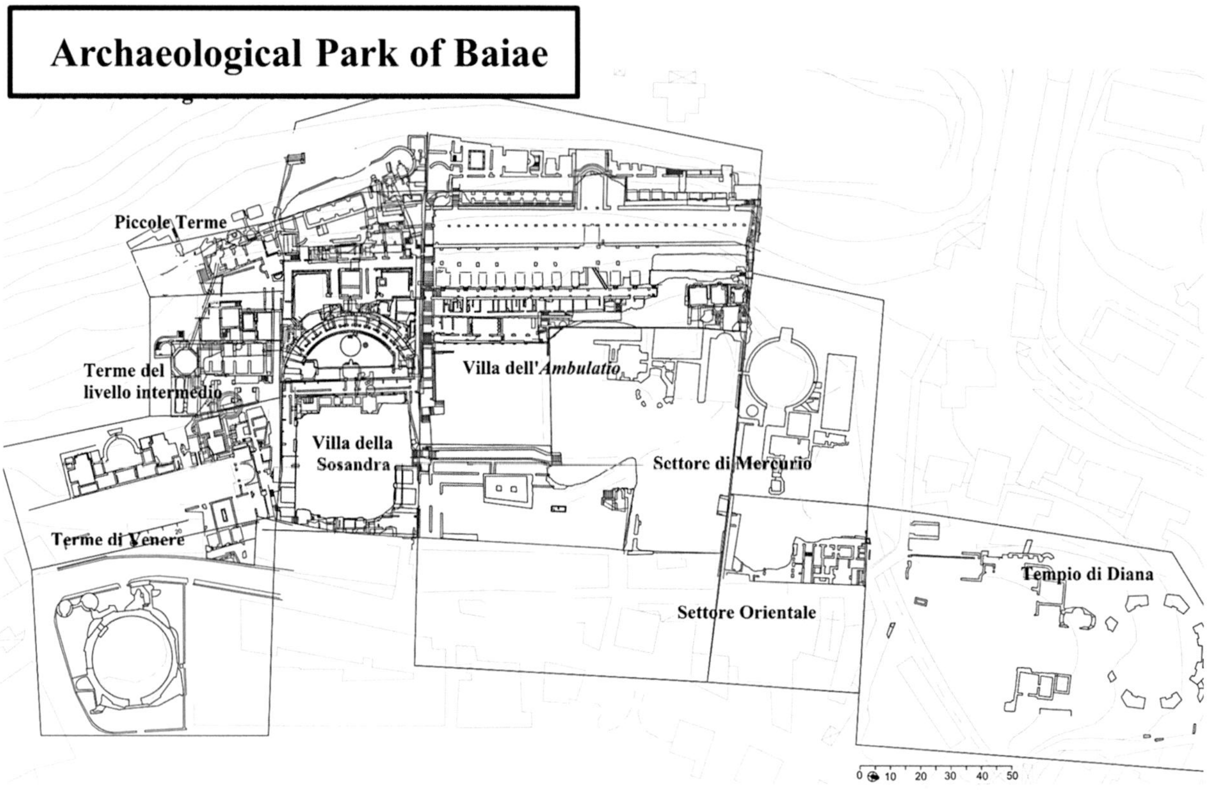

Figure 1. Baiae, Archaeological Park of Baiae. Plan. Reworked from M. Nieberle.

- *balnea* added to private houses using natural sulphurous jets;
- *balnea* in private houses heated by fire;
- bath complexes built *ex novo*, by rearranging a previous building or creating new ones.

The life of the villas on the slopes of the 'Sella di Baia' Hill changes around the second half of the 2nd century AD, when they all became part of a single large property managed by a local businessman and focused on the thermal peculiarity of the whole area: they are all built on terraces and the highest parts continued to be used as residences while the lower terraces started to be turned into bath facilities.

The only building left apart is the so called 'Villa dell'*Ambulatio*' (Giuliani 1977: 372; Di Luca 2009: 151-156 and 164; 2018: 262, 267, 269 and 272; Miniero *et al.* 2022; Di Luca and Cristilli 2023) (Figure 3), because it needs a more in-depth analysis that goes beyond the topic of this paper and for this reason remains outside of my analysis. However, it should be noted that this villa, in the past, has been considered part of the imperial estate at Baiae (De Angelis d'Ossat 1977: 274) and one of the *palatia* represented on the well-known glass flasks (Popkin 2018). But it must be reiterated, however that in Late Antiquity the terms *palatia*, praetorian and *episcopia* define buildings which house different institutions of public power, both secular and religious. In many cases, the buildings are quite similar. This longevity is, at least partially, due to the similarity of their functions: representative spaces, reception halls, baths, rooms for private use, all reflect in the layout and choices of decoration the models chosen by the new elites, according to a shared expressive language that covers the entire Mediterranean area. This is why it is possible that the 'Villa dell'*Ambulatio*' could have been used as a building of this type (Di Luca 2009: 163), escaping the massive transformations of the hill.

The so called 'Villa della Sosandra' together with the next building known as 'Piccole Terme' (Figure 4) look like the most damaged part of the hillside, or the only ones sold for public use and/or used as a public space: in fact, just here many hydraulic systems were built over the years.

The southern side of the villa was actually turned into cisterns of different size, including a very large one probably connected with the Constantinian improvement of the *Aqua Augusta* (Di Luca 2022).

The 'Sosandra' complex includes all three bath types. A private *balneum* was added to a previous vaulted corridor (very well decorated with plasterwork dating back to the late Antonine age) beside a dining

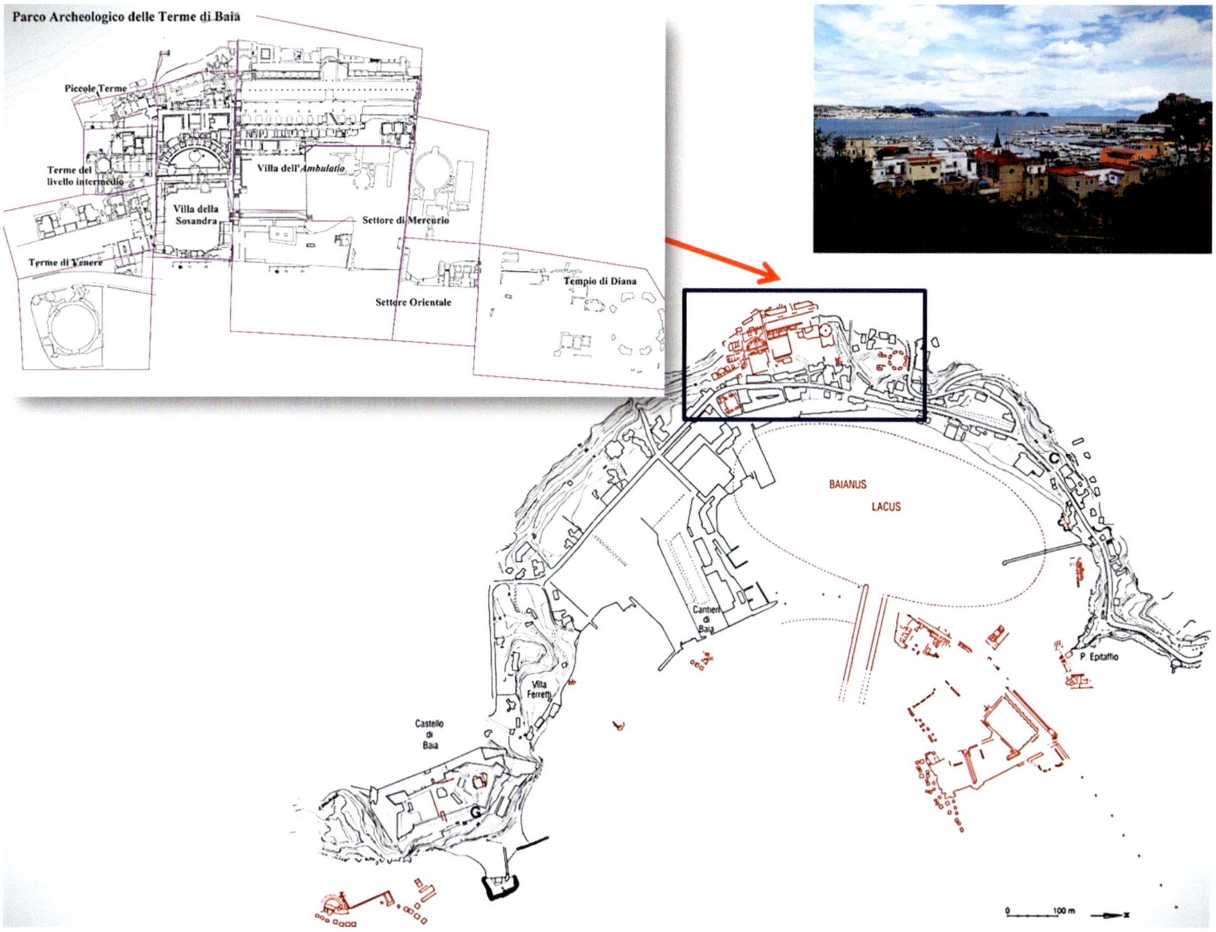

Figure 2. Baiae. The Roman *Baianus sinus*. Plan. Reworked from M. Nieberle and Gianfrotta 2011.

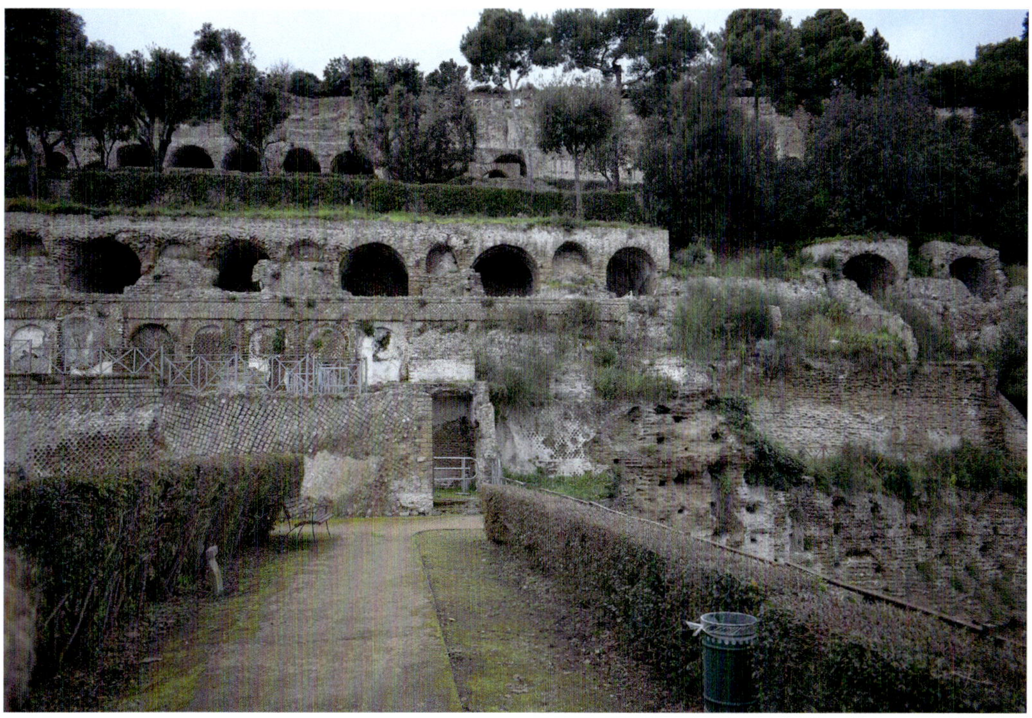

Figure 3. Baiae, Archaeological Park of Baiae. The so-called 'Villa dell'*Ambulatio*'. View of the sea front. Photo by the Author.

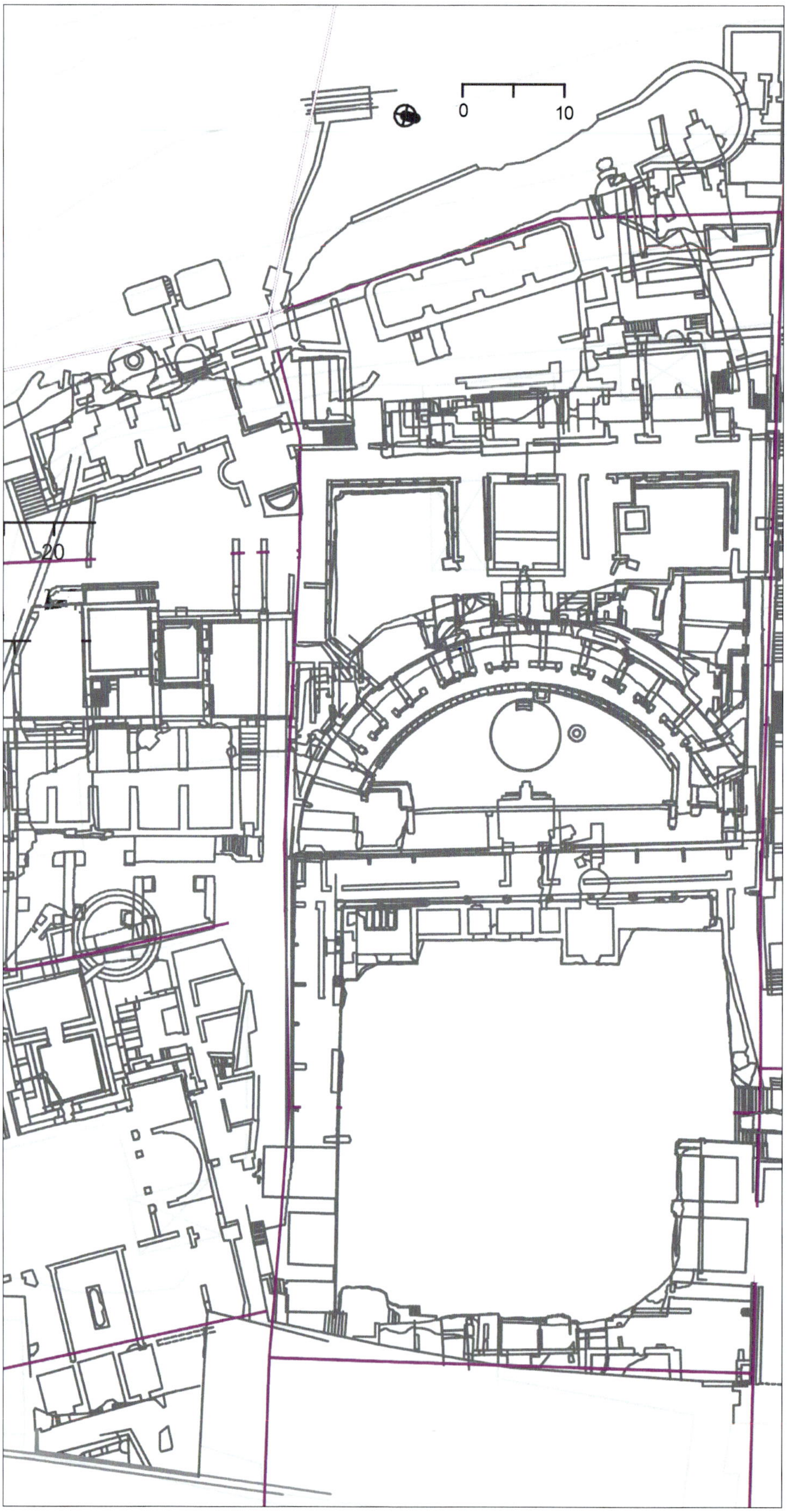

Figure 4. Baiae, Archaeological Park of Baiae. The so-called 'Villa della Sosandra'. Plan. Reworked from M. Nieberle.

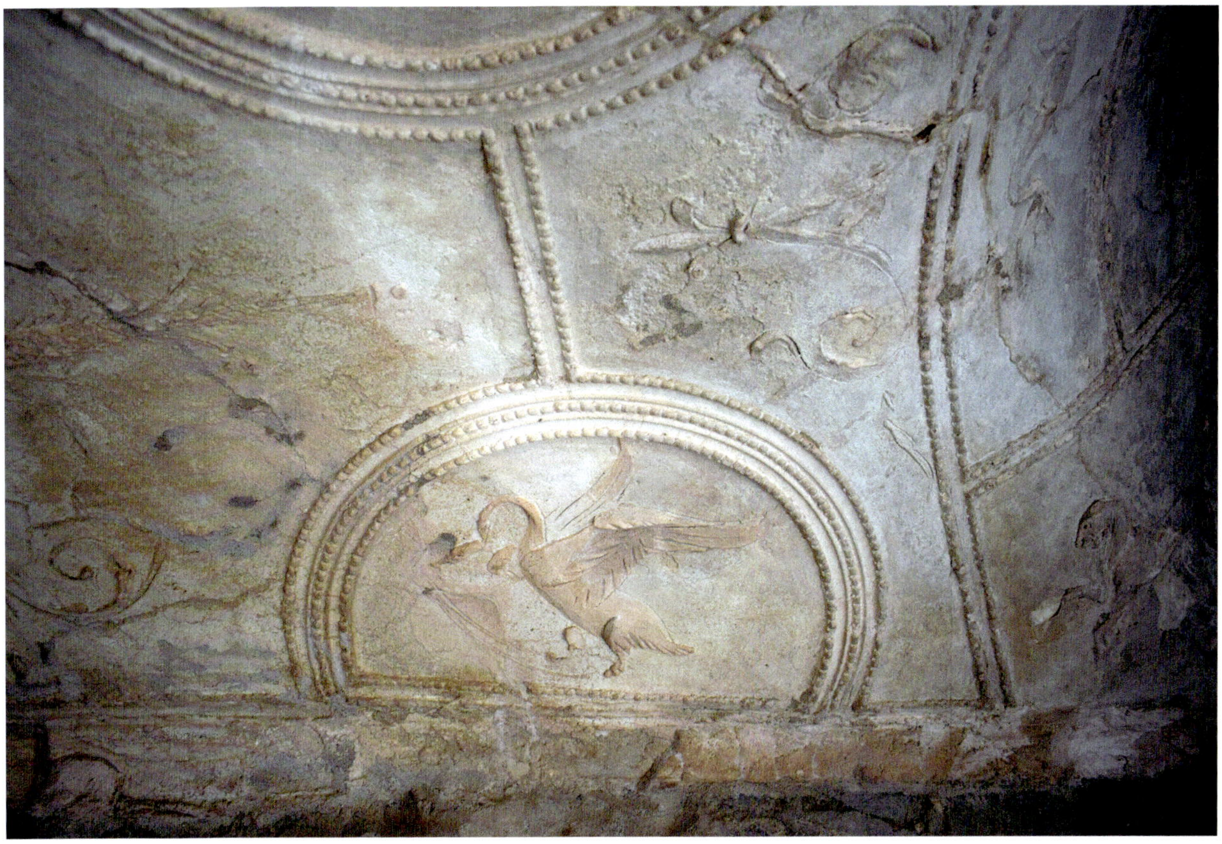

Figure 5. Baiae, Archaeological Park of Baiae. The so-called 'Villa della Sosandra'. The late Antonine plasterwork. Photo by the Author.

room with a system of *alcovae* on the opposite site (Figures 5-6). The *balneum* was heated by a natural hot sulphurous jet coming up from under the same villa where another small bath was completely renovated and enlarged at the same time (Di Luca 2009: 160-161) and maybe turned into a public place (when it belonged to the private villa there was only a *calidarium*, but later an entrance room and a *frigidarium* were added). The evidence of this renovation is still visible all around in particular along the covered corridor running along the northern side and once leading up and down, and then only down, toward the so called 'Piscina'.

At the same time, on the highest terrace, another private and independent small house (Di Luca and Narès 2022) was remodelled using part of a previous long *xystus* with the addition of a large triclinium connected with a *balneum* heated by fire coming from the nearby *culina* (Figure 7). Both rooms were finely decorated with frescoes and marble *sectilia*, including an elegant floor in marble ('Breccia nuvolata rosa'), dating to the 4th century AD (Figure 8).

Also, some extensive interventions carried out on the lower portico, once focused on a central *ninfeo* with an impressive waterfall and served by side corridors decorated with elegant painting and marble *sectilia.* Now this portico was divided into multiple rooms to house the customers of the near bathhouses, disfiguring its original arrangement (Di Luca 2009: 160) (Figure 9). Its decoration is highly elaborate and exhibits well the restoration works of the 1st, 2nd, 3rd and at least 4th centuries AD (Narès 2018; Di Luca 2023).

Beside the Villa of Sosandra a new public bath complex is known as 'Terme del Livello intermedio', because it is situated between the two oldest bathhouses. This spa was built up by demolishing and reusing the previous buildings (Figure 10): the one on the top of hill is the oldest of the whole area, dating back to the Republican age (the so called 'Piccole Terme'), while the other at the bottom is known as 'Stanze di Venere' (Figures 11-12).

The new complex rests on artificial terraces. The upper terrace, extended to the east, is supported by a system of huge substructures. The masonry is made of yellow tuff stones and bricks but only the pillars are in *opus listatum* (alternating a row of tuff stones and two rows of bricks), probably for better weight distribution and strengthening. Basically, the whole building is a scenographic scaffolding to support the upper level,

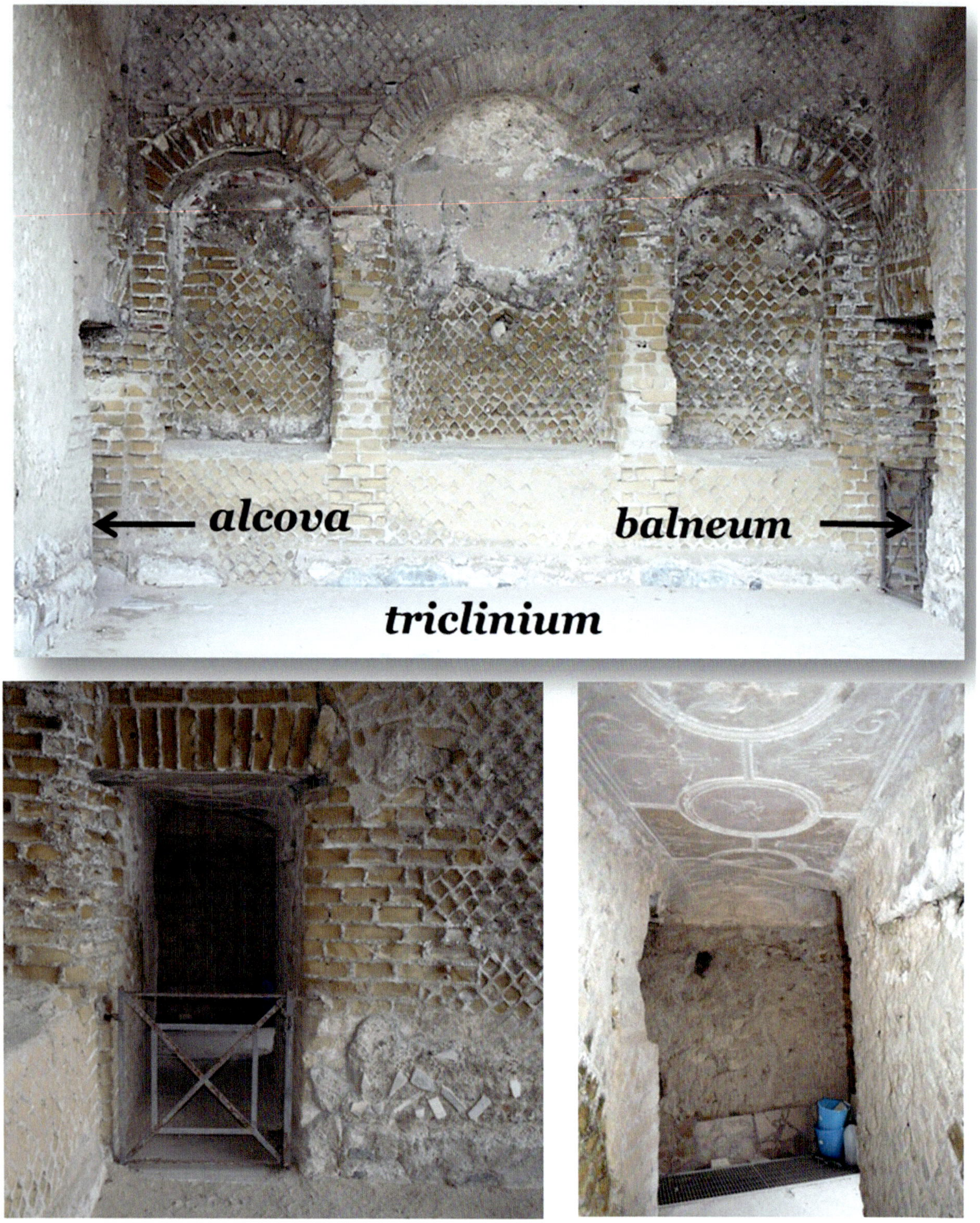

Figure 6. Baiae, Archaeological Park of Baiae. The so-called 'Villa della Sosandra'. The dining room with *alcovae* on the opposite site. Photo by the Author.

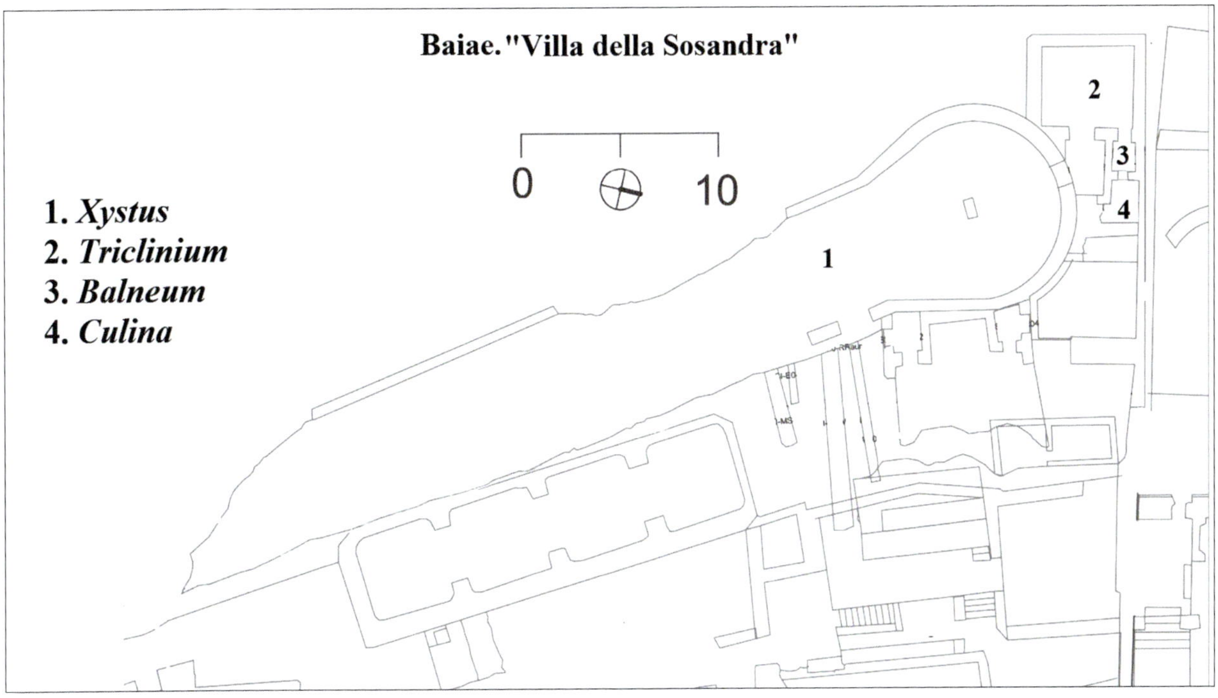

Figure 7. Baiae, Archaeological Park of Baiae. The so-called 'Villa della Sosandra'. The highest terrace. Plan. Reworked from M. Nieberle.

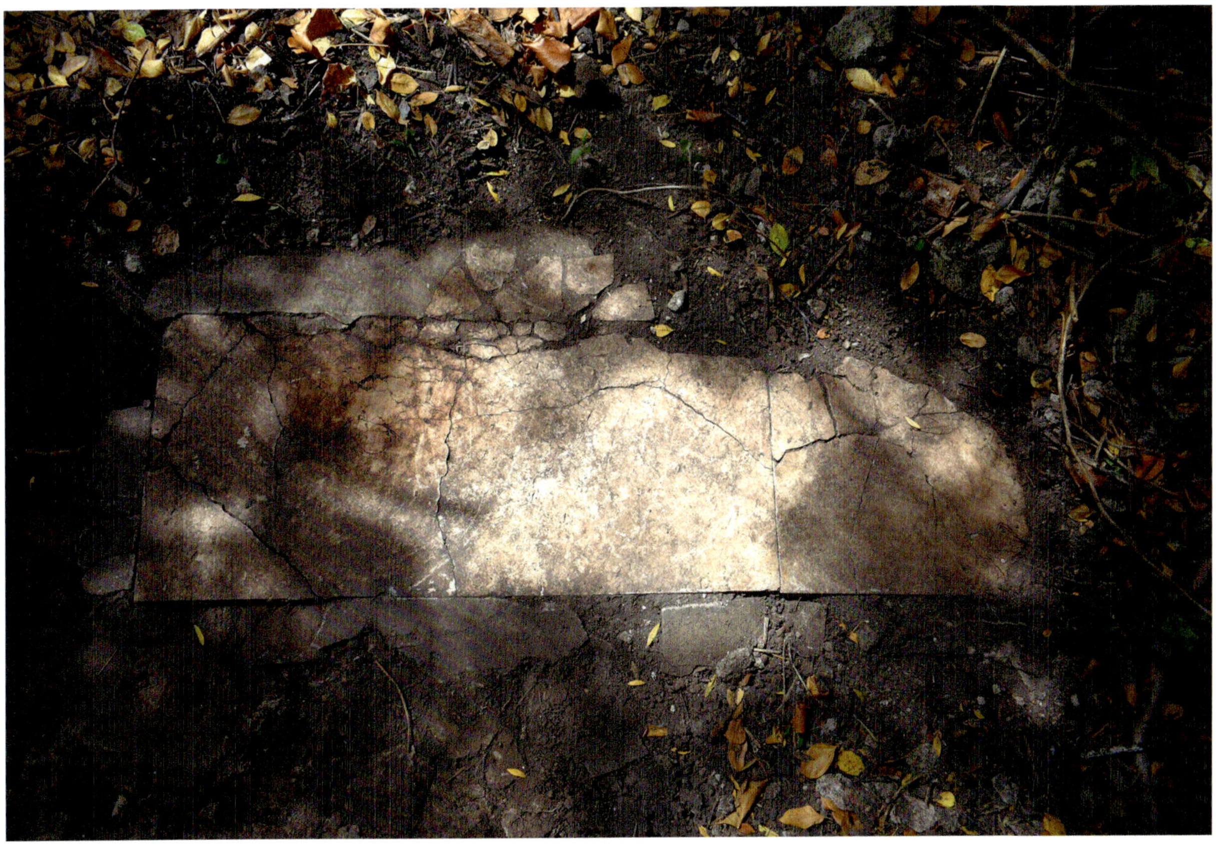

Figure 8. Baiae, Archaeological Park of Baiae. The so-called 'Villa della Sosandra'. The highest terrace (the *triclinium* floor). Photo by the Author.

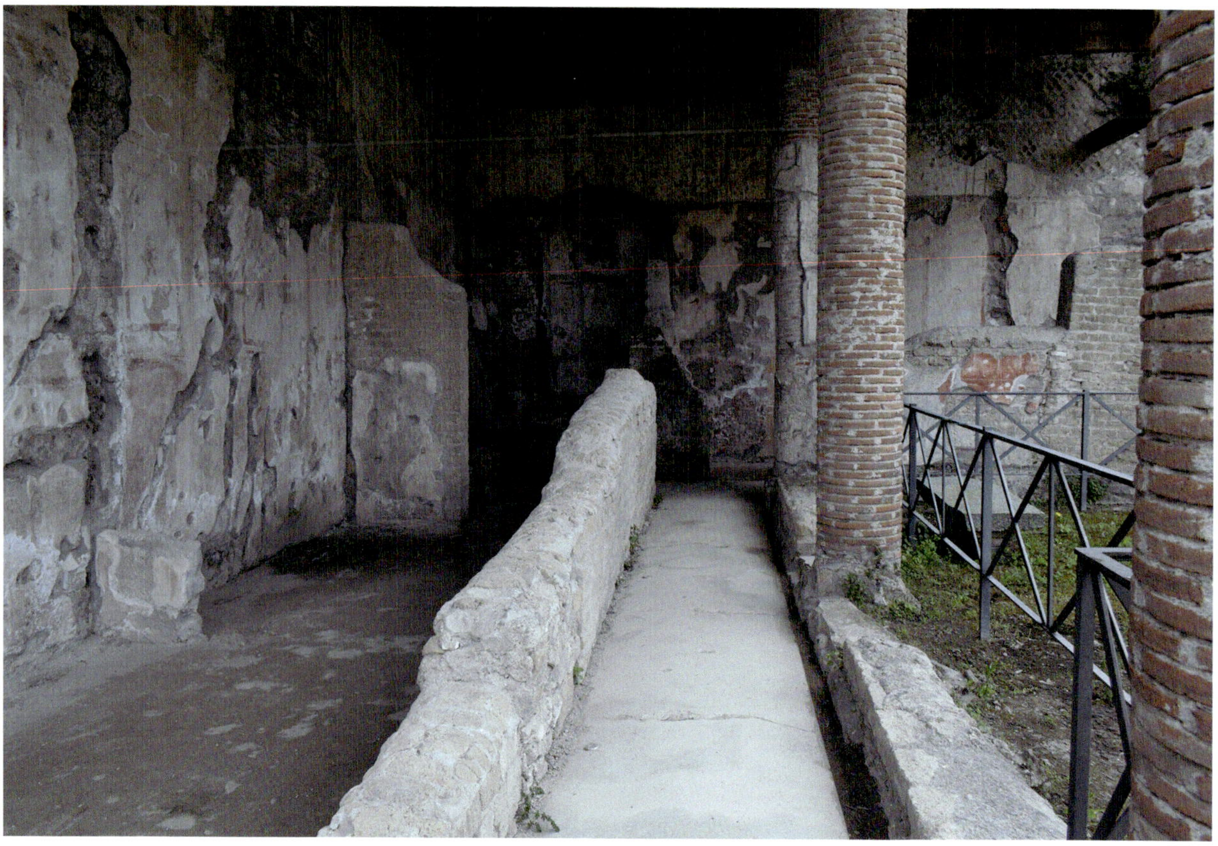

Figure 9. Baiae, Archaeological Park of Baiae. The so-called 'Villa della Sosandra'. The lowest terrace portico. Photo by the Author.

the true spa. The rooms of the lower levels are only service and storage rooms.

The so called 'Piccole Terme' (Figure 11) once comprised only two rooms (a *laconicum* and a *calidarium*) heated by the most famous hot sulphurous jet of the area. Here, heat came directly from natural volcanic underground sources. A long sloping passage explored in the 1960s and named 'Great Antrum' was used as a steam system to serve the surface bath (Medri *et al.* 1999; Di Luca 2009: 161-162; Medri 2013). The addition here of a new *frigidarium* demonstrates its transformation into a public place (Di Luca 2009: 162; Medri 2013).

The 'Stanze di Venere' (Figure 12), instead, were once a small thermal complex with a *tepidarium*, a *calidarium* and a *laconicum*, then turned into cisterns connected with the *Aqua Augusta* water (as the deep layers of limestone show). They were part of a private or public spa, but it is almost impossible to say more, because it has been partially destroyed by the 'Terme del Livello Intermedio'. We can only have an idea of when it was originally built thanks to the beautiful ceiling plasterwork, dating to the mid-1st century AD.

For many natural reasons – bradyseism, the Mount Vesuvius volcanic activity or climate change – the hot steaming jet coming from the 'Great Antrum' (Figure 13) became more powerful over the years, explaining the large number of *calidaria* built in this part of the Sella di Baia Hill (Medri 2018). Thus, in Late Antiquity there were, on the one hand *calidaria* heated by natural steam on the upper part of the hill, on the other large *natationes* of warm water coming up from mineral springs (still active) on the lower part.

Another private house (Figure 14) – the last of this short presentation – was adapted into the public area known as 'Terme di Venere', dating back to the Hadrianic age and once a luxury bathhouse then abandoned or used for different purpose. Part of it was turned into a house, with many rooms and a garden to welcome guests, including a dining room with a *balneum* heated by fire controlled from a nearby large *culina* (the same system for the *balneum* of the house with *xystus* in the upper level of the 'Villa della Sosandra'). The *sectilia* decorating floors and walls show us an elaborate residence on the model of the aristocratic houses of Ostia or Rome at the same time.

In conclusion, all these examples, in their architectural planning, purpose and use, testify to changes in local needs during the Late Antique centuries and also demonstrate innovative and interesting improvisations

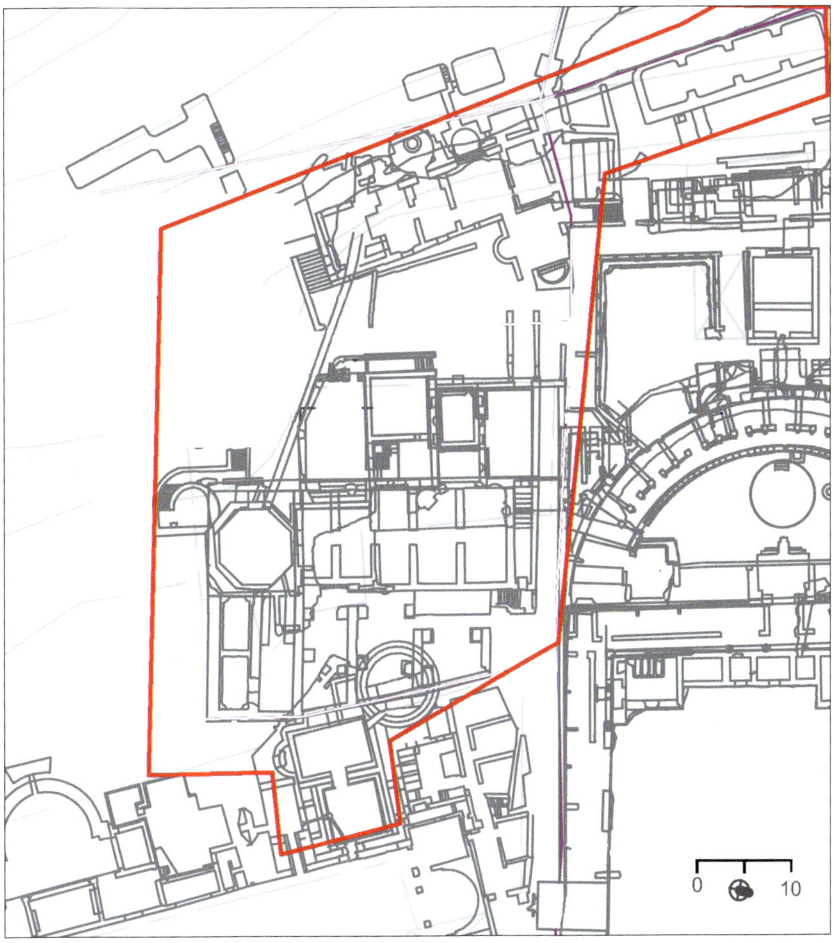

Figure 10. Baiae, Archaeological Park of Baiae. The so-called 'Terme del Livello intermedio'. Plan. Reworked from M. Nieberle.

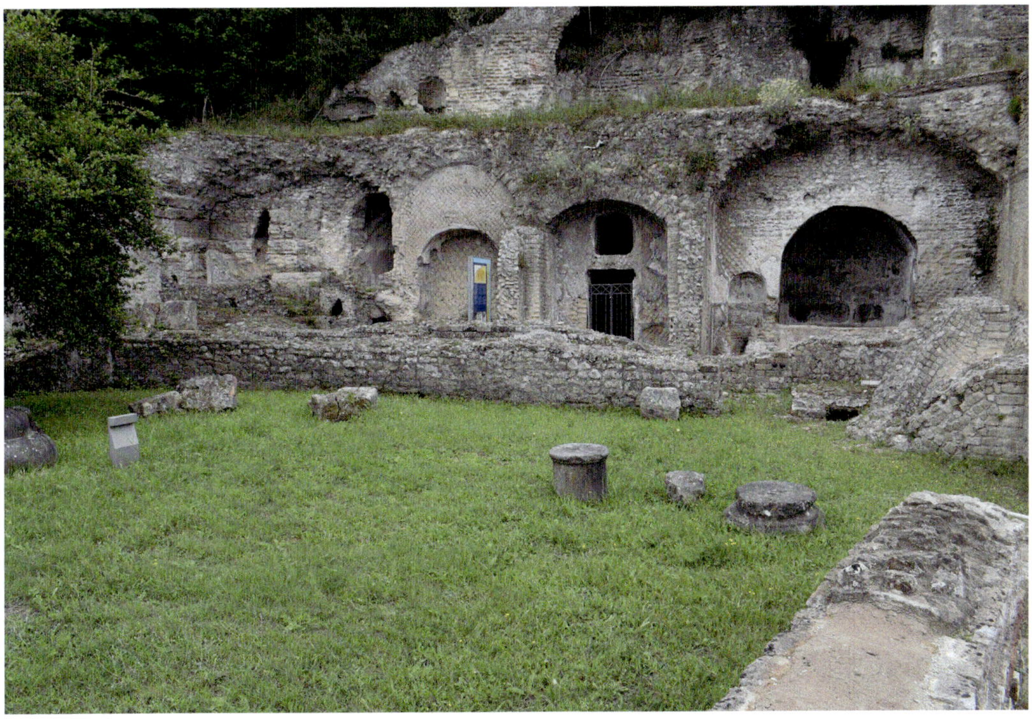

Figure 11. Baiae, Archaeological Park of Baiae. The so-called 'Piccole Terme'. View of the sea front. Photo by the Author.

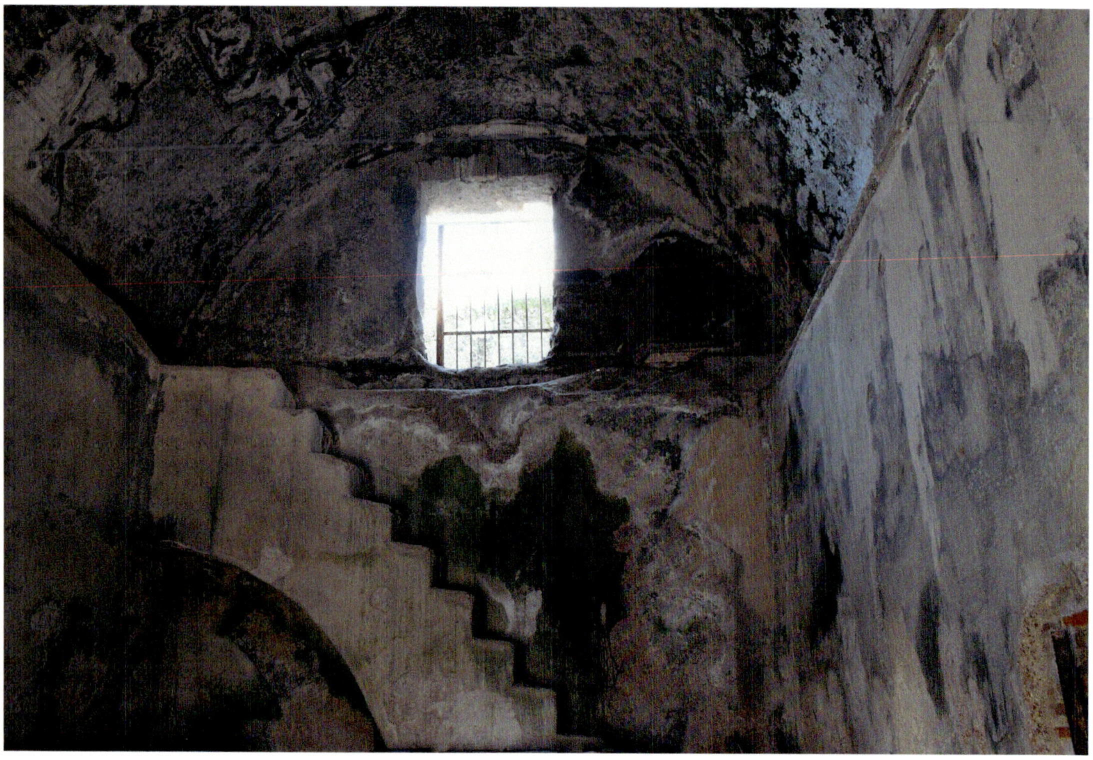

Figure 12. Baiae, Archaeological Park of Baiae. The so-called 'Stanze di Venere'. View of the interior. Photo by the Author.

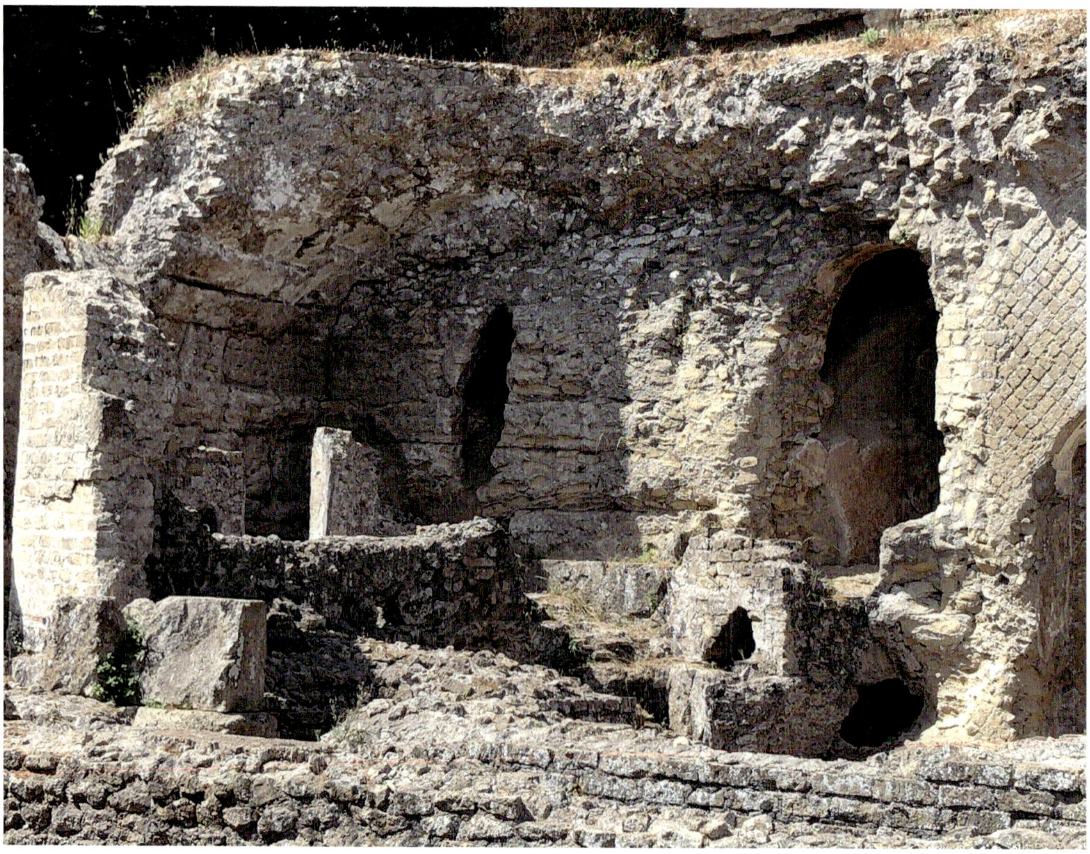

Figure 13. Baiae, Archaeological Park of Baiae. The so-called 'Piccole Terme'. The 'Great Antrum'. Photo by the Author.

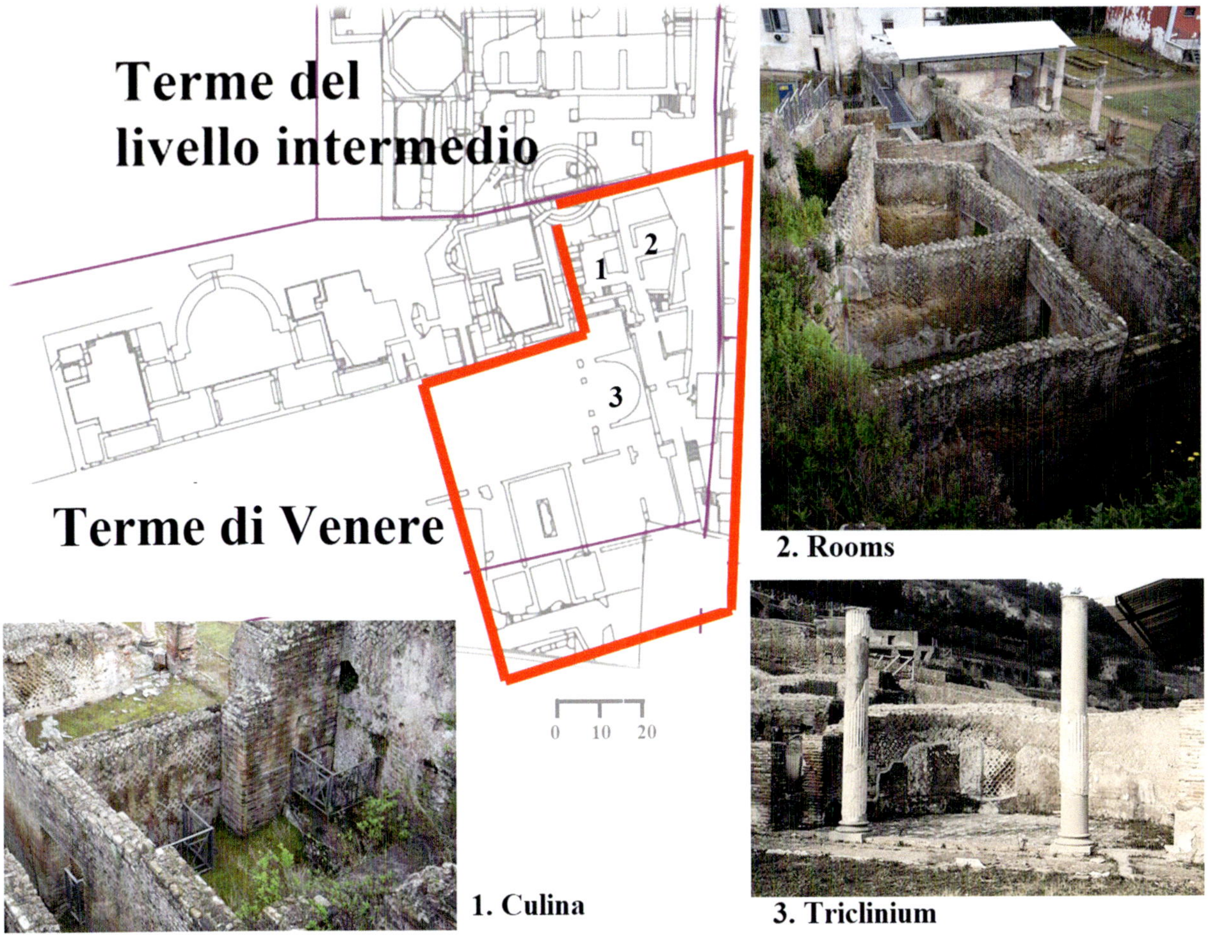

Figure 14. Baiae, Archaeological Park of Baiae. The private house remodelled into the so-called 'Terme di Venere'. Plan and some views of the rooms. Plan reworked from M. Nieberle and photos by the Author.

in the process of transformation of residential architecture into places of leisure, body care, healing and entertainment in the landscape.

So, if the heating system, typical of the Baiae style, is described by Vitruvius, Celsius, Seneca, Pliny the Elder and Dio Cassius (Medri 2018; Miniero *et al.* 2022: 325-327), the new situation and the social and architectural changes over time find an echo in the words of contemporary roman writers. And if in their words Baiae is now only a spa centre where the roman upper class have *praetoriae* and *deversoria*, actually the ruins of the ancient city give us the image of a chaotic and crowded place, full of those *filii terrae*, considered so troublesome by Symmachus when looking for a more peaceful place.

Bibliography

De Angelis d'Ossat, G. 1977. L'architettura delle terme di Baia, in *I Campi Flegrei nell'archeologia e nella storia*: 227-274. Roma: Accademia Nazionale dei Lincei.

Di Luca, G. 2009. *Nullus in orbe sinus Bais praelucet amoenis*. Riflessioni sull'architettura dei complessi c.d.'dell'*Ambulatio*', 'della Sosandra' e delle 'Piccole Terme' a Baia. *Bulletin Antieke Beschaving* 84:149-168.

Di Luca, G. 2018. Cantieri edili e modalità di costruzione di età romana nei Campi Flegrei, in R. Bosso and E. Nuzzo (eds) *Symplegmata. Studi di archeologia dedicati a Simona Minichino*: 253-282. Napoli: Giannini Editore.

Di Luca, G. 2020. Il paesaggio del *Sinus baianus* tra abbandono e riutilizzo, in A. Cristilli, A. Gonfloni and F. Stok (eds) *Experiencing the Landscape in Antiquity*: 1-8. Oxford: Bar Publishing.

Di Luca, G. 2022. The Thermal Baths Archaeological Park of Baiae and the Aqua Augusta Story: an attempt of reconstruction, in *Rome Transformed. Newcastle University colloquium, 5-6 may 2022*. (forthcoming).

Di Luca, G. 2023. Temi figurativi e sviluppo architettonico nel portico inferiore della c.d. 'Villa della Sosandra' a Baia, in *AIPMA VI. Connessioni mediterranee in età ellenistica e romana. Agrigento, 6-8 luglio 2023*. (forthcoming).

Di Luca, G. and L. Narès 2022. La decorazione parietale e pavimentale di un settore tardoantico della Villa della Sosandra di Baia (Napoli). *AISCOM*: 339-348.

Di Luca, G. and A. Cristilli 2023. La decorazione marmorea di un'esedra-ninfeo tardoantico di Baia. *AISCOM*. (forthcoming).

Giuliani, C.F. 1977. Note sull'architettura dei Campi Flegrei, in *I Campi Flegrei nell'archeologia e nella storia*: 374-375. Roma: Accademia Nazionale dei Lincei.

Medri, M., G. Soricelli, and A. Benini 1999. *In Baiano Sinu*. Le Piccole Terme di Baia, in J. Delaine and D.E. Johnston (eds) *Roman Bath and Bathing*: 207-219. Porthsmouth: University of California.

Medri, M. 2013. *In baiano sinu*: il *vapor*, le *aquae* e le piccole terme di Baia, in M. Bassani, M. Bressan and F. Ghedini (eds) *Aquae salutiferae. Il termalismo tra antico e contemporaneo*: 119-144. Padova: Padova University Press.

Medri, M. 2018. La fama di Baia e le risorse naturali tipicamente baiane nelle fonti letterari. *Archeologia Classica* 69: 549-578.

Miniero, P., D. De Simone and G. Di Luca 2022. La Villa dell'*Ambulatio* di Baia: progettare seguendo l'acqua, in A. Cristilli, F. De Luca, G. Di Luca and A. Gonfloni (eds) *Experiencing the Landscape in Antiquity 2*: 325-332. Oxford: BAR Publishing.

Narès, L. 2018. Comprendre les complexes thermaux de Baïes à partir de leurs décors : l'exemple de la dernière phase décorative du portique, in P. Giulierini, A. Coralini and V. Sampaolo (eds) *Picta Fragmenta. La Pittura Vesuviana. Una rilettura*: 279-288. Cinisello Balsamo: Silvana Editore.

Popkin, M.L. 2018. Urban Images in Glass from the Late Roman Empire: The Souvenir Flasks of Puteoli and Baiae. *American Journal of Archaeology* 122.3: 427-461.

The Roman Healing Spa of Termas de São Vicente (Penafiel, Portugal) and Its Surroundings in Roman Times and Late Antiquity

Teresa SOEIRO
CITCEM-Faculty of Letters. University of Porto (FLUP).
teresasoeiro@sapo.pt

Silvia GONZÁLEZ SOUTELO
Universidad Autónoma de Madrid (UAM) y Madrid Institute for Advanced Studies (MIAS). Facultad de Filosofía y Letras. Departamento de Prehistoria y Arqueología. Campus Cantoblanco, UAM.
silvia.gonzalezs@uam.es

Helena BERNARDO
Museu Municipal de Penafiel y CITCEM.
helena.bernardo@cm-penafiel.pt

Jorge SAMPAIO
Área Arqueológica do Freixo - Património Cultural, I.P.
jorgesampaio@patrimoniocultural.gov.pt

Abstract: This paper examines the Roman healing spa of Termas de São Vicente, located in the municipality of Penafiel (Portugal), and evaluates the latest data concerning the spatial distribution and architectural typologies of Roman settlements in the southern region of *Callaecia*. The study specifically concentrates on the communities in the area closest to the spa, which were presumably integral to its operational logistics and among those most immediately influenced by its presence.

The objective of our paper is to discern how such a distinctive establishment, a healing spa, was integrated into and interacted with the settlement network established in the area, amidst a period marked by considerable change, ultimately leading to the emergence of a novel historical landscape.

Keywords: Penafiel (Portugal); Termas de São Vicente; Roman healing spa; settlements typology in Roman times; historical landscape.

The Termas de São Vicente Roman healing spa, unearthed in 1901 amidst efforts to research and harness mineral-medicinal water sources for a contemporary spa, is situated in the heart of Penafiel municipality (Portugal). Approximately 3km north of the Douro River and 32km from the Atlantic Ocean, it forms a part of the densely populated network that epitomized southern *Callaecia bracarense* from Roman times through to Late Antiquity. Remarkably well-preserved since its discovery, the site is accessible within the leisure park of the contemporary Palace Hotel and Spa. The archaeological site was practically entirely excavated and consists of a small-sized building (± 400m2) constructed around prolific cold sulfuric water springs, now utilized by the modern spa. It was meticulously documented in 1902 by the archaeologist José Fortes, whose seminal work, complemented by photographs, provides an in-depth view of the structures, archaeological finds and contextual background (Fortes 1902). (Figure 1)

The building comprises 11 rooms organized around a central enclosure (C courtyard or vestibule) paved with large shale slabs. Rooms A and B are speculated to have served as reception and changing areas or for undetermined purposes. Rooms D and E each contain a cold water pool while the function of room F remains uncertain. Additionally, two heated rooms (H and I), feature hypocausts and are adjoined by service areas with external entrances (rooms J and K).

Despite the precision and quality of J. Fortes' 1902 descriptions and plans, gaps persist in understanding and interpreting the building's layout. Consequently, in 2020, the leader of the UAM/MIAS project *Healing spas in Antiquity*, in collaboration with the Municipal Museum of Penafiel, initiated an archaeological intervention to re-evaluate the structures and their role within the context of Roman thermal practices (González Soutelo *et al.* 2023).

In this paper we examine the contextual significance and territorial positioning of Termas de São Vicente spa, primarily dictated by a source of sulphurous water (17.8ºC). The Penafiel municipality, known for its granite subsoil, has several thermal springs, yet most remained unexploited except for the one to the

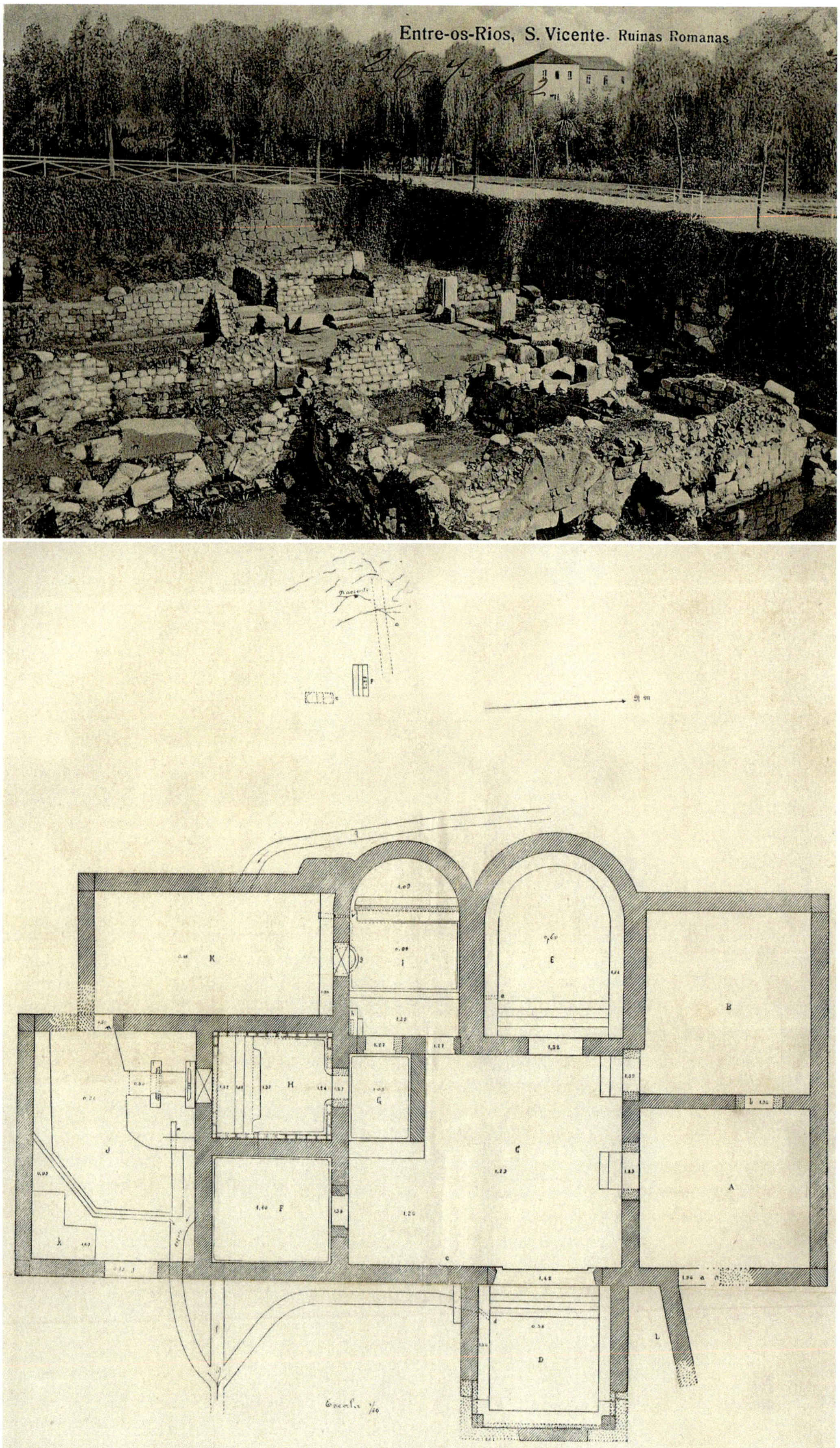

Figure 1. Roman healing spa of Termas de São Vicente: view of the ruins (Postcard edit by Bazar Soares – Porto, stamped in 1902) and Roman healing spa plan published by J. Fortes (1902).

south of São Vicente, on the same road axis, known as the Entre-os-Rios healing spa. This site, overlooked in Roman times, gained prominence in the 19th century as a therapeutic and leisure destination for the national elite. In contrast, just beyond the northeastern limit of the municipality, the Termas de Canaveses in Marco de Canaveses, located along the Roman road from *Bracara Augusta* to *Augusta Emerita* and near the bridge over the Tâmega, operated simultaneously with São Vicente.

Our aim is to elucidate how this innovative establishment -a healing spa- was integrated and interacted within the existing settlement network established in this region, during a period of profound changes, leading to the formation of a new historical landscape.

Brief geomorphological characterization

The current municipality of Penafiel is part of the Douro river hydrographic basin, bordering it to the south, and includes sub-basins of the Tâmega and Sousa Rivers, its right-bank tributaries, to the east and west, respectively. The geomorphological composition of Penafiel's north and center regions is shaped by a network of fractures and faults, likely of late-Hercynian origin, aligned NE-SW or perpendicular. This tectonic activity, which occurred in the final phase of granite mass formation (Pereira, Medeiros and Moreira 1980: 9, 24), sculpted the landscape into mountainous areas (585m max. height, Serra da Brenha), plateaus and valleys, each with their respective hydrographic network of varying scales. The region's sandy-clayey soils, conducive to agriculture, have supported farming operations at least since Roman times. This agricultural productivity correlates with the characteristic dispersed settlement patterns observed in the area. The mapped archaeological sites mostly follow the contour lines between 150 and 250 meters in elevation. The lowest point is the village of Chaves (Canelas), situated at 45 meters above sea level along the banks of the Douro, while the highest is Castro de Monte Mozinho, at an absolute elevation of 408 meters. (Figure 2)

The remaining area of the municipality is predominantly covered by granite, forming a less rugged terrain where the Tâmega river, running from NE to SW (Eastern limit of the municipality), carves a valley with steep slopes. This topography is likely influenced by a geological fault (Pereira, Medeiros and Moreira 1980: 8). The area's unique geographical features combining northern protection, intense sunlight, and abundant water sources, have historically needed labor-intensive land preparation on narrow terraces. This environment has been conducive to the cultivation of vineyards, olive groves, fruit trees and vegetables, which thrive here, yielding early and high-quality produce. This landscape, shaped over time, supported a distinct and prosperous occupation during the Roman era.

Several tributaries of the Tâmega river, including the notably linear Ribeira da Camba, exhibit geomorphological characteristics shaped by the same tectonic forces (Pereira, Medeiros and Moreira 1980: 9). This regional tectonic influence is believed to have played a crucial role in the formation of the São Vicente thermal water spring. The spring emerges in an area marked by a geological fracture running in a N/S direction, coinciding with the river's course, and is now partially buried by alluvium and sandy-clayey deposits in the bottom of the valley (Pereira, Medeiros and Moreira 1980: 39). The São Vicente thermal spring surfaces through a granitic vein within the predominant coarse-grained granite. Its waters are alkaline sulfuric, like the mineralized waters of Torre (Entre-os-Rios). The spring is situated in a Hercynian age calco-alkaline granite lithological environment, associated with ductile shear zones. This geological setting is similar to that of the thermal site of Caldas de Canaveses (Marco de Canaveses) (Oliveira and Cramez 1992; Calado 2001: 63-67, 82), immediately upstream from the Roman road and bridge.

On the western boundary of the Penafiel municipality, the predominant granite gives way to shale, intersected by quartzite ridges with areas of frequent gold metallization (Rebelo 1975; Couto 1993). These geological features attracted extensive Roman mining in the areas of Castromil-Quinta and Banjas since the first half of the 1st century (Soeiro 1984: 109-121; Lima, Mendonça and Felix 2005).

Inhabited sites and scattered finds from roman times

Current archaeological understanding indicates that the Termas de São Vicente healing spa was a prominent site, adjacent to an open settlement with a necropolis. It held a central position in the Camba river valley, a natural corridor used as a north-south route leading to the Douro, a navigable river that demarcates the boundary between the Tarraconense and Lusitania provinces. This spa forms part of an extensive network of widespread settlement, including sites of different typologies.

Notable among these is the Castro de Monte Mozinho, a large, elevated, fortified village looking over the valley. Integrated into Roman commercial networks since the Julio-Claudian era, it experienced resurgence from the late 3rd to the 5th century. Another significant site is the Cividade de Eja, strategically located over the mouth of the Tâmega river overseeing the navigation of the Douro. Additional smaller sites include late-era structures, albeit less studied, alongside numerous open settlements scattered across the *ager*. The necropolises of these settlements are better understood, and the region also features isolated rural farmhouses or

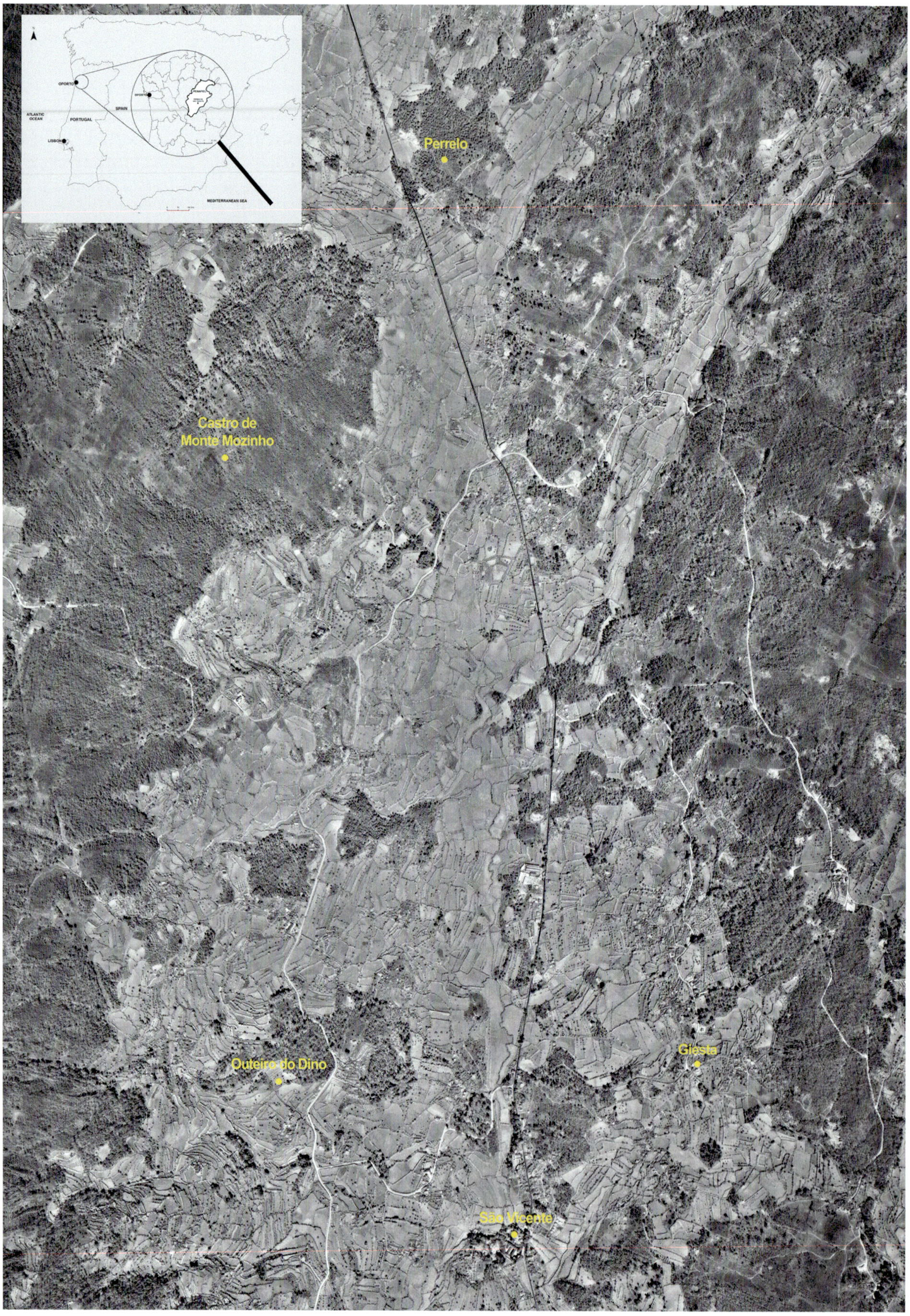

Figure 2. Aerial photography (1965) of the Camba river valley with the location of the main archaeological sites (Instituto Geográfico Cadastral, 41: 69/65, adapted by MMPNF, Ribeiro, M. 2023).

small *villae*, such as those excavated on the bank of the Tâmega river. The proximity of these settlements to the spa (< 5km) facilitated its use by the local inhabitants for daily visits, without the need of temporary residence at the spa itself.

The cartographic data obtained from the latest survey work, georeferenced using geographic information software (QGIS), has underscored the density and formal multiplicity of coexisting sites in the area. This landscape of settlements must be understood in relation to the road network, remnants of nearby mining operations and the broader political, socioeconomic and ideological transformations that persisted into the early phase of Late Antiquity.

Recent fieldwork

Between 2019 and 2022, the Cultural Heritage Management Service of the Municipal Museum of Penafiel undertook the third revision of the Heritage Charter, integral to the Municipal Master Plan, a statutory framework for territorial planning. The main objectives focused on the inspection of 163 pre-existing areas of archaeological and architectural heritage, assessing their preservation status and identifying potential threats; verifying and, if necessary, amending the recorded locations of sites and the boundaries of their respective framing areas; and seeking new archaeological evidence to refine the map of territorial occupation across various historical periods. This work led to the identification of 120 additional protected areas, bringing the total to 283, predominantly of archaeological significance. Among these, 61 sites could be chronologically classified between the Iron Age and the Roman Period, including fortified sites in commanding positions, open settlements, and necropolis. These, along with other locations not included in the Heritage Charter due to limited information and finds, are marked on the map (Figure 3).

The comprehensive survey of the territory began with meticulous preparatory work. Initially, this involved reviewing the extensive bibliography produced by generations of researchers, spanning from the end of the 19th century to the present, including brief notes, articles, and extensive monographs (Soeiro 1984). This information was documented in descriptive files for each site. Subsequently, the collected data were then cross-referenced with both historical and modern cartography, in particular the Military Maps at a scale of 1:25000 (no. 112, 123, 124, 134 and 135), which record toponyms, topographies and routes. The analysis was further enriched by examining orthophoto maps and aerial photographs, readily available online, such as the Municipal Geo-Portal, and the geological maps (no. 9-D and 13-B) and their explanatory reports (Pereira, Medeiros and Moreira 1980; Medeiros, Pilar and Fernandes 1964), among others. This approach facilitated a preliminary identification of locations most conducive to human habitation, taking into account factors such as relief, solar exposure, proximity to watercourses and accessibility. The graphic and photographic archaeological record of prior excavations and surveys was also scrutinized, including artefacts and incidental discoveries, some lacking contextual information, all held by the Municipal Museum.

The reassessment of safeguarded areas also entailed reviewing the archaeological reports from 194 municipal licensing processes for urban developments within the protected areas. This review served primarily to verify the distribution of archaeological finds in order to redefine the boundaries of occupation areas. However, this research often faced challenges, including frequent non-compliance with mandatory prior archaeological assessments, unauthorised and unlicensed projects, and notably, a lack of cooperation between the different entities responsible for territorial management. Noteworthy in this context are reforestation projects which, while requiring municipal approval, typically only involve the forestry management department, consequently overlooking the archaeological constraints outlined by the Heritage Charter. Regrettably, it was often in the process of surveying areas cleared for new plantations, particularly eucalyptus, that some archaeological sites were either identified or confirmed.

Following the preparatory phase, a thorough prospecting endeavour followed across the 212 km2 of municipal territory. This fieldwork provided not only a comprehensive understanding of the area but also fostered valuable interactions with the local community. Engaging with the residents proved to be an invaluable aspect of the research, aiding in the identification of toponyms and pathways, and enriching the study with shared ancestral stories and legends and even accounts of ancient archaeological finds.

The extensive surface prospecting was complemented by the capabilities of Geographic Information Systems (GIS), using the open-source software Quantum GIS (QGIS), which served as a repository for all the collected data. However, it was acknowledged that fieldwork remained the cornerstone of the entire process. Without systematic and accurate records of archaeological sites, the potential of these advanced technological tools remains underutilized. Although the analysis was necessarily restricted to current administrative boundaries, the flexibility of GIS environments allows for the incorporation of data from broader municipal or regional scopes, applicable to the period under study or other historical timelines. The georeferenced results, when combined with the versatility, speed, and capacity of GIS for data integration, allow for a visually rich and illustrative perspective. This is particularly evident when data is superimposed onto surfaces generated by the software, such as the Digital Terrain Model (MDT), or hypsometric map, which are based on the altimetry (Figure 3).

In summary, before delving into the details of this map, it is important to acknowledge certain limitations and challenges inherent in such representations. Firstly, the inventory of sites is a dynamic and continuously evolving task, subject to updates from ongoing fieldwork and incidental discoveries. This aspect is likely to intensify in the near future given the construction of a new road axis crossing the entire central area of the municipality and the development of new photovoltaic energy parks. Secondly, most sites are identified based on surface remains, which provide limited insights into their diachrony, size and typology. Additionally, numerous other settlements are known to us only through occasional finds submitted to the Museum, often with a near total loss of crucial information about the archaeological context. Lastly, even for the sites that have undergone urgent or programmed archaeological interventions, the excavations have typically encompassed but a fraction of the areas showing traces of occupation.

Regarding the diversity of archaeological sites

The first group of the map (Figure 3) gathers the archaeological sites that assume a dominant or strategic position over the surrounding territory. Predominantly, these sites are the characteristic *castros* (hillforts), with diverse dimensions and occupation periods starting from the Iron Age. These *castros* often exhibit overlapping stratigraphic layers that go back to Recent Prehistory and continuing the occupation beyond Antiquity. But in other cases, some sites may represent Roman establishments situated mid-slope, marking the boundaries of the *ager* and the *saltus*, a pattern also observed in subsequent historical periods. Given that our knowledge is primarily based on surface remains, it is challenging to determine the diachrony of these settlements. Notably, it is difficult to rule out the existence of earlier occupations than those evidenced by sporadic structural remnants and artefacts. In cases of medium to large-sized sites, it is necessary to consider that certain areas were preferable while others were abandoned over various epochs a phenomenon exemplified by Castro de Monte Mozinho.

Of all the inventoried sites, Castro de Monte Mozinho is the only one that has undergone significant archaeological intervention, covering approximately 10% of its area (Soeiro 2019). Located just 3.5km away from São Vicente spa, this fortified settlement is prominent in the landscape, with the *castro* at its highest point at 408m and the low river valley at 148m. Situated at the head of the Ribeira da Camba valley, on a natural route to the Douro, its strategic position offers an expansive visual range. To the north, the view stretches to the mountains of Santa Catarina, Monte Córdoba and Vandoma, beyond the Tâmega river to the peaks of Marão, and south of the Douro to the Montemuro mountains, encompassing a radius of more than 30km.

Spanning roughly 20 hectares, Castro de Monte Mozinho was densely populated and well planned from its inception. Current evidence suggests its establishment dates back to the Augustan era and could have been a strategic move during or after the wars against Astures and Cantabrians, aimed at controlling and systematically organizing the Northwest territory. With the consent (or on the initiative) of new landowners, local populations were possibly consolidated here and assigned a political-administrative structure to facilitate interaction with the Romans, potentially functioning as a *castellum* (Pereira Menaut 1998: 39). This settlement likely represented a community of *peregrini* and *stipendiari* from an ancient *populus* (possibly *Callaicus*) and later, a new civitas. This community would delineate a defined territory, essential for administrative and taxation purposes, always within the framework of the *conventus bracaraugustanus*, in the provincia *Tarraconense*.

The residents of this area largely preserved their indigenous customs and material culture, which gradually diminished over the course of the 1st century. However, archaeological excavations reveal that from the outset, there was a significant influx of goods imported from other regions of the empire. This suggests not only considerable economic resources but also integration into exchange and trade networks. There is also evidence of the adoption of new habitus, evidenced in attitudes such as mandatory burials in necropolis outside the village, the acquisition of a second language and literacy, changes in personal names, religious beliefs, and more. Additionally, there was even the possibility of working in the new nearby mining area of the Valongo and Banjas mountains, in public works or serving in the army would be easier. By the middle of the century, a shift was evident as inhabitants began to disperse into surrounding low-lying and fertile lands, establishing various types of settlements, including the open and low settlements that will be further discussed.

During the Flavian era, the Castro de Monte Mozinho continued its transition towards a Roman lifestyle. However, it appears it didn't fully transform into a classical Roman town, characterized by substantial investments in buildings symbolic of political and religious authority or meant for public recreation

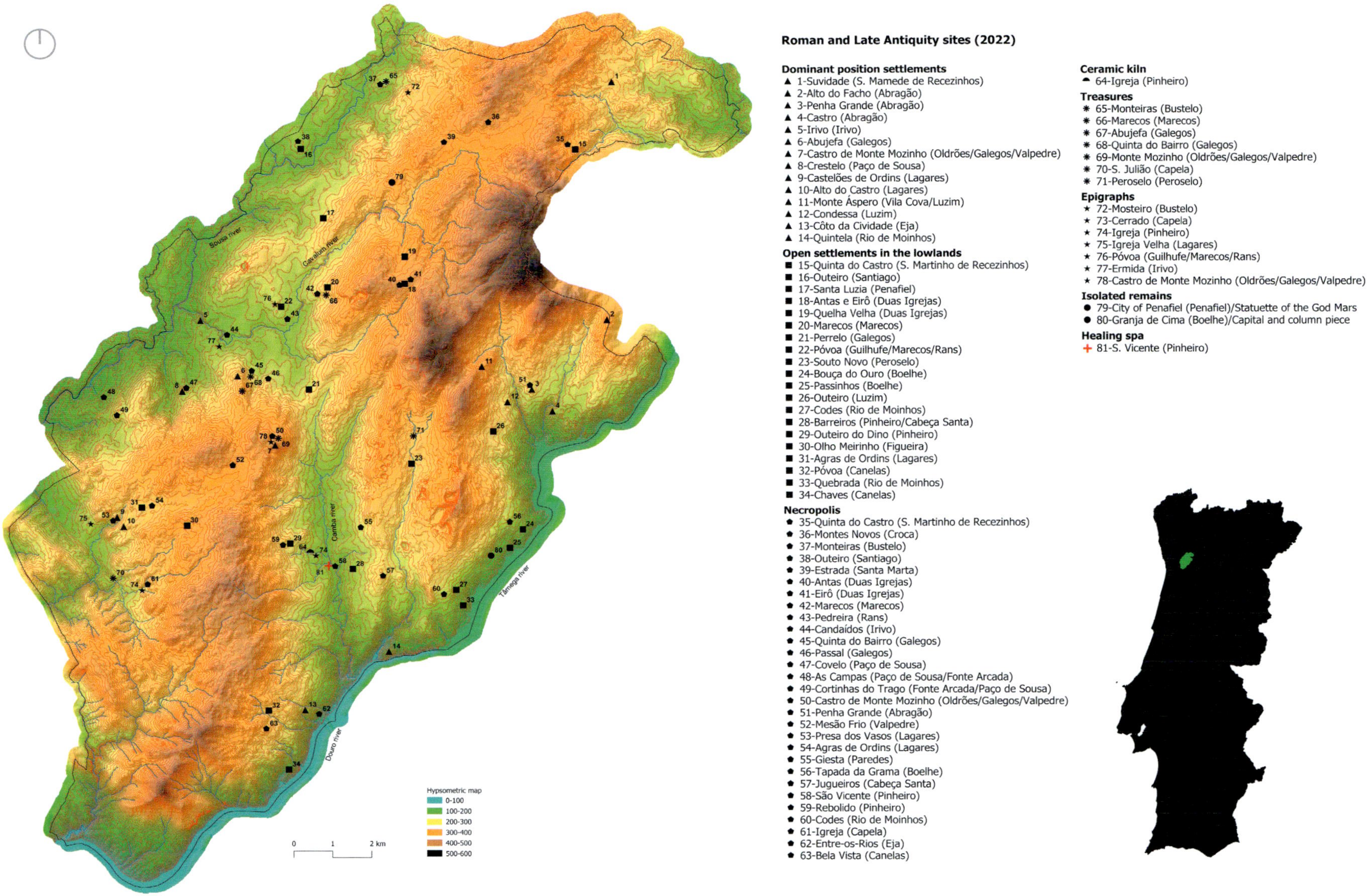

Figure 3. Municipality of Penafiel: location of the sites and archaeological remains from Roman times and Late Antiquity (MMPNF, prepared by H. Bernardo, 2023)

(Mateos *et al.* 2022). Drawing comparisons is challenging, especially given the limited 10% of the excavated area and the absence of comprehensive data about Castro's political status, the extent and nature of its administrative or economic jurisdiction, the wealth of its inhabitants or any notable individuals linked to the Roman provincial power or demonstrating *evergeta* behaviour (Carvalho, Fernandes and Lacerda 2022).

What is apparent is that in the initial blocks close to the main street, indigenous houses were demolished to build more complex residences that aligned more closely with Roman architectural tradition, occasionally encroaching upon occupying public spaces. The most exemplary of these structures comprise several compartments arranged around a central circulation area with controlled access points connecting to the public thoroughfare.

The remodelling of the elliptical enclosure at the summit of the site, which lacks any traces of residential structures within, is also traced back to this period. This is a distinct space, approximately 509m2 in size, accessible through a doorless passage from the main street, and featuring external stairs on the opposite side. The interior of the thick surrounding wall, is tapered halfway up, resembling a bench that could accommodate spectators. Interpreted as a central public space, this enclosure, possibly serving multiple functions, might have been used for markets, games, performances or even administrative tasks.

The monument erected outside the first wall, situated near the main circulation axis, clearly exhibits Roman stylistic preferences. This monument's structural remnants include a quadrangular *podium in situ*, complete with is mouldings. Additionally, the bases and shafts of columns, along with and an interesting collection of sculptural fragments – human figures and a horse, the latter with at least one front paw raised- are all carved in granite. These artefacts are currently on display at the Museum.

This architectural transformation is emblematic of the mimetic monumentalization prevalent during Flavian times, characterized by significant shifts in the design and utilization of interior spaces in small private residences and the methods of construction, notably the widespread adoption of ceramic roofing. The influx of consumer goods, both imported from other provinces and locally produced near the conventual capital *Bracara Augusta* saw a marked increase during this period, with evidence of these goods present in almost every household. However, this development and refinement coincided with a gradual depopulation of the summit of this great hillfort, particularly from the final decades of the 1st century. This trend occurred simultaneously with an increase in the establishment of open settlements in the more fertile lowlands, areas which have continued to be pivotal for agricultural activities up to the present day. These new settlements were strategically located in territories that, with appropriate cultivation techniques, would yield substantial agricultural output. (Figure 4)

These villages, devoid of defensive walls or other structural features that significantly alter the terrain's contours, nor evident monumentality in the residential areas (with the exception of some columns of Tuscan order), are often discovered fortuitously during ploughing, road and public infrastructure construction, or while laying foundations for new homes or industrial buildings. None of these sites have been excavated in a significant area. Instead, it is their necropolis that have stood out and been reported, possibly due to a culturally ingrained respect for the deceased. This respect for burial sites has occasionally allowed for archaeological interventions, at least in part. The inhabited sites, generally contiguous to these cementeries, are identified through the discovery of ceramic building materials, dressed stone, occasional hoards of coins or fragments of columns. Fieldwork evidence suggests that these settlements often comprised multiple family units, as inferred by the number of burials chronologically attributable to specific time intervals and the organized layout of the necropolis.

The necropolis of Monteiras (Bustelo), situated in the fertile lands on the bank of the Sousa, serves as an example. Here, incinerations dating back to the middle of the 1st century, which still contained indigenous ceramics, are found alongside burials that persisted until the late 4th century (Soeiro 2009-2010). Similarly, in other necropolis, such as Montes Novos (Croca) (Pinto 1998; Pinto 2021) or Duas Igrejas (Sousa and Soeiro 2020), dating from the final decades of the Empire, the typical burials are in rectangular graves carved into the gravel. Rarely are these graves lined with stone slabs or constructed from masonry. The deceased were typically enshrouded in fabric, laid on a stretcher, or, less commonly, placed in a wooden coffin. These burials were invariably accompanied by offerings, predominantly foodstuffs, deposited in coarse ware containers. Glass vessels are less frequently encountered, while decorative adornments or tools are scarce; however, coins are a prevalent find in these graves. (Figure 5)

Along the banks of the Tâmega, where the microclimate is more suitable for Mediterranean agriculture, in particular vine cultivation, another type of settlement emerges. These settlements seem to be characterized by a series of farmhouses facing the river, halfway down the slope. The significance of the surface remains was underscored by the archaeological work carried out in Bouça do Ouro (Boelhe), where, following

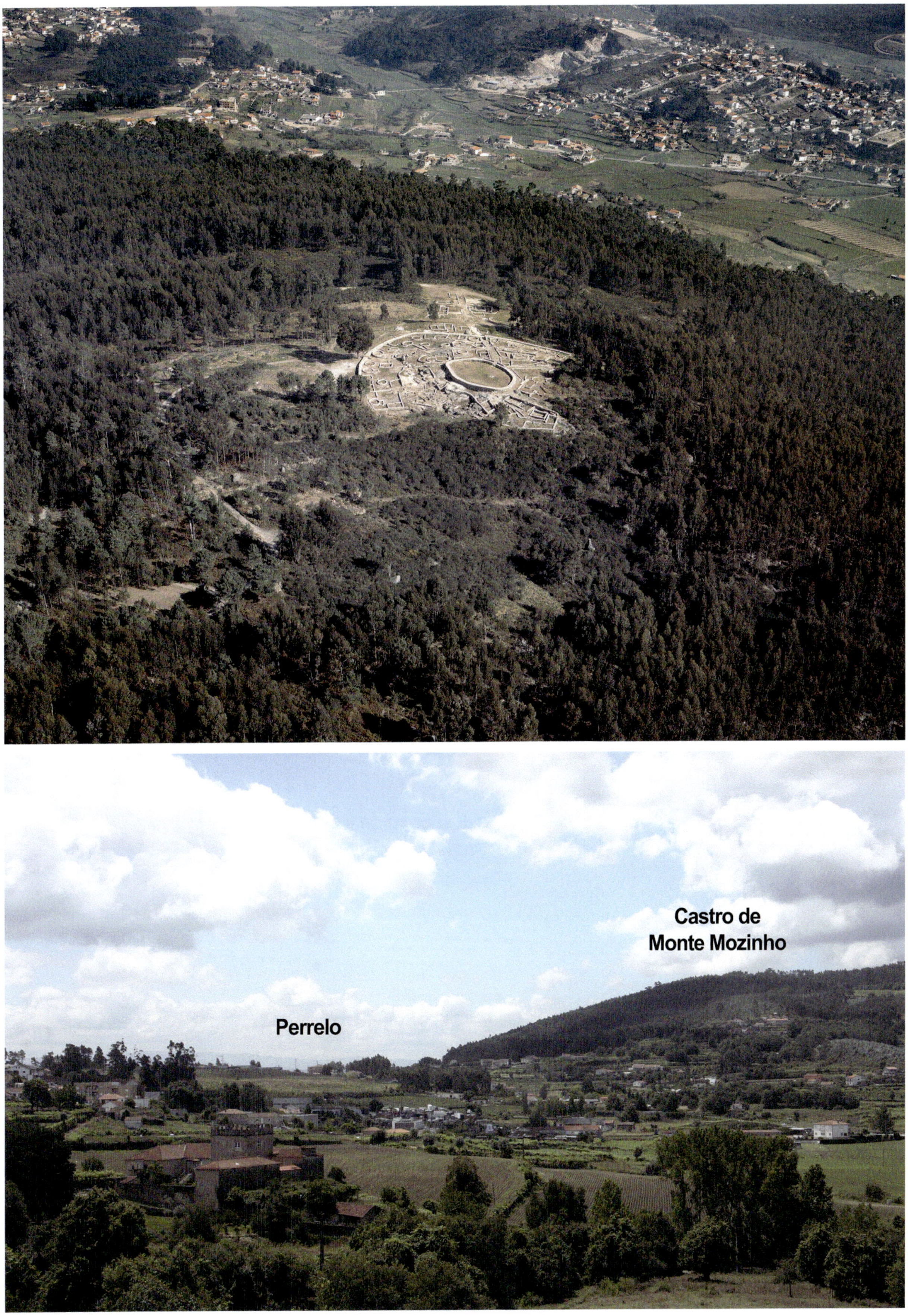

Figure 4. Aerial photography (1998) of the Castro de Monte Mozinho, overlooking the Camba river valley (MMPNF, photo capture by Penaguião and Burnay) and relative position of the Castro and the Perrelo site (Galegos), at the head of the valley (MMPNF, photo by H. Bernardo, 2022).

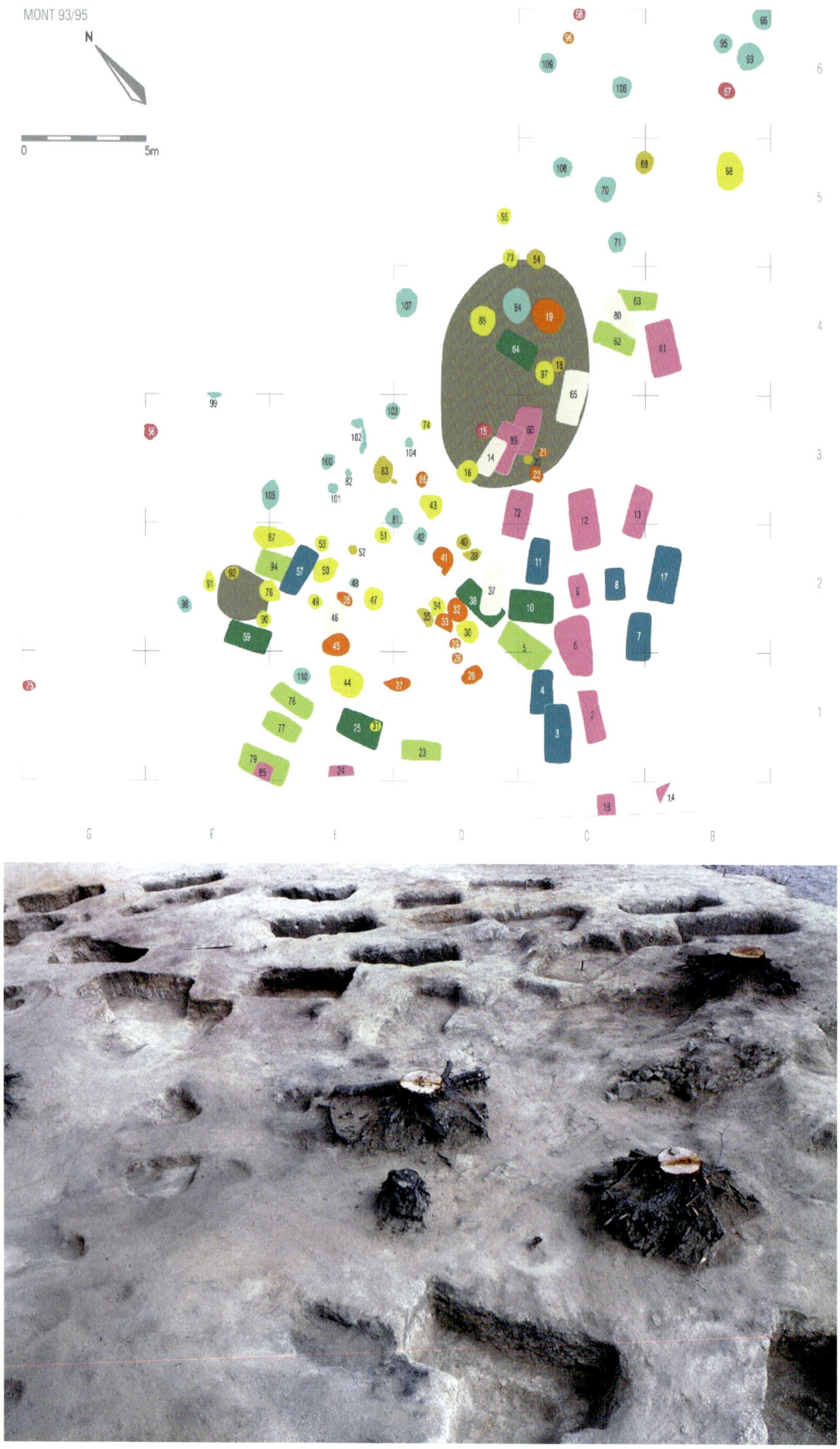

Figure 5. Plan and partial view of the excavated area in the Roman necropolis of Monteiras (Bustelo) (Soeiro 2009-2010).

incidental discoveries, two farmhouses (200m2 and 240m2) were unearthed. Separated by just a few meters, both structures were built in the second half of the 1st century AD. In the first house, Tuscan-style columns supported the roof rafters in the largest room and near the entrance. In the second house, the use of these columns was more extensive, likely forming part of a gallery overlooking the river, a feature that was later nullified during the last centuries of the Empire (Soeiro 1998). Similar sites are found in proximity, maintaining the same river-facing orientation, though these are primarily identified by sparse remains. Examples include Outeiro (Luzim), Passinhos (Boelhe), Codes and Quebrada (Rio de Moinhos). (Figure 6)

In addition to the more prominent agricultural estates, another category of habitation -poorer and more isolated rural dwellings associated with their respective farmlands- presents a viable alternative, as seen in places like Santa Luzia (Penafiel), on the slope overlooking the Sousa valley. However, a more definitive understanding of the composition of these units, which date back to the 4th-5th century, and their spatial relationship with neighbouring dwellings- whether as part of a village or as a more loosely structured entity (locus) requires an expansion of the excavation area. Such an investigation would clarify whether these dwellings formed structured settlements or more dispersed habitations, similar to those that characterized the regional settlement pattern until the last century.

It should also be noted that during the Late Roman Empire, alongside the diverse residential patterns prevalent in the plains and the lower elevations, there was a resurgence and enhancement of occupation in some high-altitude settlements, such as in Castro de Monte Mozinho and, possibly, Cividade de Eja. In Castro de Monte Mozinho, the summit of the site was vacated, with streets, dwellings and production facilities spreading across the entire slope between the upper and peripheral walls, leaving the necropolis outside the living areas. A comprehensive picture of this significant site from the late 3rd century to the 5th century awaits future excavation efforts in this extensive area (López Quiroga 2004; Soeiro 2018).

An inter-regional road network and local paths played a pivotal role in structuring the settlement, yet the absence of milestones, bridges or specific archaeological markers renders their precise documentation challenging. One exception worth noting is the axis deriving from the Roman road originating from Bracara Augusta heading southward towards the Douro, and crossing the Tâmega at the Canaveses bridge (Dias 1997: 319-320). This road, starting in the northern part of the current municipality, utilized the natural N-S corridor, which partly coincides with the Camba river valley, and passed near the São Vicente spa.

As can be seen in map 1 (Figure 3), numerous open settlements (along with their necropolis) are situated alongside this strategic road. Notably, we must emphasize the archaeological site of Marecos. Positioned on a slight elevation, adjacent to fertile farmland in the middle of the valley and near the road, this site yielded a significant altar adorned with an extensive list of offerings to both indigenous and Roman deities. The altar was dedicated by the *Danigi*, a local community (perhaps part of a *civitas*?), under the leadership of two *curatores*, individuals likely of prominent social and economic standing. The date of the ceremony is pinpointed to AD 147 (9th April), as indicated by the reference to the consular year. This discovery leads us to the hypothesis of an organized population centre in the vicinity, with political, administrative, and religious functions managed by local aristocrats (Le Roux and Tranoy 1974; Pereira Menaut 1998; Redentor 2017, v.1: 200, 275-277, 704-708; v.2: 027).

Flanking this road at the entrance of the Camba river valley, two notable landmarks distinguish this territory. On the west side sits Castro de Monte Mozinho; to the east, the intriguing archaeological site of Perrelo (Galegos) is situated, characterized by its elevated, flat terrain, sharply defined by the surrounding slopes. The scarce surface material recovered from Perrelo can be traced back to Roman times. However, the distinct position and morphology of this site set it apart from others in the region. Its features could suggest a Roman origin, but the scarcity of findings and research in this area precludes the formation of any solid hypothesis. (Figure 4)

As we will discuss further, the São Vicente thermal spa represents a distinctive case within the territory, finding its nearest counterpart in the Canaveses spa, situated along the Tâmega, in proximity to the aforementioned Roman bridge.[1]

[1] In the *Memórias Paroquiais*, national royal inquiry of 1758 (Capela *et al.* 2009: 408), the parish priest of Sobretâmega reports on the rediscovery, around three decades ago, of the thermal sulfur springs of Canaveses, which began to be recommended by doctors and sought after by patients in cases of 'rheumatism, obstructions and hysterical morbidities'. When building the bathroom, five years later, coins and a stone inscription with many letters appeared, and on the river side, also one and a half inches of clay tiles also appeared, described as arranged in the form of a staircase. At the beginning of the 20th century, the contemporary spa building continued to grow, and the construction left visible 'some old bricks and some stone gutters that were certainly used to transport mineral water from its source to the place where they were found when the foundations of the new bathing establishment were being built' (Vasconcellos 1903: 14). The news was communicated to Leite de Vasconcelos, who, in the *Arqueólogo Português* periodical, records the finding of plaster from the pools, bricks and tiles (Vasconcellos 1903: 284-285); shortly afterwards, Manuel de Vasconcelos followed new occurrences of tiles, bricks and pipes (Vasconcelos 1935: 2). Following a note by Rui de Serpa Pinto (1934: 165) on the presence of *opus signinum* in the pool in the archaeological site of Freixo (Tongobriga), Russel Cortez refers the notice of 1902 and the existence of mosaics destroyed a few decades later, during improvements in the spa area (Cortez 1946: 278), an attribution replicated by other authors (Mora 1981; Dias 1997: 309).

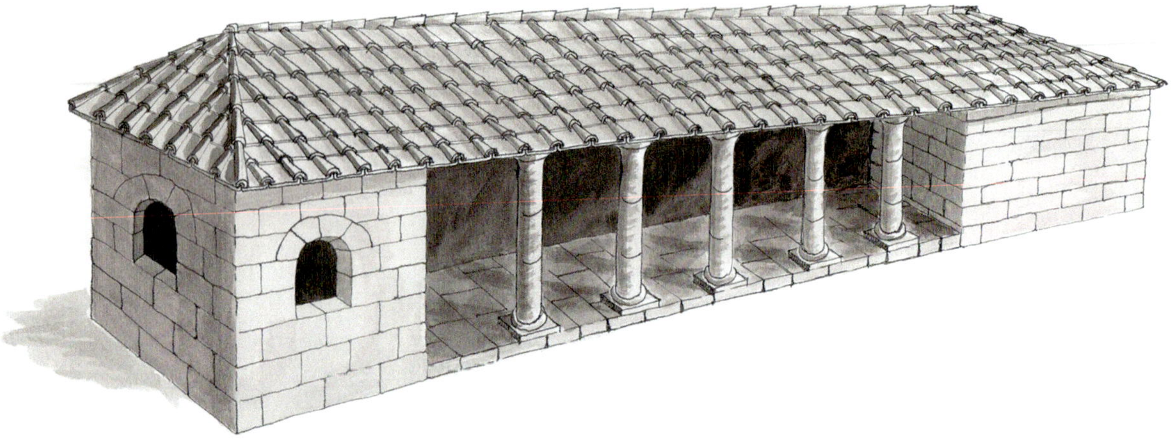

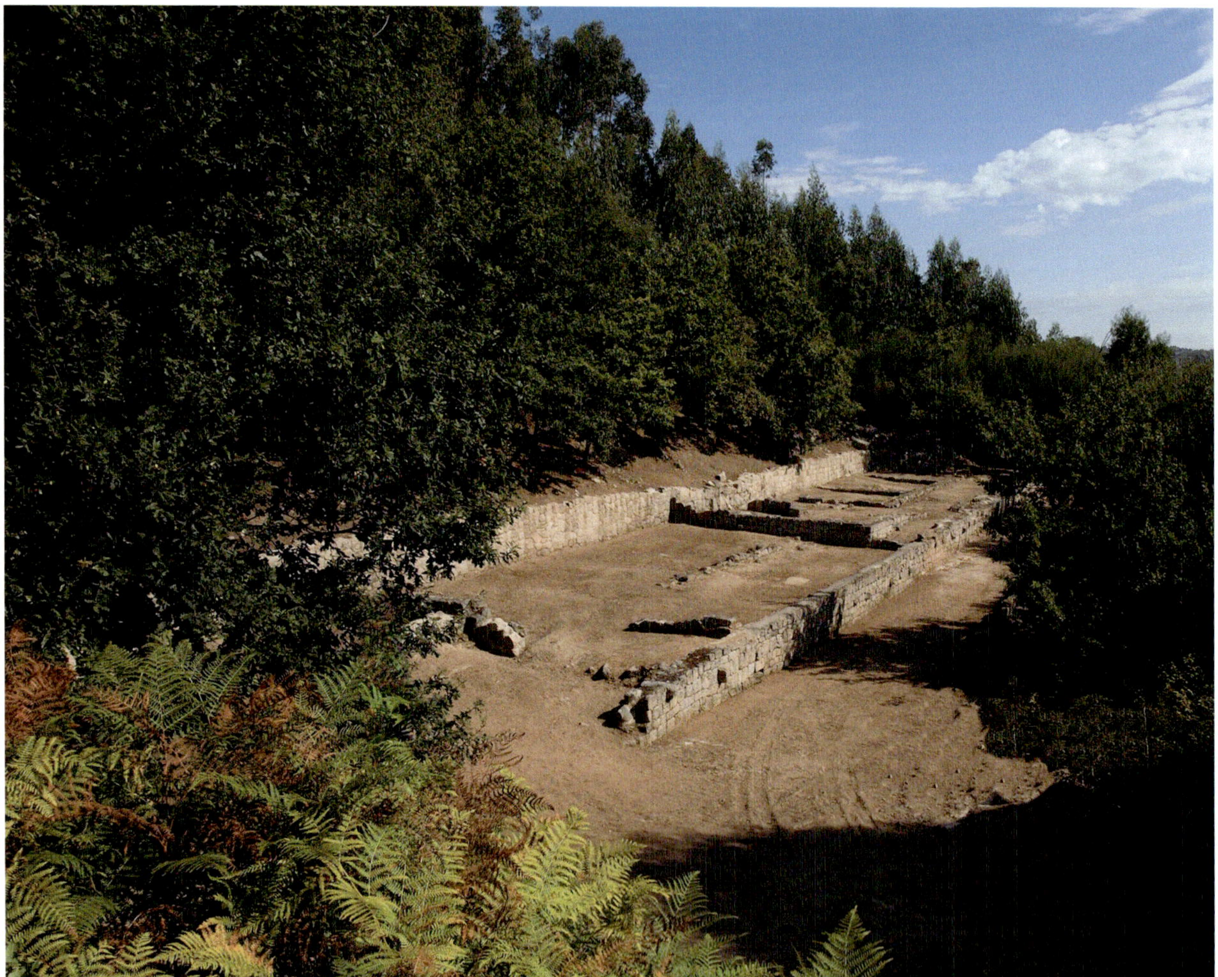

Figure 6. Essay on reconstitution of phase 1, and partial view of the phase 2 farmhouse B excavated at Bouça do Ouro (Boelhe) (Soeiro 1998).

Various artefacts, often displaced from their original archaeological context or repurposed, contribute additional pieces to the puzzle of this landscape, as is commonly observed with altars. For instance, the funerary altar dedicated to Úlpio Heracliano was repurposed in the kitchen of the Bustelo Benedictine monastery (Soeiro and Redentor 2021). In Lagares, beneath the main chapel of the parish church, an altar dedicated to the *Lares Anaeci* was discovered, sponsored by two *dispensatores*, who were likely involved in the administration of the neighbouring Banjas-Castromil gold mines (Redentor 2017, v. 1: 506-507, v. 2: 123; HEp 2016-2017, 2023: 1073). Additionally, a unique stele with a female representation was also found, albeit out of context, yet not far from a necropolis and a village where some 4th century (?) treasure was unearthed (Soeiro 2013; Santos and Pires 2014; Gutiérrez Alonso *et al.* 2021: 109-113; HEp 2014-2015, 2021: 880).

Monetary hoards are often discovered serendipitously. However, their perceived value, either as raw material or as collectible numismatic items, often leads to their sale, resulting in many such finds being reported only in the press or through anecdotal accounts. Consequently, the coins, their containers, and the archaeological context of these discoveries are frequently lost. In contrast, the Castro de Monte Mozinho stands out as an exception, where several hoards have been discovered with their context preserved and documented (Centeno 1989; Pinto 2005-2007; Ferreira 2018).

Roman-times settlements around the São Vicente spa

Concluding our exploration of archaeological Roman sites in the Penafiel municipality, we revisit the São Vicente healing spa. Conducting archaeological surveys in this area is presently challenging due to dense modern construction, and instances of archaeological monitoring have been rare in recent decades. (Figure 7)

N.º 81 Roman healing spa of São Vicente (Pinheiro, Termas de São Vicente)

In Termas de São Vicente, the spa capitalizes on cold sulphurous, sodium bicarbonate water (18,6ºC) primarily for the prevention and mitigation of respiratory ailments and is acclaimed for the efficacy of its inhalation treatments (Acciaiuoli 1940: 32; 1944, 1: 91; Cruz 1992: 75). During the works to capture and adapt the main spring for the modern spa in 1901, the ruins of a Roman building were discovered at a depth of 3m below current ground level and just a few meters away from the main spring (Fortes 1902; Soeiro 1984: 67-75; Alarcão 1988: 1/473).

The excavated structure is prominently displayed within the courtyard of the spa, enclosed by a peripheral retaining wall that showcases the remarkably well-preserved remains, including some partially standing walls. The initiation of the multi-annual archaeological research project Baln-São Vicente. PIPA, 2021-23, with an exceptional backing from the Direção Geral de Patrimonio Cultural de Portugal and by the UAM/MIAS, has facilitated a renewed study of this building. This project also has supported the re-excavation of some parts of the thermal complex (González Soutelo *et al.* 2023).

The site comprises a small bathhouse spanning approximatey 400m2. Despite using the mineral-medicinal waters native to the area, its layout diverges from that of typical bathing complexes. This difference in the construction likely stems from the low temperature of the water, the presence of different heated rooms, a central courtyard and additional chambers whose specific functions remain undetermined.

The materials unearthed during earlier excavations hold particular significance, notably a bronze vessel currently deposited in the Municipal Museum of Penafiel. This artefact was originally positioned beneath the praefurnium arch on the suspensura floor. As a working hypothesis, it is posited that this vessel may have been used to generate steam within a heated room. This theory aligns with contemporary practices of using mineral water is currently used for inhalation treatments, suggesting a historical continuity in therapeutic techniques (González Soutelo *et al.* in press).

An equally significant aspect is the isolated and enclosed nature of the building, indicated by the abscence of adjacent constructive evidence. This isolation supports the hypothesis that the facility primarily served a health related function. However, its significance probably extended beyond mere health benefits, encompassing social and public dimensions as well. It would have served the inhabitants of nearby synchronous settlements, including villages, manors, villae, and significant castros in the area, such as Monte Mozinho. The existence of such a dedicated structure suggests a need for health facilities including steam generation.

The dating of the building, determined through OSL and TL techniques corroborates this interpretation. The results indicate a chronology for the hypocaust system between the end of the 1st and early 2nd century AD. However, the architectural characteristics of the surviving structures suggest possible modifications during a later period, possibly areound the 4th or 5th century AD, though this needs further confirmation.

Therefore, the study of the surrounding territory, as detailed in this article, underscores the importance

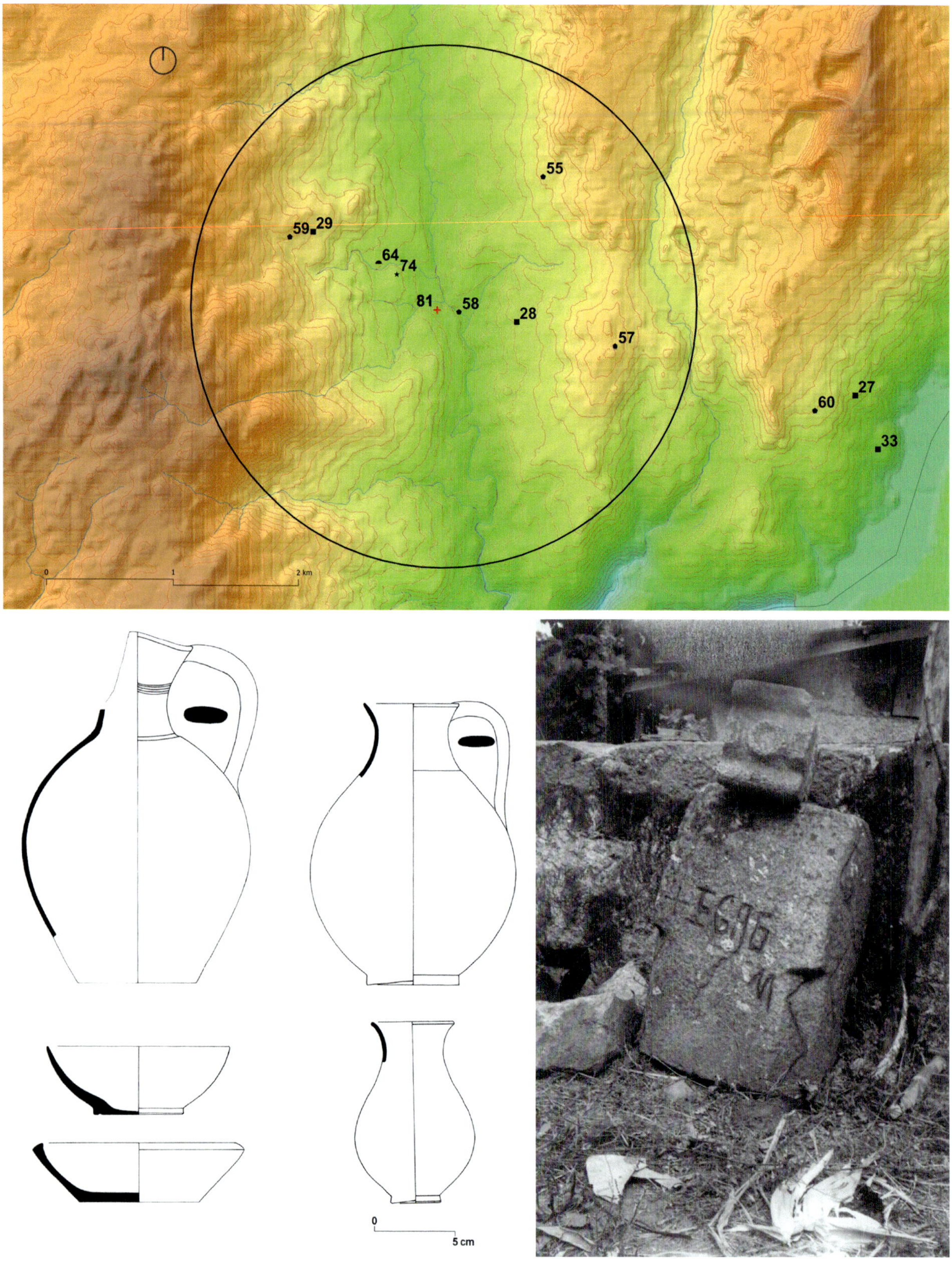

Figure 7. Archaeological sites within a radius of two kilometers of the Roman healing spa of Termas de São Vicente (MMPNF, prepared by Bernardo, H. 2023). Coarse ware from the necropolis of Giesta (Paredes) (Soeiro 1984) and Roman altar finding near the São Vicente church (MMPNF 1942?).

of contextualizing these thermal establishments. Understanding their relationship with the local environment allows for a deeper appreciation of thermalism as a strategic landmark in the territory (González Soutelo, in press).

N.º 58 Village and necropolis of São Vicente (Pinheiro, Termas de São Vicente)

In 1901-1902, José Fortes documented the discovery of Roman ceramic fragments unearthed during the construction of a bridge over the Camba river, situated 50m southeast of the Roman spa. He was also informed that 100m to the south, lamps and coarse ware were uncovered during reconstruction works on the road to Entre-os-Rios (Fortes 1902: 10; Soeiro 1984: 75; Alarcão 1988: 1/473).

Contrastingly, more recent prospecting and monitoring works in the areas south and west of the Roman baths have not yielded significant archaeological discoveries. This leads to the hypothesis of a potential village and its corresponding necropolis (justified by the complete vases and the mention of lamps) located very close to the baths. This village could have provided the necessary support for the spa's operation, the extent and seasonality of which remain unclear.

Historically, this locale would likely have been inhospitable during the winter months due to the rising and overflowing waters of the Camba river. Until the final decades of the 19th century, when the road layout was redesigned and the bridge constructed, this place was known as Lameiro dos Lodos (mud field). The combination of water from the Camba river, its tributaries and the thermal springs collectively transformed the terrain into a permanent sulphurous mud swamp.

The road itself would have faced similar problems year-round along the lower slopes of the valley. In modern times, an alternative winter route along the hillside was preferred, with the valley path being used predominantly in summer. Within the valley, no other inhabited sites have been identified as close to the river as the thermal spa and the hypothesized village and necropolis, their locations conditioned by the emergence of the medicinal water spring.

N.º 28. Village (?) of Barreiros (Paredes, Termas de São Vicente)

Within a 2km radius on the left bank, the nearest settlement to the spa is Barreiros (Paredes), situated at a locale known by the microtoponym Casal. This open site, 658m away and at a lower middle elevation of 205m, reveals fragments of tegula and coarse ware on the surface of a vineyard. The terrain here, characterized by its flatness and low altitude, seems indicative of an open settlement. However, doubts remain about the specifics of this site, including the type of occupation, its chronological framework and its spatial extension.

N.º 55. Necropolis of Giesta (Paredes, Termas de São Vicente)

Situated a little further away, approximately 1,5km and above the 200m contour line, are two necropolis, which, given their location, are likely associated with open settlements: the necropolis of Giesta (Paredes) and that of Jugueiros (Cabeça Santa). These sites were both fortuitous finds on the periphery of modern cultivated areas.

The necropolis of Giesta has been part of the historical record since as early as 1913 when Monteiro de Aguiar donated a vase from this site to the Anthropology Museum of the University of Porto. This vase was reportedly found alongside another, an "amphora", which was completely shattered (Machado 1920: 25). In a later development in 1975, a landowner, while working on his wooded land, stumbled upon the necropolis again. The burials were described as clusters of vases in the ground, accompanied by some coals, and placed without any type of protection.

The landowner contributed a collection of thirty-four coarse ware vases, albeit badly fractured, to the Municipal Museum of Penafiel. The physical nature of the discovery, coupled with the characteristics of the ceramics, suggests that these were simple incineration graves, a practice prevalent in the 2nd-3rd centuries, according to the ceramic's chronology (Soeiro 1984: 64-66; Alarcão 1988: 1/471). (Figure 7)

During the fieldwork carried out to update the Heritage Charter (2022), an octogenarian was contacted who reported having also come across burials when building his house in the 1960s. He recounted finding a bowl and a small plate of coarse ware which he collected himself, and later donated to the Museum in 2013. He described one of the graves, noting that it was surrounded by stones, and had a slab at the bottom, which he preserved in his backyard. Upon investigation, it was identified as a manually operated millstone of an older chronology, repurposed as part of the grave. This slab of rectangular shape, now also housed in the museum's reserve, suggests that the burial was a structured inhumation grave.

Furthermore, various sources indicated that an unspecified quantity of other coarse ware vases from this necropolis, particularly those that were best preserved, were extracted at the time of discovery and offered to a private collector from Maia. These artefacts likely remain in the possession of the family.

N.º 57. Necropolis of Jugueiros (Cabeça Santa)

This necropolis was first discovered in 1954 when pulling up pine roots in a forested area. Unfortunately, the specific nature of the burial and the details of the materials unearthed at that time remain unclear. Although a newspaper report from the era mentions that the artefacts were handed over to the Municipal Museum of Penafiel (O Penafidelense 1954; Soeiro 1984: 64, 67; Alarcão 1988: 1/479), we can only hypothesize that the seventeen Roman coarse ware vases, presently unattributed and stored in the Museum's reserve, may have originated from this site.

N.º 29. Village of Outeiro do Dino (Pinheiro, Termas de São Vicente)

On the right bank of the Camba river, symmetrically positioned to the previously mentioned sites, is Outeiro do Dino. This site is situated on the eastern side of a distinct flattened hill, detached from the plateau. It appears to be a more complex site, with its occupation in pre-Roman times still uncertain (Soeiro 1984: 60-61; Alarcão 1988: 1/472).

Records from 1936 by Monteiro de Aguiar indicate the presence of Roman constructions at this location, associated with tegulae, imbrexes, slate, coarse ware, dolia, column shafts and millstones (Aguiar 1936:116). Additionally, Elísio Ferreira de Sousa carried out excavations here, uncovering a quadrangular structure (Sousa 1962: 128). Unfortunately, documentation of these excavations is not available, and the artefacts recovered during these investigations were lost. However, local residents who witnessed the excavations, recall the discovery of ceramics, coins, iron tools and a piece of golden metal, which they compared with a "radiance".

Currently, there are ruins of this quadrangular buildings on the slope facing the spa, with scattered building stone and tegula fragments, all concealed beneath vegetation. In 1983, surface collection from the disturbed soil yielded Hispanic sigillate Drag. 37 (late 1st- 2nd century) coarse ware and a loom weight. Column shafts and both upper and lower millstones were also observed.

In the same area, during the early 1980s, the foundation work for a house led to the discovery of a capital. This artefact was significantly mutilated and repurposed as a sink. Crafted from coarse-grained local granite, its classification is challenging due to the extent of the alteration. However, two rows of ribbed acanthus leaves are discernible. For its transformation into a (holy water?) sink, the top surface was hollowed out, culminating in a rounded edge. On the exterior, any prominent decorative elements on the corners appear to have been pared down and smoothed to fit its new function more aptly (Soeiro 1984: 60-61). (Figure 8).

N.º 59. Necropolis of Rebolido (Pinheiro, Termas de São Vicente)

Adjacent to the area of ruins mentioned earlier, a necropolis was accidentally uncovered during tree uprooting. The graves, constructed using slates and bricks/tegulae, contained ceramic vases (Aguiar 1936: 116). It is believed that these vases are the same ones that were once displayed in the old Termas museum, given that the landowner was the same and the vases are featured in a photograph from that period.

This collection of eleven coarse ware vases, is currently deposited at the Municipal Museum of Penafiel (Soeiro 1984: 62-63; Alarcão 1988: 1/472). (Figure 9)

N.º 74. Roman altar (Pinheiro, Termas de São Vicente)

Situated between the archaeological site of Outeiro do Dino and the Roman baths, is a parish church. During renovation works at the parish residence, stone artefacts were recovered, including the upper part of a Roman altar that was reused as a frame for vines. Knowledge of this altar comes from the brief note and a photograph of the collection of finds taken during a visit of Abílio Miranda (Figure 7). The altar, crafted from granite, is positioned atop a medieval inscription. Visible elements include the top of the capital, the *cymatium* with a central *focus*, the triangular pediment and gable and the lateral *tori* or *pulvini*. It appears to have been fractured at the shaft and seems to have lost any eventual epigraph content, as this was not mentioned by the local scholar who visited the site (Miranda 1942: 3; 1944: 25-26). This small altar, like many other Roman altars in the municipality, was relocated to a church. It was possibly brought from Outeiro do Dino or even from the spa itself, both located within the parish of São Vicente do Pinheiro (Soeiro 1984: 64).

N.º 64. Ceramic kiln (Pinheiro, Termas de São Vicente)

In a note accompanying the donation of construction ceramics by Humberto Mendes Correia to the Anthropology Museum of the University of Porto, it is mentioned that the brick, along with others, originated from a ceramic firing oven that existed in a field close to the church (Museu 1926: 60). This suggests that a significant portion of the material used in the construction of the spa may have been produced in this oven (Soeiro 1984: 75; Alarcão 1988: 1/473).

Conclusions

While the evidence remains inconclusive, the nearby village (along with its necropolis) presents the most

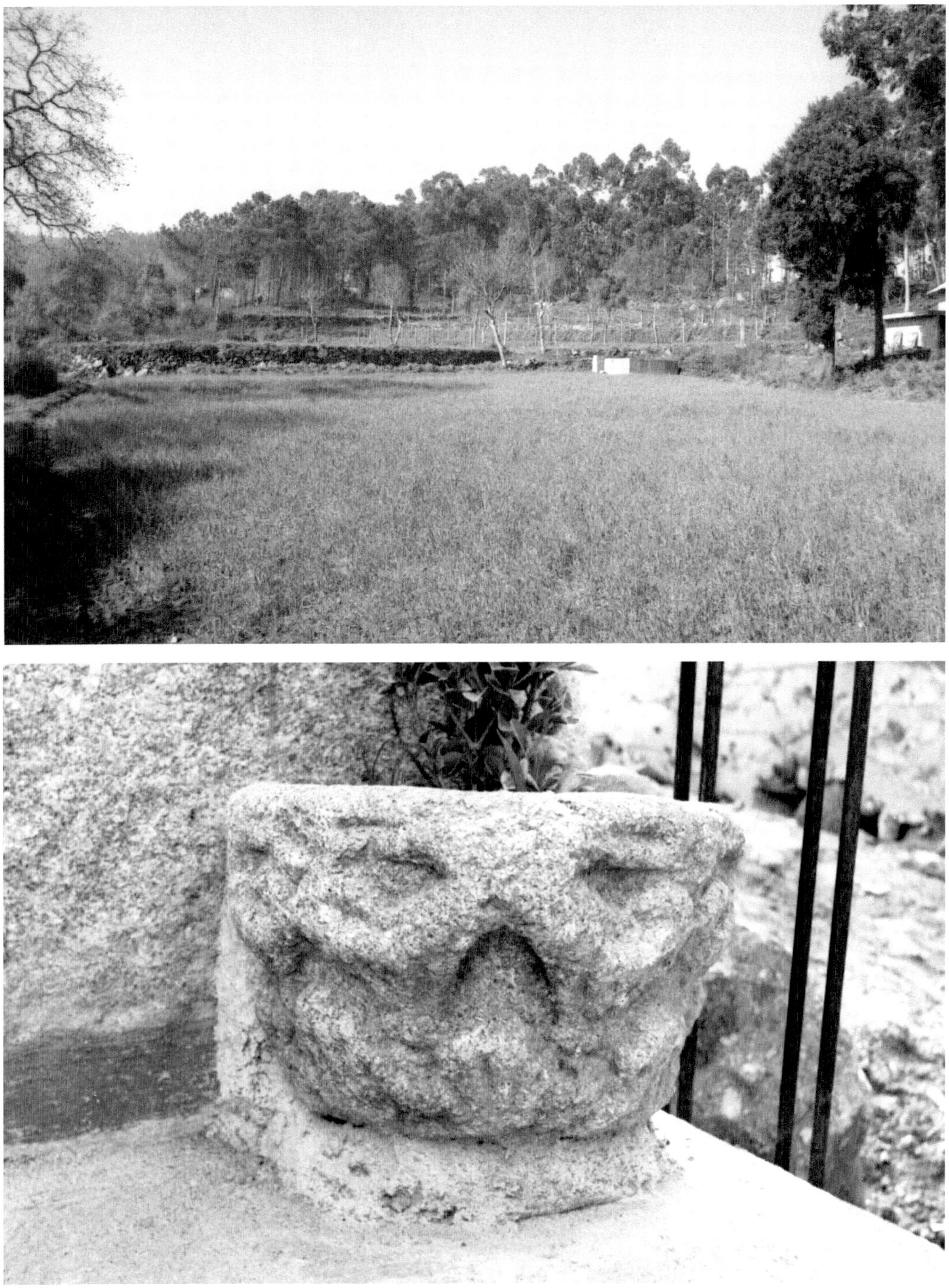

Figure 8. Outeiro do Dino (Pinheiro) Roman settlement view from East, and the reused capital found at this site (Soeiro 1984).

compelling case for being associated with the everyday operations and workforce of the São Vicente roman spa. This site (Nº 58) likely necessitated by its proximity to the spa - whose location is conditioned by the thermal springs - is unusually positioned at the bottom of the valley and close to the river, an area that poses habitability challenges for several months of the year.

Nevertheless, the strategic positioning of the healing spa on a significant natural pathway, along with the number of nearby settlements representing diverse typologies, would have likely ensured a steady influx of clientele, without the need for displacement from their places of residence.

The motivations behind the construction of the thermal establishment during the first half of the 2nd century (González Soutelo *et al.* 2023) remain a mystery. However, this timeframe corresponds with a period of significant expansion and transformation in the

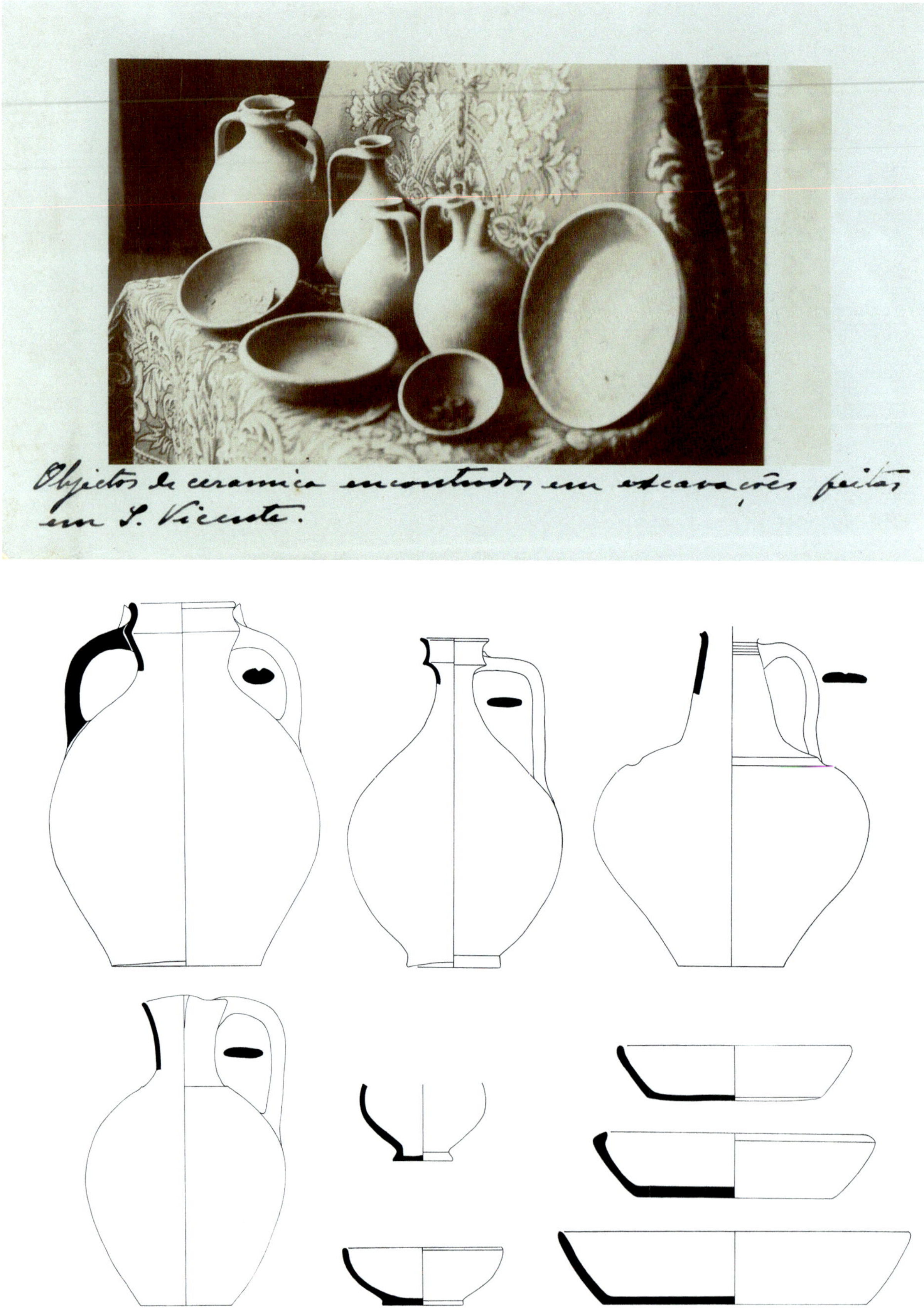

Figure 9. Photograph taken in the occasion of the findings in the necropolis of Rebolido (Outeiro do Dino, Pinheiro) and the same coarse ware kept at the Municipal Museum of Penafiel (Soeiro 1984).

southern part of the *Bracarugustanus* convent. This era was marked by a proliferation of inhabited sites, both urban and rural, and a broader integration into the Roman way of living. As previously discussed, within the present-day municipality of Penafiel, this period witnessed a restructuring of the residential areas in Castro de Monte Mozinho, meticulous attention to communal spaces, and the erection of a monument. Simultaneously, rural communities expanded throughout the territory, venturing into new lands for innovative agricultural practices.

Yet, numerous questions persist. Who oversaw the operation of the spas? Who were the clients and what were their reasons for frequenting these establishments? While these inquiries remain unanswered, it is plausible to surmise that the thermal spa served its clients up until the demise of the Roman Empire, possibly even extending into Late Antiquity, before being lost beneath layers of mud until its rediscovery in early 20th century.

Bibliography

Achados arqueológicos. 1954. *O Penafidelense* 77.16: 10th Augst.

Alarcão, J. 1988. *Roman Portugal: volume II Gazetteer: Fascicule 1*. Porto. Warminster: Aris & Phillips LTD.

Aguiar, J.M. 1936. Zeidoneses, in *Câmara Municipal de Penafiel*: 113-121. Penafiel: Câmara Municipal.

Aguiar, J.M. 1945. Penafiel antiga, in Câmara Municipal de Penafiel: 49-135. Penafiel: Câmara Municipal.

Calado, C.M.A. 2001. A ocorrência de água sulfúrea alcalina no Maciço Hespérico: quadro hidrogeológico e quimiogénese. Unpublished PhD dissertation. Lisboa: Universidade de Lisboa.

Capela, J.V., H. Matos and R. Borralheiro 2009. *As freguesias do distrito do Porto nas Memórias Paroquiais de 1758: Memórias, história e patrimonio*. Braga.

Carvalho, P.C., L. Fernandes and S. Lacerda 2022. Towns and small towns in the north of Lusitania: Singular images of the city as a symbol of power, in P. Mateos, M. Olcina, A. Pizzo and T.G. Schattner (eds) *Small towns, una realidad urbana en la Hispania romana*: 177-193. Mérida: Instituto de Arqueología.

Centeno, R.M.S. 1987. *Circulação monetária no Noroeste da Hispânia até 192*. Porto: Sociedade Portuguesa de Numismática.

Cortez, F.R. 1946. Mosaicos romanos da Estremadura. *Boletim da Junta de Província da Estremadura*, 2nd serie, 13: 273-279.

Couto, H. 1993. As mineralizações de Sb-Au da região Dúrico-Beirã. Unpublished PhD dissertation, Faculdade de Ciências da Universidade do Porto.

Dias, L.T. 1997. *Tongobriga*. Lisboa: IPPAR.

Ferreira, H. P. 2018. Um tesouro monetário Baixo-Imperial do castro do Monte Mozinho (Penafiel). *Nvmmvs*, 2nd serie, 41: 39-108. Porto.

Fortes, J. 1902. *Balineum luso-romano de S. Vicente do Pinheiro (Penafiel)*. Porto.

González Soutelo, S. In press. Roman Healing Spas in Context. Considerations about some Examples from the Western Provinces. In G. Wiplinger (ed.) *Bathing culture in Budapest. International Conference of the Frontinus Society*. Baesch.

González Soutelo, S., T. Soeiro, J.D. Carmona Barrero, J. Sampaio, H. Bernardo and C. Seara Erwelein 2023. Balneário romano de São Vicente (Penafiel): projeto de revisão das estruturas construídas e do contexto histórico-arqueológico do sitio. *Arqueologia em Portugal 2023. Estado da questão*: 771-785. Lisboa: Associação dos Arqueólogos Portugueses.

González Soutelo, S., T. Soeiro, J.D. Carmona Barrero, I. Donate Carretero and Cl. Seara Erwelein (in process). A new interpretation of a bronze object from the Roman spa of Termas de São Vicente (Penafiel, Portugal).

Gutiérrez Alonso, A., A. Redentor, M. Farjas Abadía, M. González Herrero and J. Encarnação 2021. Ingeniería y epigrafía caminan de la mano: aplicaciones de análisis digital en epígrafes latinos de difícil lectura (FE 510, IRCP 339 y CPIL 221), in K. Lennartz (ed.) *De falsa et vera Historia 4: Engaños e invenciones. Contribuciones multidisciplinares sobre pseudoepígrafos literarios y documentales*: 107-121. Madrid: Ediciones Clásicas.

Hispania Epigraphica 2014-2015. 2021. Madrid: Ediciones Complutense.

Hispania Epigraphica 2016-2017. 2023. Madrid: Ediciones Complutense.

Le Roux, P. and A. Tranoy 1974. Contribution à l'étude des régions rurales du NO hispanique au Haut Empire: deux inscriptions de Penafiel, in *Actas do III Congresso Nacional de Arqueologia*: 249-258. Porto: Ministério da Educação Nacional.

Lima, A., A. Mendonça and N. Félix 2005. As Minas de Ouro de Castromil (Norte de Portugal), in *Actas del VI Congreso Internacional de Patrimonio Geológico y Minero*: 237-250. Madrid: SEDPGYM.

López Quiroga, J. 2004. *El final de la antigüedad en la Gallaecia. La transformación de las estructuras de poblamiento entre Miño y Duero (siglos V al X)*. A Coruña: Fundación Pedro Barrié de la Maza.

Machado, F.S.L. 1920. *Uma cidade Morta no Monte Mòsinho ou Castro de Santo Estevão de Oldrões: Estudo de arqueologia*. Coimbra: Imprensa da Universidade.

Mateos, P., M. Olcina, A. Pizzo and T.G. Schattner (eds) 2022. *Small towns, una realidad urbana en la Hispania romana*. Mérida: Instituto de Arqueología.

Medeiros, A.C., L. Pilar and A.P. Fernandes 1964. *Notícia explicativa da Folha 13 - B Castelo de Paiva (Carta Geológica de Portugal escala 1: 50 000 - Penafiel)*. Lisboa: Direcção-Geral de Geologia e Minas, Serviços Geológicos de Portugal.

Medeiros, A.C., E. Pereira and A. Moreira 1980. *Notícia explicativa da folha 9 - D (Carta Geológica de Portugal escala 1: 50 000 - Penafiel)*. Lisboa: Direcção Geral de Geologia e Minas, Serviços Geológicos de Portugal.

Miranda, A. 1942. Uma notável descoberta arqueológica. Penafiel.

Miranda, A. 1944. Ara zoomorfa. *Douro Litoral* 2nd serie, 2: 25-26.

Mora Rodríguez, G. 1981. Las termas romanas en Hispania. *Archivo Español de Archeologia* 54: 37-90.

Museu Antropológico do Porto 1926. Trabalhos de Antropologia e Etnologia 3: 60.

Oliveira, J.M.S. and P. Cramez 1992. Caracterização geoquímica dos granitóides. In E. Pereira (coord.). *Notícia Explicativa da Folha 1 da Carta Geológica de Portugal, na escala 1:200.000*: 39-46. Lisboa: Serviços Geológicos de Portugal.

Pereira Menaut, G. 1998. Reflexións en clave histórica sobre Monte Mozinho. *Cadernos do Museu* 2: 37-50.

Pinto, A.R.S. 2021. Estudo do espólio numismático da Necrópole de Montes Novos (Croca, Penafiel) (unpublished master dissertation, Faculdade de Letras da Univerdade do Porto).

Pinto, G.C. 1998. A necrópole romana de Montes Novos/ Croca. *Cadernos do Museu* 2: 187-240.

Pinto, J.M.S.M. 2005-2007. Tesouros monetários Baixo-Imperiais entre Douro, Ave e Tâmega. *Nvmmvs* 2nd serie, 28-30: 7-299.

Pinto, R.S. 1934. Inventário dos mosaicos romanos em Portugal. *Anuario del Cuerpo Facultativo de Archiveros Bibliotecarios y Arqueologos* 1: 161-179.

Rebelo, F.M.S. 1975. *Serras de Valongo. Estudo de geomorfologia*. Coimbra: U. Coimbra – Faculdade de Letras.

Redentor, A. 2017. *A cultura epigráfica no* conuentus Bracaraugustanus (pars occidentalis): *percursos pela sociedade brácara da época romana*. Coimbra: Imprensa da Universidade de Coimbra.

Santos, M.J.C. and Pires, H.A.M.P. 2014. A estela funerária de Capela, Penafiel *(conventus Bracaraugustanus). Ficheiro Epigráfico* 119: n.º 510.

Soeiro, T. 1984. Monte Mozinho. Apontamentos sobre a ocupação entre Sousa e Tâmega em época romana. Penafiel. *Boletim Municipal de Cultura* 3rd serie, 1: 5-232.

Soeiro, T. 1998. O sítio romano da Bouça do Ouro, Boelhe. *Cadernos do Museu* 4: 5-62.

Soeiro, T. 2009-2010. Necrópole romana de Monteiras (Bustelo-Penafiel). *Cadernos do Museu* 12/13: 5-221.

Soeiro, T. 2013. Notícia sobre uma nova estela romana figurada de Capela, Penafiel (Portugal), in F. Acuña Castroviejo, R. Casal García and S. González Soutelo (eds), *Actas da VII Reunión de escultura romana en Hispania*: 335-348. Santiago de Compostela: Universidad de Santiago de Compostela.

Soeiro, T. 2015. A preferência pela inumação nas necrópoles romanas dos sécs. III - IV d.C. do Município de Penafiel (Norte de Portugal), in Branco, G., L. Rocha, C. Duarte, J. Oliveira and P. Bueno-Ramirez (eds) *Actas do II Congresso Internacional sobre Arqueologia de Transição*: 159-174. Évora: Universidade de Évora/Centro de História de Arte e Investigação Artística.

Soeiro, T. 2018. O Castro de Monte Mozinho (Penafiel, Porto) e o seu aro em época tardo-romana e tardo-antiga, in López Quiroga, J. (coord.) *In tempore sueborum*: 211-216. Ourense: Deputación Provincial de Ourense.

Soeiro, T. 2019. *Castro de Monte Mozinho: roteiro. Penafiel*: Museu Municipal de Penafiel.

Soeiro, T. and Redentor, A. 2021. Um altar funerário romano em Bustelo (Penafiel, Porto, Norte de Portugal). *Portugalia* 42: 85-109.

Sousa, E.F. 1962. A citânia (cidade morta) situada no Sul do concelho de Penafiel e os seus castros. Studium Generale 9.1:126-132.

Sousa, L. and T. Soeiro 2020. A Necrópole Romana do Eirô, Duas Igrejas (Penafiel): intervenção arqueológica de 2016, in J.M. Arnaud, C. Neves and A. Martins (coords) *Arqueologia em Portugal 2020 - Estado da questão*: 1439-1455. Lisboa: Associação dos Arqueólogos Portugueses e CITCEM.

Vasconcellos, J.P.S. 1903. *As águas sulfurosas de Canavezes: estudo sucinto das suas propriedades physiologicas e therapeuthicas baseadas na composição chimica e na observação clinica*. Porto: Officinas do «Commercio do Porto».

V[asconcelos], J.L. 1903. Noticias várias: 4. Balneario romano de Canaveses. *O Archeólogo Português* 7: 284-285.

Vasconcelos, M. 1935. *A vila de Canaveses. Notas para a sua história*. Lisboa: Imprensa Nacional.

The Exploitation of Natural Resources at *Aquae Flauiae* (Chaves, Portugal)

Sérgio CARNEIRO
UNIARQ – Centre for Archaeology. School of Arts and Humanities. University of Lisbon. Alameda da Universidade, 1600-214 Lisboa, Portugal;
CCDR-LVT - Commission for Regional Development and Coordination of Lisbon and Tagus Valley, Department of Culture.
sergio.carneiro@ccdr-lvt.pt

Abstract: In light of the data provided by the waterlogged remains exhumed at the excavations of the healing spa of *Aquae Flauiae* and the previous research into its territory in antiquity, we analise the settlement strategies and natural resources exploitation in this Roman city and the role played by the bathing complex in its development, integrated in the larger provincial framework.

Keywords: Roman Healing Spas; Northwestern Hispania; Natural resources in Iberian Antiquity; Spa Cities in Roman Iberia

Introduction

A recent spatial analysis of the so-called 17th road in the Antonine Itinerary concludes that, "Besides the two terminal, obvious nodes (*Bracara* and *Asturica*), the analysis suggests that the locations later occupied by *Aquae Flauiae* and *Petauonium* were also *a priori* nodes for the road" (Fonte *et al.* 2017: 182). In the case of *Aquae Flauiae* (Chaves, Portugal) (Figure 1) this detour from the Least Cost Path (LCP) determined by the authors between *Bracara* and *Asturica Augusta* may have been due to the unique presence, in this area, of natural resources that were of crucial value to the settlement of the new power, these were: first grade agricultural land; the control over gold and tin ores; and medicinal waters.

"The long and winding road"

The building of the early Roman road network in Northwestern *Hispania* is inextricably linked to the aftermath of the cantabrian wars. Four milestones of Augustus found along the road, two of them in the vicinity of *Ad Aquas*, prove the early date of its building (Rodríguez Colmenero 1999a: nº387-390) (and hence its political context). after the hard fought victory, the maintenance of an enduring peace, the effective occupation of the territory and the exploitation of its resources, demanded means of quick and easy access. Although the first segment of the *Tabula Peutingeriana*, comprising the Iberian Peninsula and most of Great Britain is missing,[1] this is an invaluable source of knowledge for the study of ancient healing spas. As Allen puts it (1998: 8): "One of the symbols depicted most prominently is a 'birds-eye' view of a square building with a central, open courtyard filled in with blue colouring which represents water. The front of the building is shown with one or more entrance doors flanked by two towers. On the structure's left side, there is a series of openings which probably represent an enclosed portico or colonnade. Of the 52 examples of this symbol, 28 are labelled with a form of the word *aquae*"[2]. The prominence given to this conventional representation of healing spas and the large number of its occurrence, demonstrate the importance given by the romans to this valuable natural health resource. The presence of medicinal water springs would, therefore, be a deciding factor for the establishment of a settlement, and, as shown by the conclusions of Fonte *et al.* (2017), one that would justify the extra mileage in the planning of a road. Further studies would, of course, be needed to confirm this pattern elsewhere in the Empire.

As the settlement of *Ad Aquas* grew in importance and became the *municipium* of *Aquae Flauiae*, new roads were built to connect with the new itinerary from *Bracara* to *Asturica Augusta*, the *Via Nova* (XVIII, in the 19th. century classification of the Antonine Itinerary) and leading to the mining districts to the North and South of the city (see bellow). In fact, eight secondary roads can be identified, turning *Aquae Flauiae* into a major crossroad in regional terms (Lemos 2010: 89)

The paleoecological evidence

The excavation of the Roman healing spa of *Aquae Flauiae* (Chaves) revealed a vast set of waterlogged archaeobotanical remains, ascribed to the late fourth

[1] The reconstruction by Miller (1916) being a spurious attempt, based on roman written itineraries and generally disproved by further investigation (Talbert 2010: 189-192, with notes at 330-331), even with all its many mistakes, gives us an idea of how the full map would have looked like.

[2] Peréx Agorreta and Rodríguez Morales (2011:155), state, based on Talbert (2010:120), that there are only 35 instances of the symbol in the *Tabula*.

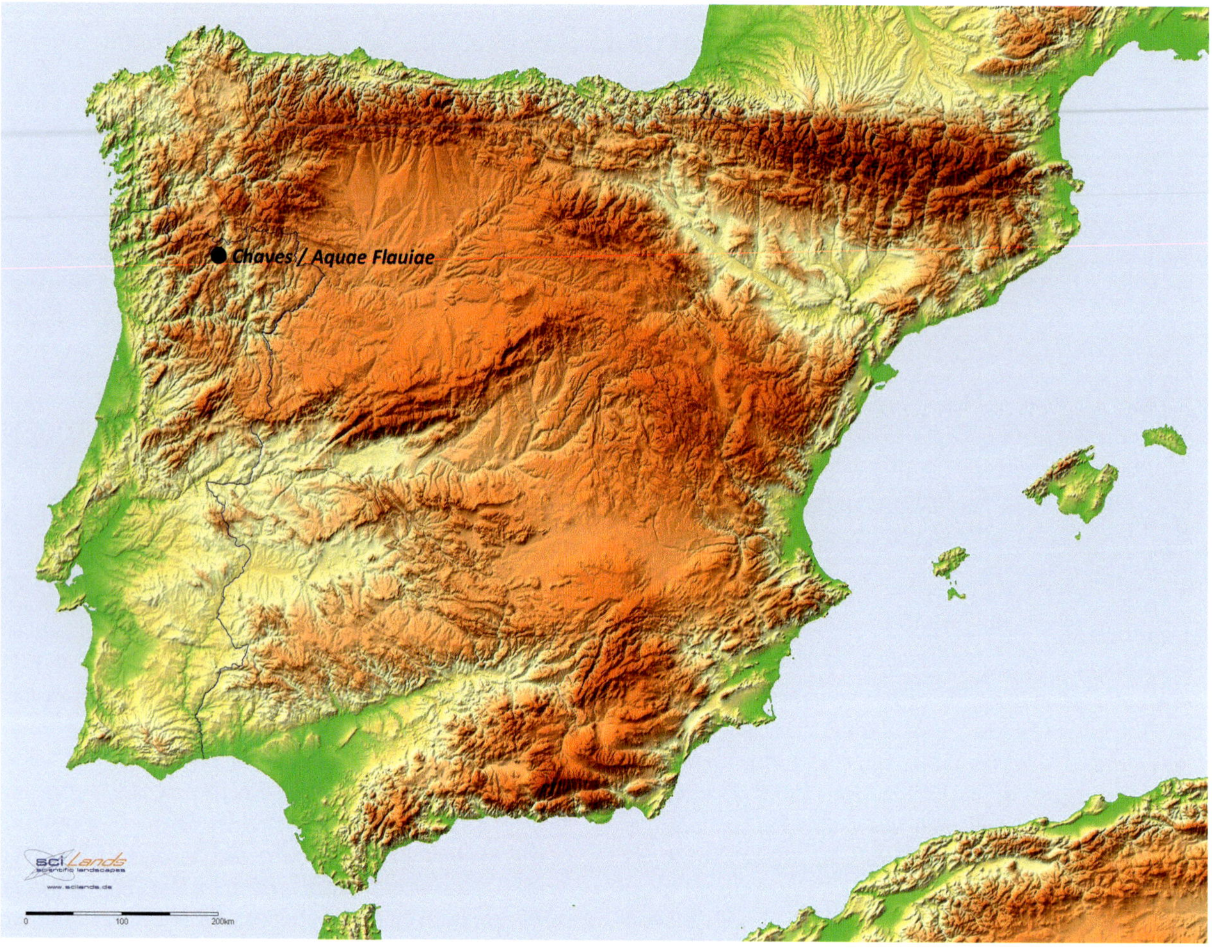

Figure 1. Location of Chaves / *Aquae Flauiae* in the Iberian Peninsula. By author.

century AD. This material included varied timber pieces, diverse small wooden objects and macro carpological remains (Vaz *et al.* 2016).

Among the carpological assemblage, the presence of non-native species, such as peach (*Prunus persica*) and Plum (*P. domestica*), attests their introduction and cultivation by the Roman settlers. Sweet cherry (*P. avium*) and sloe (*P. spinosa*) stones were also found, but since these species were already present in the wild before the Roman conquest, it is not certain whether they were cultivated or picked from wild trees. Other native species to Northwestern Iberia found in this assemblage, that were probably cultivated in Roman times, include: chestnuts (*Castanea sativa*), walnuts (*Juglans regia*), olives (*Olea europaea*) and pine (*Pinus pinaster* and *P. pinea*). The size of the endocarps of these species strongly suggest that they were indeed cultivated. The second oldest presence of cypress tree (*Cupressus sempervirens*) during Roman times in western Iberia (Vaz *et al.* 2021) was also identified, possibly an evidence of the use of this tree as an ornamental species in the surroundings of the Healing spa, although we may not exclude the possibility of its use as a medicinal plant. In fact, Pliny lists no less then 23 medicines made from cypress (*HN* 24.10). (Figure 2).

The archaeobotanical study of wooden remains, aside from the identification of technical and technological features of each typology, revealed a selection of species for specific purposes, such as *Quercus deciduous* and *Pinus pinaster* in beams, formwork stakes and planks used to build concrete walls, and *Acer* sp., *Buxus sempervirens* and in *Pinus pinaster* in several types of objects such as containers, combs and needles.

As we have already published the wooden artifacts elsewhere (Vaz *et al.* 2022), we will concentrate on the conclusions reached for the wood employed in construction materials, which are more relevant for the subject of the present work, not without referring, for its cultural meaning, the fact that all of the wood container fragments large enough for their types to be identified, were perfect matches to *Late Terra Sigillata Hispanica* counterparts from the Douro and Ebro river valleys. It is also noteworthy to refer the presence of a wooden *ampulla* with a christian inscription engraved in its body which reads: (crux) *lla* [---] *uita.* although

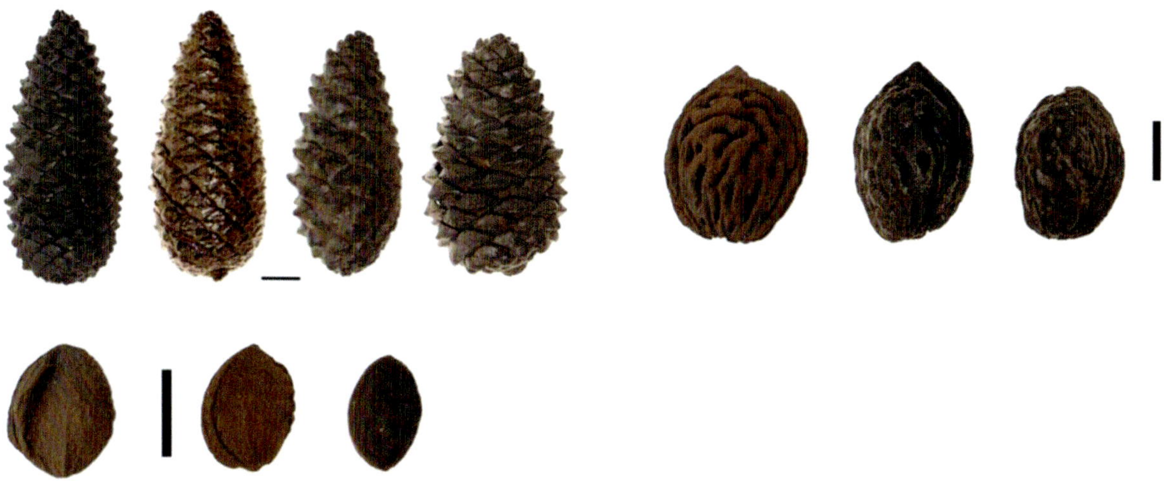

Figure 2. Carpological remains from the Healing Baths of *Aquae Flauiae*, from Vaz *et al.* 2016: Figure 7.

the defformation of the wood renders the reading extremelly difficult, it is clear the presence of a greek cross at the beginning of the remaining inscription, most common in christian inscriptions of this time and later, followed by a double l and an a or δ. bearing in mind that the cross precedes a double consonant, it is possible that this symbol has, here, the double function of establishing the christian character of the inscription and the phonetic value of *ti*. The inscription would, then, read: *tilla*, the end of many feminine Roman names. There are many examples of this double usage of the christian cross as a symbol and digraph, for instance, in an inscription from Medina Sidonia in the *conuentus Gaditanus*, a cross-crismon replaces the inicial *h* in a word (Del Hoyo Calleja 2016: 64). The second word of the readable part of the inscription could also be the fragment of a female name (*Auita*, *Vitalis*, etc.), among many other possibilities. as for the typology of this vessel, *ampullae* are relatively rare but recurring in *terra sigillata* assemblages, from the *marmoratae* (SIG-SG De63) and South gallic (Hermet 13; SIG-SG De63) productions to claire B (CLAIR-B 90, CL-REC 24a).

As for the wooden building materials, we will highlight for its rarity the presence of three fragments of wooden glazing bars. These were employed in framing window glass to allow sunlinght to enter the building while keeping the hot air inside. These elements were all made of pinewood (*pinus pinaster*) and are almost identical to the ones found at *vindonissa* (Amrein 2015: figs. 15.1, 15.2, 15.3, 15.4). The most common category is that of the wooden planks, most of them retrieved from pool B, where indirect evidence led us to conclude that a wooden floor was employed to insulate the feet of the bathers from the very hot spring water at the bottom of the pool (Carneiro 2017: 76). elsewhere in the complex, most of the building was made of concrete walls, which required a large quantity of formwork planks some of which were left behind after the construction. Most of the planks were made of oak, although pine and chestnut wood were also present.

Most relevant to the present work, the study of the architectural woods revealed the constant presence of sinuous rings, consistent with the practice of trimming the trees by cutting down all of the branches, in order to obtain longer beams and planks, more suitable for architectural purposes (Bernard *et al.* 2006). This shows a consistent planning in woodland resources management and exploitation.

The unworked twigs and branches accumulated, mostly in the *cloacae* of the bath complex and in the pools in the short period between the collapse of the covering vault and the filling of the space, give us a much wider array of plant species and provide a most interesting sample of the paleoecology of the surroundings. In this group we find maple (*acer sp.*), alder (*alnus sp.*), strawberry tree (*arbutus unedo*), european box (*buxus sempervirens*), heather (*erica spp.*), laurel (*laurus sp.*), bean (*Fabaceae*), pine (*pinus pinaster / pinea*), deciduous and evergreen examples of the Oak genus (*quercus*), apple tree (*rosaceae maloideae*) and moschatel tree (*Viburnum sp.*).

Soldiers and peasants

The valley of the Tâmega river is one of the few fluvisoil regions in Portugal and the largest example in the Northwestern Iberian hinterland (see figs. 1 and 2). These are extremely valuable soil types for ancient agriculture as is proven by the emblematic cases of the Mesopotamian region and the Nile river valley. Roman mastery of floodplains and their advantages are in the very origin of the city-state (Brock 2017: 169) (Figure 3). In a study of the territory of La Carència, Valencia, Spain, the authors found evidence

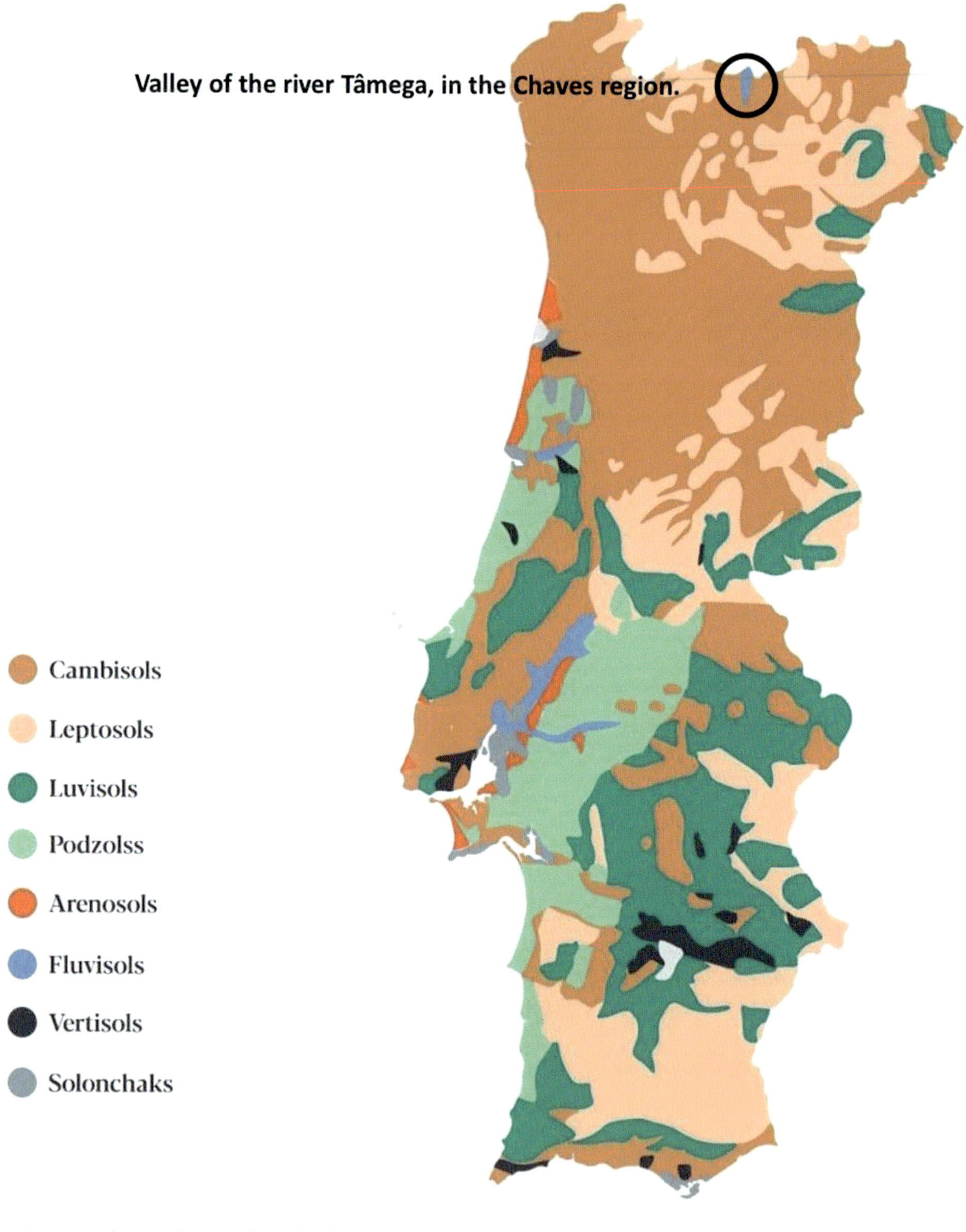

Figure 3. Soils map of Portugal: simplified from *Carta dos Solos de Portugal*, Serviço de Reconhecimento e de ordenamento Agrário, Secretaria de Estado da Agricultura, 1971. https://www.agroportal.pt/o-estudo-do-solo-a-pedologia-e-as-cartas-de-solo-em-portugal

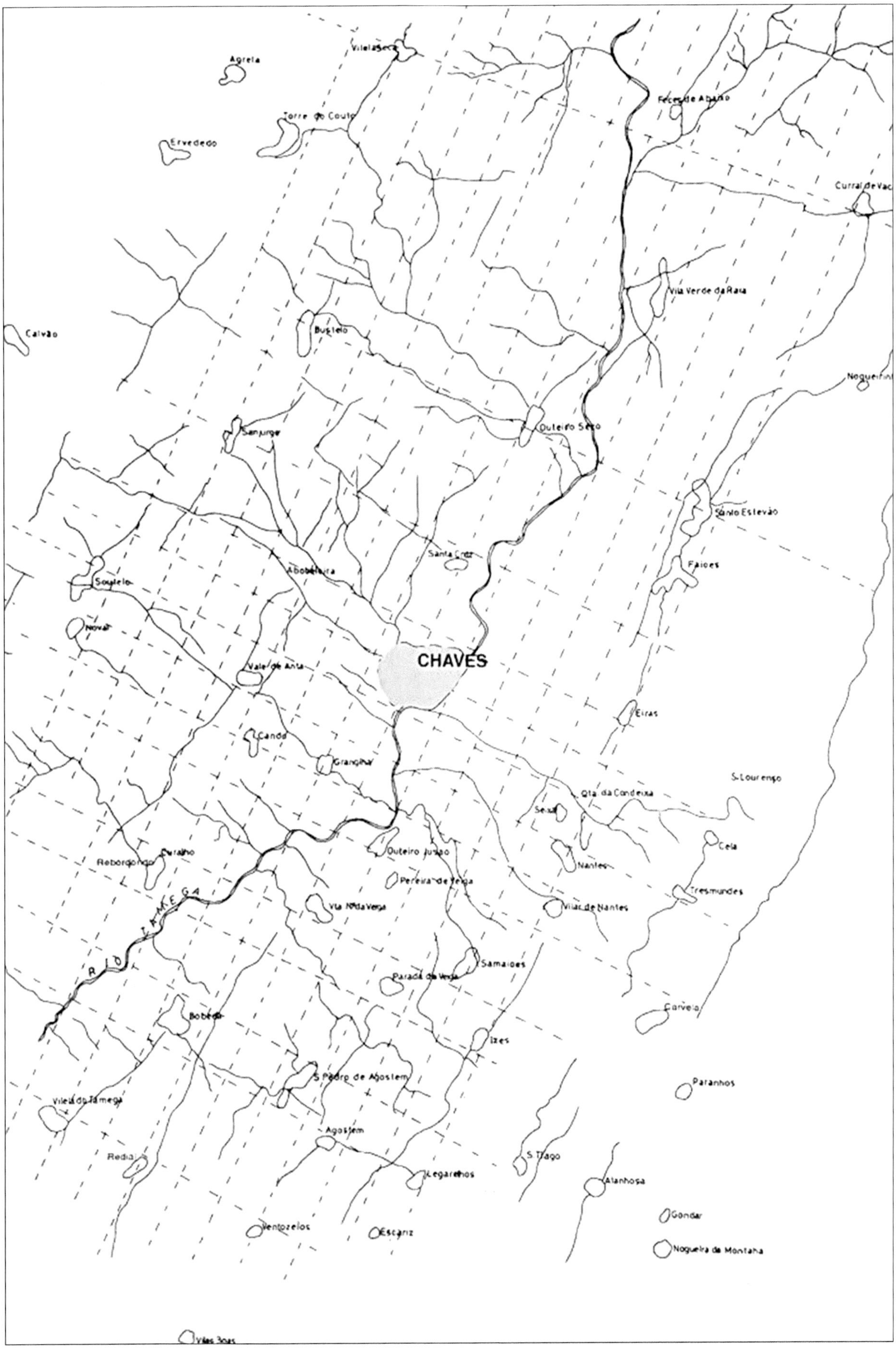

Figure 4. Remains of centuriation in the valley of Chaves, from Rodríguez Colmenero 1999: Figure 133.

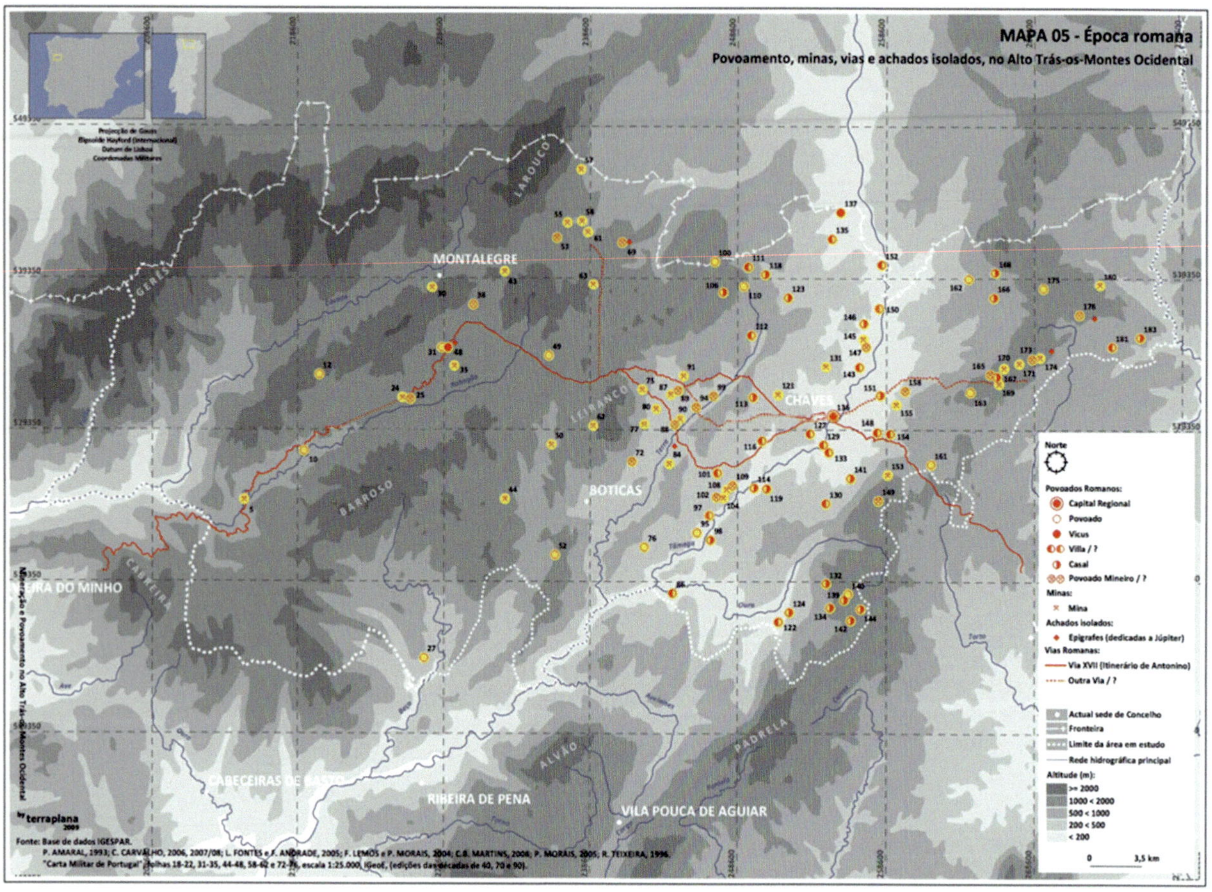

Figure 5. Roman mining evidences in the area of *Aquae Flauiae*. From Martins 2010: map 05.

of Roman settlements at the edges of flooding areas, concomitant with a shift in settlement patters from the previous Iron Age models. According to them, "this shift is closely related to Roman water management practices, as it is suggested by the habitation of areas that required complex technical skills and an in-depth environmental knowledge in order to be effectively exploited" (Orengo *et al.* 2014: 274). The same phenomenon seems to have happened in the Chaves region, where the Iron Age hilltop settlements, based on a small-scale Agro-Pastoral Production system, was replaced by the roman settlement near type A soils that indigenous peoples were unable to exploit, due to their usage of more rudimentary agricultural techniques. Furthermore, Roman settlements seem to follow the limits of the flooding zone, as in the case of La Carència. In 1721, Thomé de Távora e Abreu, a Portuguese Army Engineer who was rebuilding the defenses of Chaves, wrote in his memoirs that Roman remains were almost continuous along the road that runs by the right bank of the river Tâmega, across from the floodplain, but in higher ground (Machado 1989: 19).

A study of the floodplain of Chaves (Rodríguez Colmenero 1999) managed to identify – based on the road network of the earliest 20th century topographical surveys, the RAF and USAF aerial photography of 1947 and 1958, respectively, and the dispersion of villages with Roman remains – what seems to be traces of centuriation (Figure 5).

Given that *Ad Aquas* (only later to be given the qualificative *Flauiae*) was established immediately after the end of the Cantabrian wars, it is possible that this centuriation served the purpose of distributing land among army veterans. A network of *villae* has been identified in archaeological survey, all of them of Julio-Claudian foundation (Teixeira 1996, quoted by Lemos 2010: 97).

The gold rush

The mineral richness of northern Spain, already praised by Strabo (*Geo.* III, 3, 5), was among the main reasons for the waging of the Cantabrian wars. After the pacification of the Astur-Cantabrian area, heavy mining operations were carried out in places like Las Médulas (Lewis *et al.* 1970); Southwestern Asturias (Álvarez Muñoz *et al.* 2020); Fucochicos (Matías Rodríguez 2006), in the Astorga area; and O Sil and O Courel in Lugo (Sánchez-Palencia *et al.* 2009).

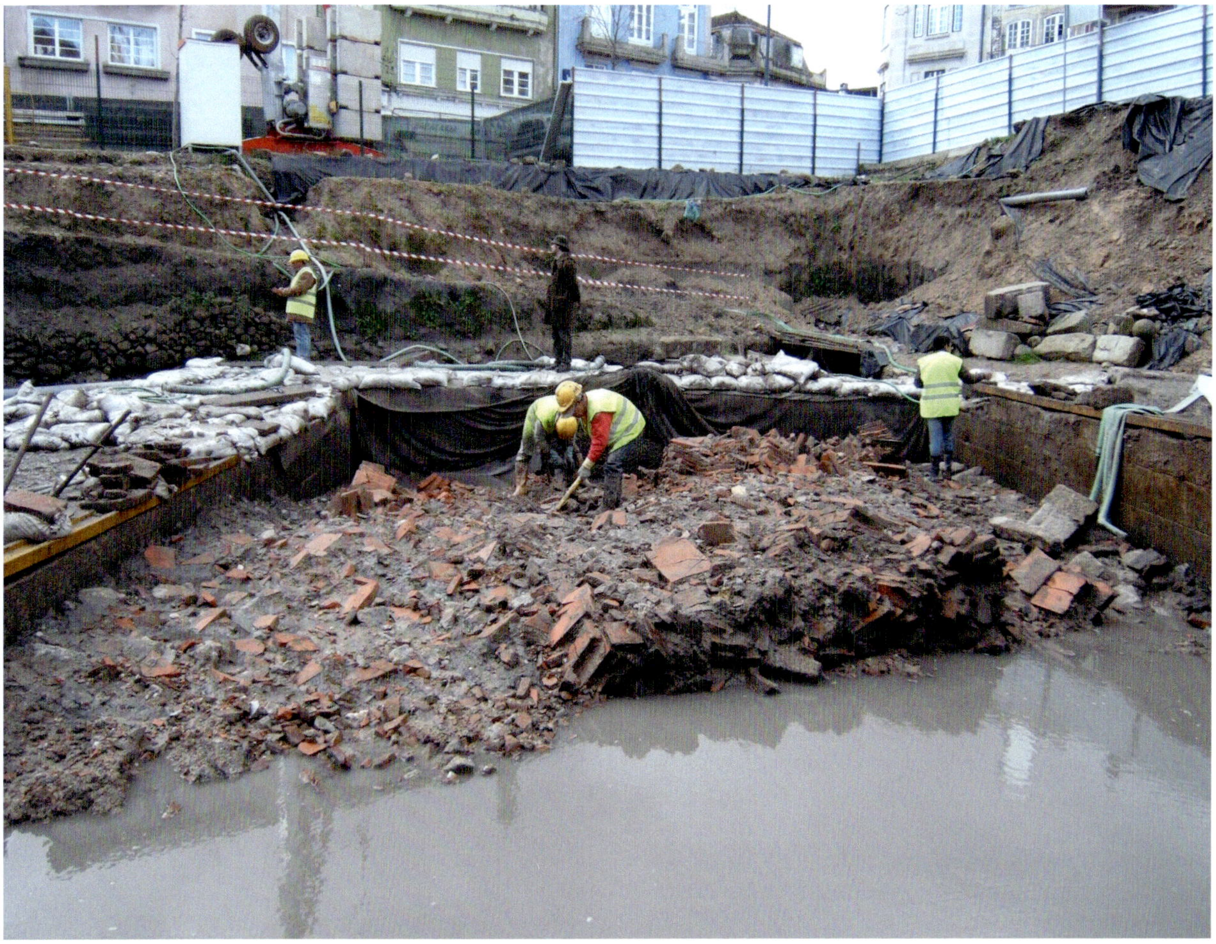

Figure 6. Excavation of the waterlogged deposits in Pool A at the healing baths of *Aquae Flauiae*. Photo by Rui Lopes.

Near *Aquae Flauiae* several Roman mining areas can be identified, such as those in Serra da Padrela (Três Minas and Jales) to the South (Martins *et al.* 2005: 269). Closer to the city, Poço de Freitas, Carvela and Outeiro Machado, where a large granitic rock, filled with engravings representing anthropomorphic figures with ladders and mining tools, bear vivid witness to the extraction activity (Júnior 1982). The transformation of the landscape is still to this day quite striking as in another site, by the banks of the river Tâmega, a mere kilometer and a half to the North of the city (Runcal / Montes Claros, Outeiro Seco) in association with large quantities of roman brick ovens that probably exploited the clays resulting from the mining operations and provided the city with ceramic building materials. fig. 6

Martins (2010) identifies an impressive number of mining sites in the area of influence of *Aquae Flauiae* (see fig 4). Even if the role of the *municipium* in the administration of the mining district is still open to debate (Lemos and Martins 2010: 80, 85), it is clear that, being, as we have seen, a pivoting regional crossroad it must have been of crucial importance in controlling the outflow of the metals.

A biased view

The development of modern Medicine and pharmacy, especially since the second half of the 19th century, brought about the need for scientific studies in order to prove the validity of medical treatments and, in time, a growing attitude of general suspicion towards healing spa treatments. In France, where there is a long tradition of going to *stations thermales* (spa cities) for treatments and the state supports 65% to 100% of the costs with these therapies, it has been argued in recent years, that the studies conducted so far have failed to prove beyond doubt that these treatments provide an actual cure, independent from the placebo effect[3]. In Portugal, state funding of spa treatments was suspended in 2011, following the financial crisis, only to be reinstated in July 2023, in response to strong lobbying by regional authorities with minero-medicinal facilities. It is as if the usage of minero-medicinal water treatments is a remnant of a time when

[3] "Cures thermales : bienfaits douteux, lobbying puissant" in *Sciences et avenir* https://www.sciencesetavenir.fr/sante/cures-thermales-bienfaits-douteux-lobbying-puissant_167367, AFP, 28.10.2022:9h42

magical thought still lived side by side with science and the modern world, focused on cost/benefit equations and the interests if large pharmaceutical companies is unforgiving with this *ancient régime* habit. And yet, wherever human communities came across minero-medicinal water springs, the supposed healing properties of these resources were exploited, invariably connected to religious cults. From Southern Africa (Ncube *et al.* 2020) to South Corea (Byoung 1999) from India (Chandrasekharam 1999) to New Zeland (Severne 1999), people have always turned to thermal spring for health benefits.

The question of the *actual* healing power of thermal-mineral waters is, of course, irrelevant. What we are trying to establish is if Romans valued it as a health resource and therefore a very important one, to exploit in the new areas annexed to the Empire, and of this we have ample proof, both in the archaeological record (most of the springs exploited in modern day Portugal have evidences of use in Roman times (Frade 1993), in epigraphical sources: the overwhelming quantity of votive inscriptions thanking the deities connected with health for specific cures that we can find associated with a vast majority of Roman healing spas (for our area of study see Redentor 2017) and in literature, for instance, Pliny the Elder (*HN* 31.32), who, besides listing a number of medicinal water springs with the specific ailments they cure, states their widespread usage throughout the Empire. One literary example that vividly illustrates the importance given to healing spas both by common people and Roman authorities, Procopius of Cesarea in his panegyric of Justinian's public buildings program *Περὶ Κτισμάτων* (III, 7), writes that

> There is a certain city on the coast of the Euxine Sea, inhabited by Thracians, Anchialus [Modern day Ankhialo, near Burgas in Bulgaria] by name (...). At that place, then, natural springs of warm water bubble forth, not far from the city, providing natural baths for the people there. The Emperors of earlier times used to allow this place to remain unwalled from ancient times, though such a host of barbarians dwelt near by; and sick persons used to visit the place, gaining relief at the cost of danger. Therefore, the Emperor Justinian made it a walled city, as it now is, and thus made the cure free from danger. (Dewing 1940: 219).

Another clamorous example of the belief in the healing power of minero-medicinal waters is the poem by Aelia Eudocia, wife of the emperor Theodosius II, found in an inscription from the Roman spa city of Hamat Gader, in the Golan Heights:

> *Of the Empress Eudocia*
> *In my life many and infinite wonders have I seen,*
> *But who, however many his mouths, could proclaim, o noble Clibanus,*
> *Your strenght, having been born a worthless mortal? but rather*
> *It is just be called a new fiery ocean,*
> *Paeanand life source, provider of sweet streams.*
> *From you is born the infinite swell, here one, there another,*
> *On this side boiling, but there in turn cold and tepid.*
> *You pour forth your beauty into four tetrads of springs.*
> *Indian and Matrona, Repentinus, Elijah the holy,*
> *Antoninus the Good, dewy Galatia and*
> *Hygieia herself, the large warm (baths) and the small warm (baths),*
> *The Pearl, the old Clibanus, Indian, and also another*
> *Matrona, Briara and the Nun, and the (spring) of the Patriarch.*
> *For those in pain your mighty strength (is ever constant).*
> *But (I will sing) of god, famous for wisdom...*
> *For the benefit of men and...* (Green and Tsafir 1992: 80)

And yet, many authors insist on referring to healing spas in the Roman Empire as a mere convenience for travelers to bathe away the fatigue of the journey and clean the road dust. This flaw of interpretation may be a form of presentism projecting modern undervaluation of healing spa tratments into the analysis of the Roman attitude towards it and thus failing to correctly evaluate Roman strategies in the exploitaition of this natural resource.

Bibliography

Álvarez Muñoz, E., B. González Fernández and B. Menéndez Casares 2020. Morteros mineros antiguos de la cala del Figo (Salave, Asturias). *Nailos* 7: 35-55.

Amrein, H. 2015. Two wooden glazing bars found in *Vindonissa* (Switzerland) from the collection of the Swiss National Museum in J. Bayley, I. Freestone and C. Jackson (eds) *Glass of the Roman World*: 165–169. Oxford: Oxbow Books.

Bernard, V, S. Renaudin and D. Marguerie 2006. Evidence of trimmed oaks (Quercus sp.) in north western France during the early Middle Ages (9th–11th centuries AD) in A. Dufraisse (ed.) *Charcoal analysis: new analytical tools and methods for archaeology*, BAR Int. Series, 1483: 103-108.

Byoung, Y. 1999. Historical review of hot spring waters in the Republic of Korea" in R. Cataldi, S. F. Hodgson and J. W. Lund (eds) *Stories From a Heated Earth: Our Geothermal Heritage*, Geothermal Resources Council Special Report 19: 378-391.

Brock, A. L. 2017. Floodplain occupation and landscape modification in early Rome. *Quaternary International* 460: 167-174.

Carneiro, S. 2017. New data from the roman healing spa of *Aquae Flauiae* (Chaves, Portugal) in G. Matilla Séiquer and S. González Soutelo (eds) *Termalismo antiguo en Hispania: un análisis del tejido balneario en época romana y tardorromana en la península ibérica*, Anejos del Archivo Español de Arqueología 78: 65-94. Madrid: Consejo Superior de Investigaciones Científicas.

Chandrasekharam, D. 1999. A prehistoric view of the thermal springs of India in R. Cataldi, S. F. Hodgson and J. W. Lund (eds) *Stories From a Heated Earth: Our Geothermal Heritage, Geothermal Resources Council*, Special Report 19: 357-365.

Del Hoyo Calleja, J. 2016. Fórmulas singulares en la epigrafía cristiana de la Bética occidental, in J. Carbonell Manilsand and H. Gimeno Pascual (eds) *A Baete ad fluvium Anam: Cultura epigráfica en la Bética Occidental y territorios fronterizos*, Alcalá de Henares: 51-66.

Dewing, H. (ed. and trans.) 1940. Procopius. *On Buildings*. Loeb Classical Library 343. Cambridge.

Fonte, J, C. Parcero-Oubiña and J. Costa-García 2017. A gis-based analysis of the rationale behind Roman Roads. The case of the so-called Via XVII (NW Iberian Peninsula). *Mediterranean Archaeology and Archaeometry* 17, 3: 163-189.

Frade, H. 1993. As termas medicinais de época Romana em Portugal in *Actas do II Congresso de Peninsular de História Antiga:* 873-916.

Green, J. and Y. Tsafir 1982. Greek Inscriptions from Ḥammat Gader: A Poem by the Empress Eudocia and Two Building Inscriptions. *Israel Exploration Journal* 32, 2/3: 77-96.

Lemos, F. and C. Martins 2010. Povoamento e rede viária no território de influência de *Aquae Flaviae* In C. Martins (ed.) *Mineração e Povoamento na Antiguidade no Alto Trás-os-Montes Ocidental.* Porto: 79-106.

Lewis, P. G. and G. Jones 1970. Roman gold-mining in north-west Spain. *Journal of Roman Studies* 60: 169-185.

Machado, J. 1989. Notícias Geographicas e Históricas da Província de Trás dos Montes (transcrição da crónica do mesmo título de Távora e Abreu). *Revista Aquae Flaviae* 2, 9-76.

Martins, C. (ed) 2010. *Mineração e Povoamento na Antiguidade no Alto Trás-os-Montes Ocidental.* CITCEM, Porto.

Martins, M., F. Lemos and F. Pérez Losada 2005. O povoamento romano no território dos Galaicos bracarenses. In C. Fernández Ochoa and P. García Díaz (eds) *Unidad y diversidad en el arco atlántico en época romana. III Coloquio Internacional de Arqueología en Gijón (Gijón, Septiembre 2002)*: 259-276. Oxford: BAR International Series 1371.

Matías Rodríguez, R. 2006. La minería aurífera Romana del Noroeste de Hispania: ingeniería minera y gestión de las explotaciones auríferas romanas de la Sierra del Teleno (León, España) in I. Moreno Gallo (coord) *Nuevos elementos de ingeniería Romana. III Congreso de las Obras Públicas Romanas.* Astorga: 213-263.

Miller, K. 1916. *Itineraria romana: Römische Reisewege an der Hand der Tabula peutingeriana.* Stuttgart: Strecker und Schröder.

Ncube, S., N. Mlunguza, S. Dube, S. Ramganesh, H-Ogola, M. Nindi, L. Chimuka and L. Madikizela 2020: Physicochemical characterization of the pelotherapeutic and balneotherapeutic clayey soils and natural spring water at Isinuka traditional healing spa in the Eastern Cape Province of South Africa, *Science of The Total Environment* 717, 137284. https://doi.org/10.1016/j.scitotenv.2020.137284

Orengo, H. A., A. Ejarque and R. Albiach 2014. Water management and land-use practices from the Iron-Age to the Roman period in Eastern Iberia. *Journal of Archaeological Science*, 49: 265-275.

Peréx Agorreta, M. and J. Rodríguez Morales 2011. Las *stationes* con *aquae*... en la *tabula* de Peutinger, *Espacio, Tiempo y Forma, Serie I, Nueva época. Prehistoria y Arqueología* 4: 153-170.

Redentor, A. 2017. Práticas epigráficas e termalismo terapêutico no Noroeste da Hispânia na época romana" in G. Matilla Séiquer and S. González Soutelo (eds) *Termalismo antiguo en Hispania: hacia un nuevo análisis del tejido balneário en época romana y tardorromana en la Península Ibérica.* Madrid: CSIC (Anejos del Archivo Español de Arqueologia; 78), pp. 467-483.

Rodríguez Colmenero, A. 1999a. *Aqvae Flaviae, I: Fontes epigráficas da* Gallaecia *meridional interior,* Câmara Municipal de Chaves.

Rodríguez Colmenero, A. 1999b. ¿Existem indícios de centuriação Romana na Veiga de Chaves? in *Aqvae Flaviae II: O Tecido Urbanístico Da Cidade Romana*, Câmara Municipal de Chaves. pp. 125-143.

Sánchez-Palencia, F., I. Sastre, B. Currás and D. Romero 2009. Minería romana en la cuenca meridional de los ríos Sil y Miño, *Revista Aquae Flaviae* 41: 285-301.

Santos Júnior, J. 1982. "As gravuras rupestres de Outeiro Machado (Val d'Anta - Chaves)", *Trabalhos de Antropologia e Etnologia*, 23, 2-3: 207-234.

Severne, C. 1999. Traditional Use of Geothermal New Zealand Maori in *Stories From a Heated Earth: Our Geothermal Heritage*, Geothermal Resources Council Special Report 19, pp. 435-449.

Talbert, R. 2010. *Rome's World. The Peutinger map reconsidered*, Cambridge University Press.

Teixeira, R. 1996. *De Aquae Flaviae a Chaves. Povoamento e organização do território entre a Antiguidade e a Idade Média.* Masters Dissertation, University of Oporto.

Vaz, F., C. Braga, J. Tereso, C. Oliveira, L. Carretero, C. Detry, B. Marcos, L. Fontes and M. Martins 2021. Food for the dead, fuel for the pyre: symbolism and function of plant remains in provincial Roman cremation rituals in the necropolis of Bracara Augusta (NW Iberia) *Quaternary International* 593-594: 372-383.

Vaz, F., M. Martín-Seijo, S. Carneiro and J. Tereso 2016. Waterlogged Plant Remains from the Roman Healing Spa of *Aquae Flaviae* (Chaves, Portugal): Utilitarian Objects, Timber, Fruits and Seeds. *Quaternary International* 404 A: 86-103.

Vaz, F., S. Carneiro, M. Martín-Seijo and J. Tereso 2022. Os materiais arqueobotânicos preservados em água das termas de *Aquae Flauiae*: madeiras de construção, objetos, frutos e sementes. *II Symposium Aquae: Cidades Termais no Império Romano - Atas 2022.* Chaves, 58-109.

3. Healing Spas and Ancient Roads.
Pilgrims and visitors to thermal sites.

Ad Aquas...
Some Observations on the Correlation between Accessibility and Development of Thermal Sites in Roman Thrace[1]

Mariya AVRAMOVA
National Archaeological Institute with Museum – Bulgarian Academy of Sciences
avramova.m@gmail.com

Abstract: Archaeological evidence attests that mineral springs were a significant element of Thracian culture both in the pre-Roman and the Roman periods. The discovered finds reveal that the interest in some healing sites popular in Roman times was in place earlier as well, clearly indicating an indigenous tradition.

Thermal sites in Roman Thrace demonstrate significant diversity in size and architectural appearance. As scholars have argued, the position and accessibility of a thermal site are crucial to its development and popularity (Bassani and Fusco 2019). While roads undoubtedly existed in Thrace before the province's establishment in AD 46 (Torbatov 2004: 84), the Roman infrastructure significantly facilitated travelling, making it comfortable and affordable to a broader audience. Advanced road networks, in turn, improved the accessibility to rural and mountain areas, where many mineral springs are situated. Furthermore, it enhanced the popularity of existing sites by allowing for easier and more convenient travel, especially for sick individuals searching for a cure – the most common visitors to spas.

The new roads made healing sites easily accessible to inhabitants of neighbouring cities, whose population looked for a place to relax and ease their ailments. Compared to their village counterparts, the cities' overall wealthier population was another impulse for the development of spas, which now had to cater to a more demanding clientele.

The paper explores the development of thermal sites through their correlation with the road network and infrastructure in Roman Thrace. The chronology of each site is juxtaposed with relative historical sources and the current knowledge of the road system to explain the changes in the appearance and the expansion observed in thermal settlements. Given the limited volume, the subject is explored based on case studies of settlements, i.e. *Skaptopara*, *Aquae Calidae* (Burgaski mineralni bani) and *Germania*.

By presenting the evolution of the described healing sites in connection to the road network, the author explores their relationship to better understand the development of Thracian spas in the Roman period.

Keywords: Roman thermal sites, road network, accessibility, Roman Thrace

Introduction

Without question, the Roman Empire could not have achieved its extensive territorial expansion without the benefit of an advanced road network that spanned all of its provinces, allowing communication and trade to flourish throughout its vast territories. While a spa's primary feature and fundamental component is a mineral water spring, an investigation of thermal sites shows notable variations in their size and amenities, such as bathing areas, temples, and more. As previously stated, the location and accessibility of a thermal site play a crucial role in its growth and appeal (Bassani, Fusco 2019). This study explores the thermal sites in Roman Thrace, their positioning in the province's road network, and how the latter affected their growth. As specific sites display distinct dissimilarities and numerous particular features, this subject is examined via three case studies; precisely the thermal sites at *Skaptopara* (near modern-day Blagoevgrad[2], Bulgaria), *Aquae Calidae* (Burgaski mineralni bani, Bulgaria), and *Germania* (Sapareva banya, Bulgaria) (Figure 1).

The road network in Roman Thrace: state of research

The Roman routes in Thrace have been a subject of study since the end of the 19th century.[3] Among contemporary scholars investigating the Roman road system is S. Torbatov, who presented an extensive study of the Roman road system, published in the first volume of the compendium "Archaeology of the Bulgarian Lands" (Torbatov 2004). The most comprehensive analysis of the Roman routes in Thrace to date is M. Madzharov's monograph "The Roman Roads in Bulgaria" (Madzharov 2009). He has also authored pieces on specific routes and road stations, along with a book focusing on one of

[1] This work was supported by the Bulgarian Ministry of Education and Science under the National Research Programme "Young scientists and postdoctoral students -2" approved by DCM 206/07.04.2022.

[2] All transliterations from Cyrillic follow the Official Bulgarian system for romanization introduced in 2006.

[3] For a thorough overview, see Torbatov 2004: 83-84.

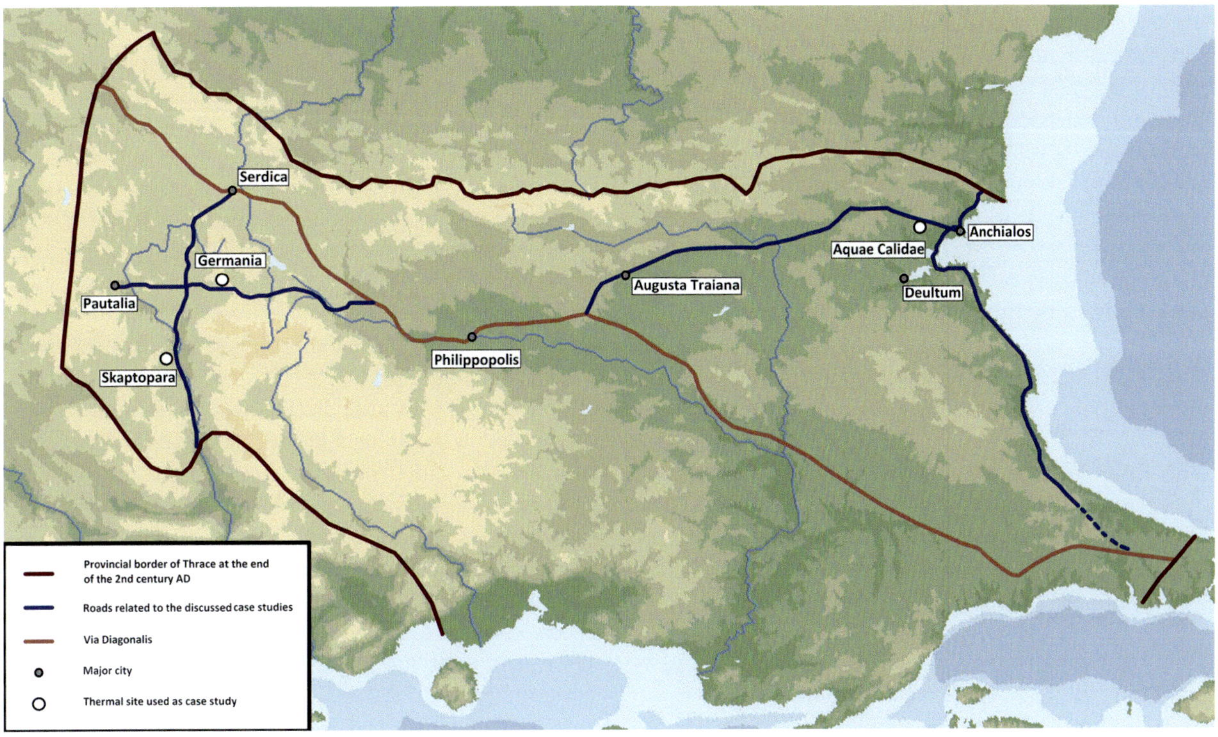

Figure 1. Map including *Skaptopara*, *Aquae Calidae* and *Germania*, as well as other Roman settlements in Thrace referred to in this text, and relevant elements of the road network (by the author).

the primary roads in the area between *Oescus* in Lower *Moesia* and *Philippopolis* in Thrace (Madzharov 2004).

Roman roads are also depicted on the maps compiled as part of the *Tabula Imperii Romani* in parts K-34, K-35/1, and K-35/2. Nevertheless, the body of the text does not discuss the roads.

Sources

The sources available for studying the road system in Thrace are plentiful and entail archaeological, epigraphic and historical monuments. The most abundant archaeological evidence consists of the remains of the Roman roads themselves, sections of which are being discovered to this day. In addition, we have the remains of other infrastructure components, such as excavated road stations (*mansiones*, *mutationes*, etc.) and road markers (*miliaria*). The inscriptions on the latter are crucial for comprehending the processes of construction and maintenance of roads. S. Torbatov observes that *milliaria*, established by emperors Diocletian (AD 284-305) and Constantine I (AD 306-337), are particularly abundant in Thrace, highlighting the region's significance during this period (Torbatov 2004: 86). Epigraphic evidence also comes from road stations located on public roads (*viae publicae*), indicating the emperor who built or reconstructed the given stop. For example, the *stelae* from Mihiltsi (station *Viamata*) on the *Oescus-Philippopolis* road show that *tabernae et praetoria* were built in AD 61 by Nero (AD 54-68) and were reconstructed by Marcus Aurelius (AD 161-180) at some point in AD 175-176 (Madzharov 2004: 92-95).

Historical sources on the Roman road system in Thrace predominantly entail *itineraria*, such as the *Itinerarium Antonini Augusti* and the *Itinerarium Burdigalense*, and probably the most famous source of ancient Roman geography – the Medieval copy of a Late antique map known as the *Tabula Peutingeriana*. These resources necessitate careful interpretation due to their particularities. As this work does not centre on the subtleties of each source, they will not be extensively examined here.

Routes in pre-Roman Thrace

Communications in pre-Roman Thrace are a topic that has received fairly little attention. This can be attributed to the absence of tangible evidence of roads from this period. Nonetheless, pre-Roman routes are believed to follow natural topographical features, such as primary rivers and mountain passes. Some scholars propose that Roman roads adhered to earlier Thracian pathways (Velkov 1979: 310). However, it is viable that Romans utilised pre-existing routes but modified them to suit their demands. For instance, the many collective discoveries of coins dating back to both the Hellenistic and Roman periods have been unearthed at various points along the central road through the Rhodope Mountains. This suggests that this route was frequented for an extended period (Madzharov 2009: 272-274). On the other hand, the many occasions where existing rock formations were cut through make it clear that the Roman road did not precisely adhere to the earlier route and introduced modifications that shortened the journey (Madzharov 2009: 278). M. Madzharov also notes the proximity of Roman and Early Byzantine settlements to those of the pre-Roman era in the *Oescus-Philippopolis* road area (Madzharov 2004: 110).

Development of the road network in Thrace

The building of the Roman road network in the territory, ultimately forming the province of Thrace, commenced in the mid-2nd century BC with the creation of *Via Egnatia*, which linked the Adriatic coast to *Byzantion* (present-day Istanbul) on the Bosphorus. The route followed the northern coast of the Aegean, and was designed mainly with the aim of facilitating the army's mobility.

The expansion of the road network was accelerated by the annexation of the Thracian vassal kingdom in AD 46. New thoroughfares such as *Via Diagonalis* and the *Oescus-Philippopolis* road were built, as were numerous roads linking the military settlements and legionary camps along the Danube with Thrace. M. Madzharov identifies the reign of Emperor Trajan (AD 98-117) as a crucial period in the evolution of the road network, with the construction of secondary roads. Roughly two decades later, under the reign of Antoninus Pius (AD 138-161), a multitude of fortifications were built. Milestones were constructed beside primary routes and in the mountain passes (Madzharov 2009: 64).

As evidenced by inscriptions, the first major reconstruction of the road infrastructure dates back to the reign of Marcus Aurelius (AD 161-180). Additional restorations were carried out by the emperors Diocletian (AD 285-306) and Constantine the Great (AD 306-337). Consequently, due to the rising unrest within the Empire and the barbarian raids, more fortifications were erected along the roads (Madzharov 2009: 64-65).

Roman roads in Thrace

The road crossing the Balkan peninsula, in use for thousands of years, was named the *Via Diagonalis*. During Roman times, it connected *Singidunum* (modern Belgrade) on the Danube with *Bysantium*. Inscriptions discovered along this route indicate that emperor Nero ordered the construction of road stations in AD 61 (Torbatov 2004: 87). The construction of roads soon after the establishment of the province held significant strategic importance. Primarily, it facilitated the rapid movement of troops to the East (Torbatov 2004). Furthermore, well-constructed roads with road stations were crucial for the mail service known as *cursus publicus*. This enabled the fast transmission of news and information between all corners of the Empire.

The Black Sea coast settlements were mainly ancient Greek colonies, e.g. *Mesambria*, *Apollonia Pontica*, etc., and aquatic passages were most likely the primary mode of transportation between them. While a West-Pontic route on land likely existed, there is no reference to it in ancient Roman itineraries. As S. Torbatov has pointed out, the only clear evidence of its use dates from the late 4th century AD. The road appears on the *Tabula Peutingeriana*. However, according to S. Torbatov, the distances indicated on the map correspond to those measured by sea and not by land, so this source probably used information from an ancient *periplous* rather than a Roman itinerary, and the route was actually travelled by water (Torbatov 2002: 42-43, 443).

Other strategically essential routes in the region were those that linked the Danube coast, otherwise known as the Danube *limes*, with the Thracian interior. One such path was the *Oescus-Philippopolis* road, previously mentioned, which was constructed by Emperor Nero, a fact confirmed by the inscription found in the *Viamata* road station near the modern village of Mihiltsi (*CIL* III 6123=1420734). Another road that connected *Ratiaria* and *Montana* to the *Via Diagonalis* at *Serdica*, a thermal site situated on an important crossroad, was constructed, likely during the same period (Torbatov 2004). A road linking *Oescus* to *Serdica* is believed to have existed, although its route is not documented in ancient sources (Gerov 1967: 89-90).

In the eastern part of the province, there are two identified roads: one connecting the legionary camp at *Novae* to *Augusta Traiana* and another leading from *Durostorum* to *Anchialos*. The latter was likely constructed at the start of the 2nd century AD when *Durostorum* was established as a legionary camp (Torbatov 2004: 89).

These roads extended over multiple provinces of the Empire. Nevertheless, there is also documented evidence of key routes solely within the province. One of the routes in *Tabula Peutingeriana* connects *Anchialos* on the Black Sea coast to *Philippopolis*, passing through *Kabyle* and *Augusta Traiana*. This route holds significance in this study, as *Aquae Calidae* served as the initial road station approximately 19 Roman miles[4] from the starting point of *Anchialos*.

Two roads led south of *Philippopolis* – one through the Rhodope mountains to the Aegean coast and another

[4] The indicated 19 Roman miles are measured following the shortest contemporary road. *Tabula Peutingeriana* lists the distance as 12 Roman miles. This is confirmed by the Gothic historian Jordanes, who places *Aquae Calidae* on the 12th milliar column from *Anchialos* (Jord. *Get*. 109).

one to the Southwest to *Nicopolis ad Nestum* and probably further to the Aegean coast.

In Western Thrace, a road led from *Serdica* through *Pautalia* to *Heraclea Lynkestis* and joined *via Egnatia* (Torbatov 2004: 91).

The aforementioned main roads were entwined with numerous local routes, of which many are not attested in written sources and are known only through the discovery of their sections. Among them is a road following the *Strymon* (modern Struma) river. Evidence indicates that this path was regularly travelled as early as the Bronze Age, potentially earlier.

Furthermore, it can be reasoned that paths and local roads must have traversed the mountains, connecting various settlements located in mountainous areas with the world. Nevertheless, accessing these settlements was likely more challenging. In actuality, numerous segments of the Roman road pavements remain apparent and in use today. Certain sections of these pavements have even become a point of interest for tourists (Madzharov 2009: 64-65).

Impact of the road network on the development of spas

The expansion of the road network undeniably facilitated travel and enhanced accessibility to inland Thrace and its thermal sites. However, was mere accessibility sufficient to make a spa a popular destination, and what other factors were involved? Primarily, the properties of the mineral water were the main reason for the existence of a spa. It is conceivable that tales of healing circulated through word of mouth and served as the primary form of advertising for the waters.

The extent to which the reputation of a site spreads is a significant factor to be considered. It can be assumed that thermal springs located near a busy road would have gained more widespread recognition. The presence of a major town near a spa is another important consideration. For instance, in *Diocletianopolis*, situated near *Philippopolis*, a thermal complex was built, subsequently expanded and had an additional bath constructed during the Late Roman period. This indicates an increased interest in the spa. The diverse range of room types highlights the varied options available. However, there are exceptions, such as the lack of significant finds from the mineral source at Krasnovo (Tsonchev 1948), despite its proximity to *Diocletianopolis* and, therefore, to *Philippopolis*. Starozagorski mineralni bani, located near *Augusta Traiana*, was likely extensively utilised and widely popular, as evidenced by the numismatic material spanning from the 4th century BC to the 12th century AD (Nikolov 1968: 43). However, due to the lack of thorough publication of the finds, a more detailed analysis is not possible.

On the contrary, a site with scarce architectural features may suggest the restricted geographic range of said site. Local thermal facilities are equally compelling and significant as the lavish and opulent spas. They provide an exceptional understanding of the life and beliefs of a section of society that is inadequately represented in epigraphic and written sources. Furthermore, the study of thermal waters in Roman provinces, Thrace included, allows for an exploration of their usage dynamics. By identifying pre-Roman vestiges, we can investigate thermalism as a local phenomenon before the Romans arrived. Analysis of findings enables the creation of a tentative chronology of the spring's usage.

Case studies

Skaptopara

The village of *Skaptopara* is attested to by the infamous *Skaptopara* inscription (*IG Bulg* IV 2236) (Figure 2), discovered in 1861 near modern-day Blagoevgrad. The text comprises a plea from the inhabitants of *Skaptopara* to Emperor Gordian III (AD 238-244), along with a speech given by *Aurelius Pyrrus*, a member of the praetorian guard born in *Skaptopara*, in front of the provincial governor. The villagers requested the Emperor's intervention due to the decline of their once-prospering village. The constant visits of soldiers and officials demanding free food and shelter as part of their rank's privilege were the cause. The main reason for people to stop in the village, as indicated in the text, was the thermal springs located nearby (*IG Bulg* IV 2236, lines 50-53). The village's pleasant surroundings and proximity to the sources were among its primary charms for visitors. Additionally, a famous fair occurred in the area (*IG Bulg* IV 2236, lines 122-138).

The location of the village has been a subject of debate among archaeologists and historians. According to the inscription, *Skaptopara* was situated near a road and mineral springs and between two military camps (*IG Bulg* IV 2236, lines 26-30, 50-53). Several scholars have associated *Skaptopara* with various archaeological sites near the area where the inscription was discovered. S. Hisarlashka-Tanova (1990) presents a synopsis and appraisal of earlier arguments and introduces new potential locations based on archaeological discoveries. Notably, some suggested sites, such as the one in proximity to modern Riltsi village, are not located in the vicinity to mineral springs, albeit the discovery of pipe fragments. In this case, the probable

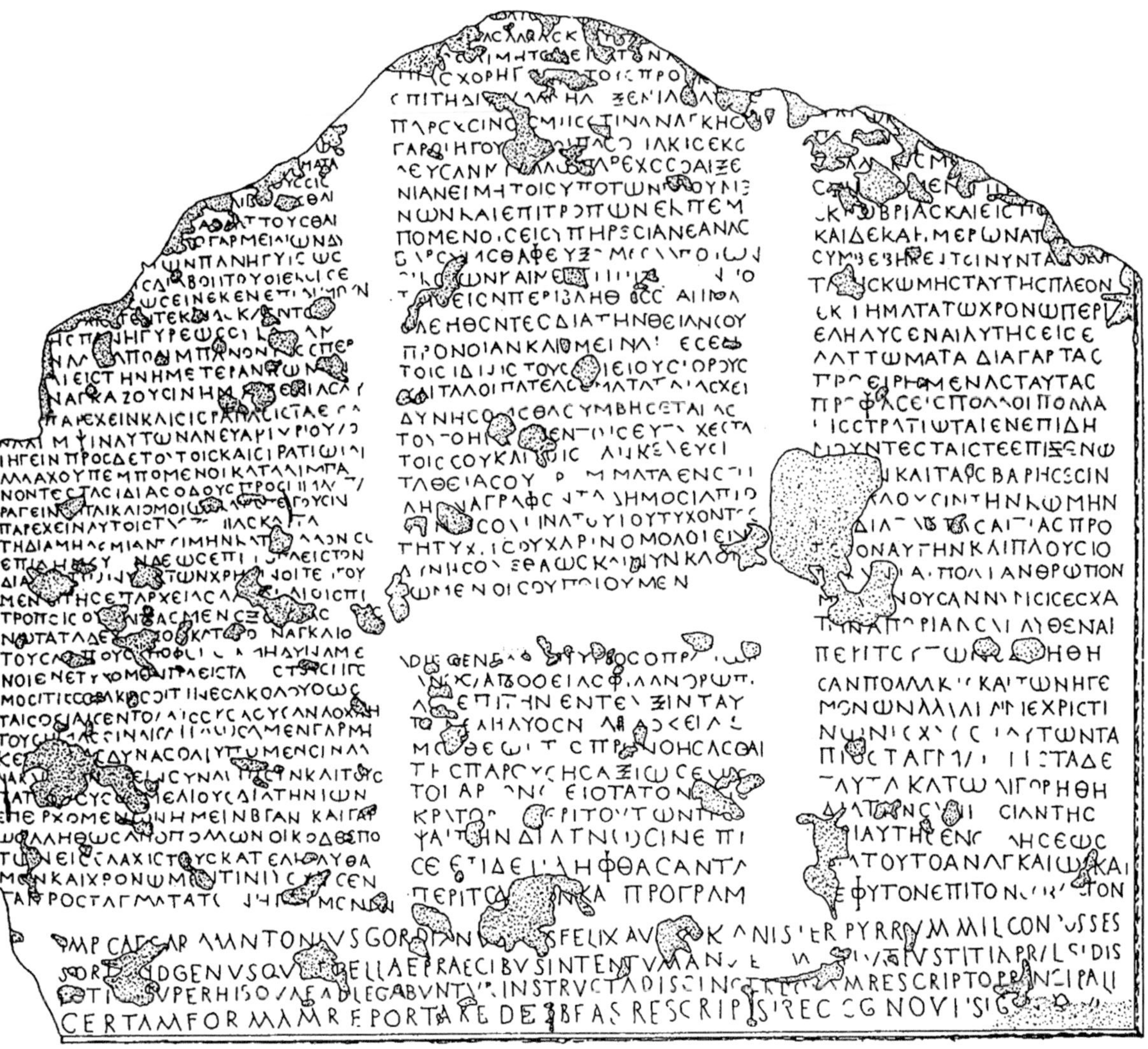

Figure 2. Fragment of the *Skaptopara* inscription (IG Bulg IV 2236, drawing, from Wikimedia Commons).

identification is corroborated by the chronology of the site (Hisarlashka-Tanova 1990: 37).

As of the time of writing, the location of *Skaptopara* remains unestablished. Contrary to public opinion and information published by several media outlets, the structures discovered during the rescue excavations west of Blagoevgrad, near the villages Pokrovnik and Zelen dol in 2017 and 2018, do not belong to ancient *Skaptopara*.[5] The location indicated in Figure 1 is the area where the inscription was discovered.

The *Skaptopara* inscription and the springs' popularity have led some to believe that *thermae* existed at *Skaptopara*. For example, the *Tabula Imperii Romani* K-34 authors place a bath on the site (TIR K-34: 82). Nevertheless, no baths have been unearthed in any of the excavated settlements. Nonetheless, there are many instances of thermal sites that prove how constructing bathing facilities is not an absolute requirement for bathing in mineral springs (Yegül 1992: 110-112). Therefore, it is imperative to confirm if a certain spring was utilised during the Roman period, even if no baths were uncovered.

Due to the area's geomorphological characteristics, over 20 minor springs with a low flow rate emerge. A geological survey carried out in 1940 revealed that they all originate from a common underground source. While working on the XXVth spring, the engineer overseeing the project, B. Radoslavov, observed a "primitive"[6] construction of Roman bricks without

[5] I would like to express my gratitude to the excavations director, Assoc. Prof. Dr. Zdravko Dimitrov, for providing me with information regarding the site.

[6] While discussing catchment installations, B. Radoslavov utilises the term "primitive" to distinguish them from modern installations, rather than an evaluation of their quality.

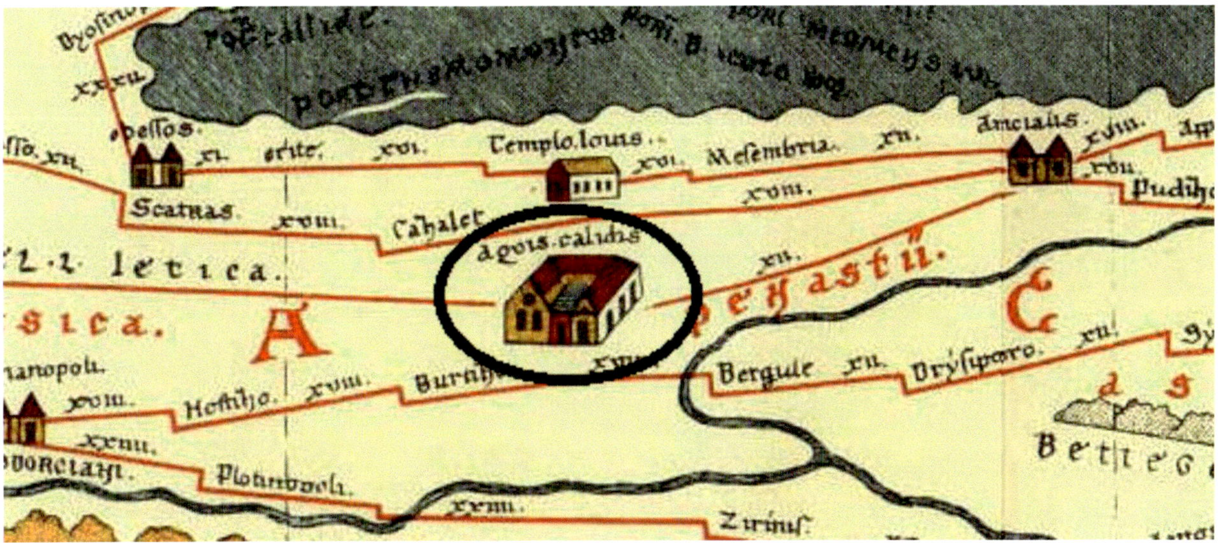

Figure 3. *Aquae Calidae* (Burgaski mineralni bani) on *Tabula Peutingeriana*, section 7 (from Wikimedia Commons).

mortar, which was neither efficient at retaining the mineral water nor preventing contamination. Several Hellenistic, Roman, and Ottoman coins were discovered in the catchment area (Radoslavov 1941: 4). Despite the fact that the numismatic evidence points to the site's use in Antiquity and the Roman period, the described catchment cannot be attributed to Roman engineering. Additionally, there are no references to water conduits, and it is safe to assume that this spring did not supply water to any *thermae*.

Aquae Calidae

Aquae Calidae is the sole thermal site in Thrace to be designated as a spa by the special vignette on the *Tabula Peutingeriana* (Figure 3). Additionally, it is the only spa in the province with a common nomenclature composed of the word *aquae* and an adjective; in this case, *calidae* indicating the high water temperature. Byzantine sources refer to the site as *Thermī*, which is either a Greek version of the Latin name or a commonly used Greek equivalent. It is worth remembering that the population in Thrace predominantly spoke Greek, especially on the Black Sea coast, which was colonised in the 7th century BC.

Archaeological evidence shows that the site was frequented long before the Roman period. The unearthing of prehistoric artefacts suggests habitation of the region surrounding the springs dating back to the Neolithic era. The site was occasionally visited in the 1st millennium BC before seeing more frequent use beginning in the 7th century BC (Momchilov and Klasnakov 2021: 45-46). There is evidence of a bath constructed during the reign of emperor Nero, as revealed by a fragment of a building inscription unearthed in 2015 (Figure 4) (Sharankov 2016: 971).

Aquae Calidae is located 28 km (approximately 19 Roman miles) from *Anchialos*, a colony of *Apollonia Pontica*, established in the late 5th or early 4th century BC. *Anchialos* was granted city status by emperor Trajan and became significant in the area during the Roman period (Dimova 2015). *Aquae Calidae* was also situated on the West Pontic route, passing along the Black Sea coast and on the road leading inland from the coast to *Augusta Traiana* and ultimately to *Philippopolis*. Being located within the boundaries of a prosperous city and on significant routes is an ideal setting for increasing the prominence of the site. Nevertheless, as pointed out by S. Torbatov, the coastline in the Roman era contrasted considerably from the current one. Also, the West-Pontic road overland was less commonly used, in preference for cabotage sailing along the coast (Torbatov 2004: 87). Even though the land route was less popular, the location was still reachable within one day's journey from *Anchialos*. Assuming an average

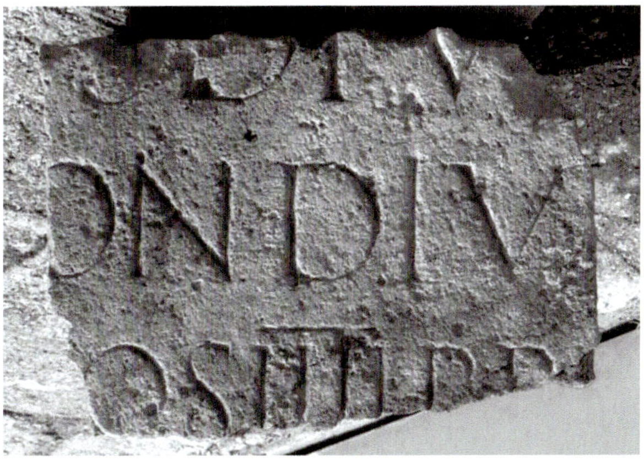

Figure 4. Fragment of the building inscription from the *thermae* at *Aquae Calidae* (Burgaski mineralni bani) (after Sharankov 2016, fig. 2).

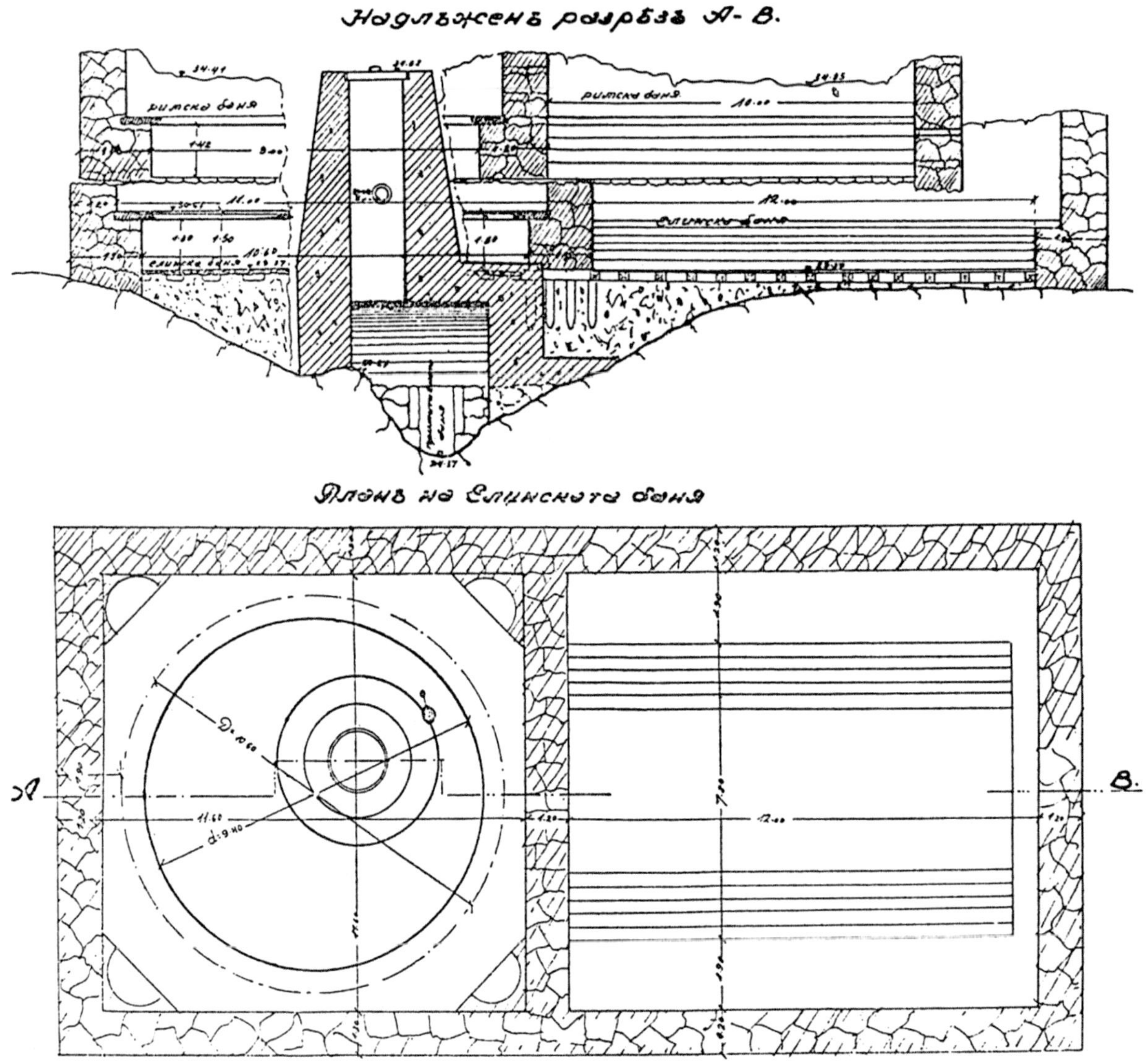

Figure 5. Section of the pools at *Aquae Calidae* discovered in 1910 and the modern catchment installation (above) and floorplan of the pools (below); the mineral spring is situated directly under the circular pools (from Angelov 1939: 5).

traveller would cover roughly 17 Roman miles a day (Torbatov 2004: 83).

The construction of the bath during Nero's reign is supported by the coin assemblage found in the spring. E. Paunov's analysis reveals a considerable decline in the number of coins around the time the water source became less accessible after being covered by a circular basin (Figure 5) (Paunov 2015: 250-251). Furthermore, the construction of the baths during the same period as other significant roads in Thrace, such as *Via Diagonalis* and the *Oescus-Philippopolis* road, supports the theory that *Aquae Calidae* was integrated into the Roman transportation system. This allowed its popularity to expand beyond the local region, attracting not only visitors seeking relief by the waters but also travellers who were unaware of the existence of the sacred spring.

Approximately 4000 coins were found in the sacred spring on two separate occasions: firstly, during spring head cleaning in 1910 (Filow 1911), and later during a cleaning effort in 1994 (Momchilov and Klasnakov 2021: 20). According to the study by E. Paunov, Roman soldiers made up the largest group of visitors to *Aquae Calidae* during the late 1st century BC-1st century AD. He identifies the visitors as originating from Thrace and *Moesia*, as well as *Macedonia*, mainland and island Greece, and Asia Minor (Paunov 2015: 249-250). The coins discovered in the baths (but not the spring!) during excavations between 2013 and 2015 further support the presence of soldiers. The recovered issues, minted in Pergamon between 23 and 15 BC by Augustus (27 BC-AD 14), were used for paying the military stationed in Asia Minor and the Balkans (Dotkova 2021: 316).

The military's affinity for mineral springs is evidenced by the numerous coins minted at the veteran *Colonia Flavia Pacis Deultensium*, which was established around AD 70 (Dotkova 2021: 317) and located about 40 km to the south of *Aquae Calidae* (approximately 27 Roman miles). The *fibulae* recovered from the sacred spring in 1910 also confirm the soldiers' presence at *Aquae Calidae* in the 1st century AD (Gencheva 2004: 29, 34, 38-39).

The mineral water from the *Aquae Calidae* spring is beneficial for the musculoskeletal, digestive, urinary and nervous systems (Vladeva *et al.* 2001: 38). Ailments of the bones, muscles, and joints can be defined as occupational diseases for the Roman military. As a result, the high number of soldiers taking the waters is not surprising. However, it is not possible to ascertain definitively if the trips to the spa were prearranged, resulted from pilgrimage, or constituted a stop *en route* to other places. Considering the location of *Aquae Calidae* on the major route from the coast to inner Thrace and the regular movements of troops, it is highly likely that the numerous visits were not premeditated.

The coin struck at *Primnessos* in Phrygia, dating to the reign of Antonines, is the one minted at the greatest distance from the site in the 2nd-3rd century AD coin assemblage. M. Dotkova interprets it as a remnant of the movement of military units previously stationed in Phrygia. However, the predominant amount of coins from the period originated from the nearby *Anchialos* (Dotkova 2021: 317).

Most of the coins from the 4th century AD were minted in *Nicomedia* and Constantinople, and were mainly used within the region of Thrace. However, few coins were struck in far-off mints, such as *Arelate* (presently Arles, France) and *Ticinium* (modern Pavia, Italy) (Dotkova 2021: 318). It is possible that these coins were brought by distant travellers, probably during a pilgrimage. It is clear, however, that the proximity of the port in *Anchialos* made *Aquae Calidae* accessible to pilgrims travelling by sea from all parts of the Empire.

Pilgrims are not attested in the inscriptions unearthed at the site. The votive reliefs recovered from the spring reveal names of dedicants, which are of local Thracian origin. Their presence is supported by the coins minted by the Thracian king Rhoemetalces I (12/11 BC- AD 12/13) (Dotkova 2021: 316).

Numismatic and epigraphic evidence should not be the sole source used to examine spa visitors. Items such as hairpins and combs (Filov 1910: 216) suggest that women also visited the site. Such votives unfortunately do not reveal what illnesses they suffered from. Infertility may have been one, as the spring's water is believed to be beneficial for this condition (Vladeva *et al.* 2001: 38).

On the *Tabula Peutingeriana*, *Aquae Calidae* appears as a road station. The decision to construct a road station in this location was likely a pragmatic one. Firstly, the springs facilitated a steady supply of water, which was a necessity for each road station. Additionally, the existence of thermal water permitted the provision of enhanced travel amenities, whereby voyagers could enjoy a hot bath whilst recuperating from their journey. The convenience of a roadside bath required minimal effort – the water was readily available and did not need to be sourced elsewhere. Although we cannot determine the exact flow rate of the mineral spring during the Roman era, the mere existence of a bath facility is evidence that the quantities were sufficient for its operation.

D. Momchilov disputes the view that *Aquae Calidae* functioned as a road station as early as the mid-1st century AD. According to him, the settlement that was already in existence was transformed into a road station during the 3rd quarter of the 2nd century AD by the provincial governor *Gaius Pantuleios Graptiacus*, whose building activity in *Aquae Calidae* is confirmed by an inscription found in 2016 (Momchilov and Klasnakov 2021: 50). Nevertheless, this theory fails to clarify Nero's construction of the bath, which is a reasonable act given the emperor's attested efforts in developing the road system in Thrace.

Germania

The thermal site of *Germania* is another interesting example of the relationship between the road network and the development of a thermal site. The site is located beneath the modern spa of Sapareva Banya and has not been fully excavated. The Roman settlement is situated at the crossroad of two roads: the *Pautalia-Philippopolis* road connecting the western and eastern parts of the province and the route from *Serdica* along the *Strymon* River, linking the *Via Diagonalis* with *Via Egnatia*. The location was chosen primarily for its strategic importance. Nevertheless, the proximity to the springs, providing a constant and plentiful water supply similarly to *Aquae Calidae*, was also an essential factor.

The Romans valued the location for its strategic significance. This is evident from the deployment of the auxiliary *Cohors II Lucensium* in AD 198-199 under the reign of Septimius Severus, as attested by discovered inscriptions (*CIL* III 12337, *CIL* III 12338 and *CIL* III 12339). The cohort continued to occupy *Germania* throughout the 2nd and 3rd centuries AD. In the 4th century AD, *Germania* became a civil settlement which existed until the Middle Ages. Archaeological excavations to date have not uncovered any evidence indicating military presence in the area prior to the late 2nd century AD or a topographical connection between the *castellum* and a preceding Thracian settlement. It is commonly believed that *Germania* constitutes one of the two military camps referenced in the *Skaptopara* inscription (for example, Staykova-Aleksandrova and Staykova 2003: 203).

The spring at *Germania* was explored during rescue excavations in 1948, yielding votive reliefs depicting healing deities *Asclepius*, *Hygieia* and *Telesphorus*, the Nymphs, the Thracian hero some with inscriptions, a gold ring (Dremsizova 1952), as well as coins primarily from the 2nd and 3rd centuries AD (Gerasimov 1950).

The dedicants' names on the reliefs suggest Thracian origin, leading some scholars to suggest that Romans did not worship in the sanctuary (Staykova-Aleksandrova and Staykova 2003: 204). Nonetheless, the discovery of coins, particularly those from the era of *Cohors II Lucensium*'s arrival and presence, indicates otherwise. Considering the military's affinity for thermal water, as evidenced, for example, by the finds from *Aquae Calidae*, it is difficult to believe that they would have ignored the springs at *Germania*.

The site's name, *Germania*, likely originates from the Thracian language and means "hot" – a reference to the thermal springs. This suggests that the Romans were not the first to settle around the spring. Therefore, it is possible that they integrated with the locals in worshipping the water source and, in this manner, increased its popularity (Ivanov 1957: 230). The degree and nature of the locals' veneration of the springs before the arrival of the auxiliary unit is underresearched. On the one hand, the exact chronology of the deposited votive reliefs cannot be determined. Nevertheless, it is incorrect to perceive the reliefs as the sole manifestation of devotion. Marble votives were undoubtedly expensive, and deities were most likely offered more affordable gifts. For instance, discoveries made at *Diocletianopolis* (modern-day Hisarya) show that fruits, eggs and small animals were also offered to the gods (Tsonchev 1937: 151).

The construction of the *thermae* did not occur until *Germania* became a civil settlement. According to T. Ivanov's observations, the bath was erected in the 3rd-4th century AD as a significant structure, complete with a minimum of two chambers featuring hypocaust installations (Ivanov 1957: 215-216). Regrettably, the excavations yielded scant information regarding the structures from the camp period. Therefore, it is currently impossible to determine if the spring water was used for bathing by *Cohors II Lucensium*. However, it is unlikely that the Romans would have avoided using it, given their ingrained practicality.

Germania is a clear example of how the military presence led to the development of a thermal site. If not for the disposition of *Cohors II Lucensium* predetermined by the location's strategic importance, the site likely would have been one of many known through a very limited number of artefacts.

Conclusion

By building an extensive network of roads, the Roman Empire and its culture spread throughout every part of Thrace, affecting the daily lives of the local population in a lasting manner. Even the hot springs of Thrace were not immune to their influence, as demonstrated by the case studies presented. They reveal that the accessibility of a site could have various impacts on the neighbouring communities.

Aquae Calidae is a renowned pre-Roman site that gained even more recognition with the rise in Roman influence and may have directly profited from the construction of the Roman road. The initial bath was constructed during emperor Nero's rule, which corresponded with the creation of the province's key roads. Most likely, the spring played a noteworthy role in the choice of this location.

Skaptopara offers a juxtaposing example. The popularity of the once prosperous village, with stunning scenery and plentiful natural resources, resulted in adverse effects as inhabitants were compelled to depart in pursuit of a peaceful existence. However, this perspective is only conveyed to us through the villagers' petition to emperor Gordian. Only by locating *Skaptopara* will we be able to reconstruct the actual evolution of the village. Nevertheless, the case of *Skaptopara* serves as a reminder that popularity is not always beneficial.

Like *Aquae Calidae*, *Germania* was situated near a road; however, it never attained the same level of popularity, perhaps because of its inland, mountainous location. The spring was visited by Thracians, judging by the findings. Nevertheless, numismatic evidence indicates an increased frequency of acts of piety since the arrival of the Roman military at the end of the 2nd century AD.

To conclude, the expansion of the road network in Thrace had a noticeable impact on pre-existing thermal sites in the newly integrated province. Roman roads were not only built to integrate the new territories with the Empire but also to connect the people themselves and provide access to places that were previously reserved for locals. As such, Thracian thermal sites became part of the Empire's thermal network.

Bibliography

Abbreviations

CIL III = T. Mommsen (ed.) 1873. *Corpus Inscriptionum Latinarum. Vol. III: Inscriptiones Asiae, provinciarum Europae Graecarum, Illyrici Latinae*. Berolini: Reimer.

IG Bulg IV = G. Mihaylov (ed.) 1966. *Inscriptiones Graecae in Bulgaria repertae. T. 4: Inscriptiones in territorio Serdicensi et in vallibus Strymonis Nestique repertae*. Sofia: Balgarska akademia na naukite.

TIR K-34 = J. Šašel (ed.) 1976. *Tabula Imperii Romani: K 34: Naissus - Dyrrhachion - Scupi - Serdica - Thessalonike*. Ljubljana: Slovenska Akademia Znanosti in Umetnosti.

TIR K-35/1 = Avramea, A. 1993. *Tabula imperii Romani: K 35/1 Philippi*. Athènes: Académie d'Athènes.

TIR K-35/2 = R. Ivanov (ed.) 2012. *Tabula imperii Romani: K 35/2 Philipopolis*. Sofia: Tendril.

Publications

Angelov, B. 1939. Hidrologichni i arheologicheski belejki za okolnostta na gr. Anhialo. *Vodosnabdyavane i kanalizacia* 3, 1: 1–11.

Bassani, M. and Fusco, U. 2019. Methodological Aspects, in M. Bassani, M. Bolder-Boss, and U. Fusco (eds) *Rethinking the Concept of 'Healing Settlements': Water, Cults, Constructions and Contexts in the Ancient World*, 3–8. Oxford: Archaeopress Publishing.

Dimova S. 2015, *Aquae Calidae* i Anhialo, *Izvestia na Burgaskia muzej*, 5: 43–47.

Dotkova, M. 2021. Numizmatichniat kompleks otkrit po vreme na razkopkite v Aquae Calidae prez 2013-2015 g., in D. Momchilov and A. Nakeva (eds) *Aquae Calidae* 1: 316–371. Burgas: Regionalen istoricheski muzey Burgas.

Dremsizova, T. 1952. Edna nahodka ot Sapareva banya. *Izvestia na Archeologicheskia Institut* 18: 353–358.

Filov, B. 1910. Nahodki ot Ajtoskite bani (Aquae Calidae). *Izvestia na Balgarskoto arheologichesko druzhestvo* 1: 216–217.

Filow, B. 1911. Bulgarien. Aquae Calidae. *Archäologischer Anzeiger: Beiblatt zum Jahrbuch des Archäologischen Instituts* 26: 349–370.

Gencheva, E. 2004. *Rimskite fibuli ot Bulgaria: ot kraya na I v. pr.n.e. do kraya na VI v. na n.e.* Veliko Tarnovo: Faber.

Gerasimov, T. 1950. Arheologicheski vesti. *Izvestia na Arheologicheskia institut* 17: 321–322.

Gerov, B. 1967. Prouchvania varhu zapadnotrakiyskite zemi v rimsko vreme. Chast 2. *Godishnik na Sofiyskia universitet. Fakultet po zapadni filologii* 61(1): 1–102.

Hisarlashka-Tanova, S. 1990. Za mestopolozhenieto na Skaptopara. *Arheologia* 32(3): 36–41.

Ivanov, T. 1957. Arheologicheski prouchvania pri Sapareva banya. *Izvestia na Arheologicheskia institut* 21: 211–232.

Madzharov, M. 2004. *Rimskiat pat Oescus-Philippopol. Patni stantsii i selitshta*. Plovdiv: Natsionalna akademia na arhitekturata.

Madzharov, M. 2009. *Rimski patishta v Bulgaria. Prinos v razvitieto na rimskata patna sistema v provintsiite Mizia i Trakia*. Veliko Tarnovo: Faber.

Momchilov, D. and M. Klasnakov 2021. Burgaskite mineralni bani (Aquae Calidae – Therma, Thermopolis) – presechna tochka na epohi, narodi, kulturi, in D. Momchilov and A. Nakeva (eds) *Aquae Calidae*: 9–210. Burgas: Regionalen istoricheski muzej.

Nikolov, D. 1968. Stroitelen nadpis ot rimska banya kray Stara Zagora. *Arheologia* 10(1): 43–47.

Paunov, E. 2015. The coin assemblage from the sacred spring of Aquae Calidae in Thrace: main problems, patterns and conclusions. *Izvestia na Burgaskia muzej* 5: 245–255.

Radoslavov, B. 1941. *Geologichesko, petrografsko, tehnichesko i hidrolozhko izuchavane i kaptirane na mineralnite izvori pri gr. Gorna Dhzumaya*. Sofia.

Sharankov, N. 2016. Epigrafski otkritia prez 2015 g. In *Arheologicheski otkritia i razkopki prez 2015 g*: 970–972.

Staykova-Aleksandrova, L., and Staykova, I. 2003. Germania (Germania, Sapareva banya), in R. Ivanov (ed) *Rimski i rannovizantijski gradove v Balgaria*: 202–214. Sofia: Ivray.

Torbatov, S. 2002. *Ukrepitelnata sistema na provintsia Skitia: kraya na III-VII v.* Veliko Tarnovo: Faber.

Torbatov, S. 2004. Patna mrezha v Trakia i Mizia (I-III v.), in R. Ivanov (ed) *Arheologia na balgarskite zemi*: 76–95. Sofia: Ivray.

Tsonchev, D. 1937. Hisarskite bani: geografski, istoricheski i arheologicheski ocherk. *Godishnik na Plovdivskata narodna biblioteka i muzej* 1935–1936: 53–210.

Tsonchev, D. 1948. Krasnovo, *Godishnik na Narodnia arheologicheski muzej Plovdiv* 1: 187.

Velkov, V. 1979. Razvitie na gradskia zhivot. Patna sistema, in V. Velkov, H. Danov, T. Ivanov and A. Fol (eds) *Istoria na Bulgaria. T. 1. Parvobitnoobshtinen i robovladelski stroj. Traki*: 304–312. Sofia: Izdatelstvo na Balgarskata akademia na naukite.

Vladeva, L., Krasteva, D., Yordanov, Y. and Kostadinov, D. 2001. *Spravochnik za balgarskite mineralni vodi. Osnovni danni, fiziko-himicheski harakteristiki, pokazania za lechenie I drugi prilozhenia*. Stara Zagora.

Yegül, F. 1992. *Baths and Bathing in Classical Antiquity*. New York: The Architectural History Foundation; Cambridge (Massachusetts), London: The MIT Press.

Thermalism and Road System in the African Roman Provinces. A Focus on Roman Algeria

Paola ZANOVELLO
Department of Cultural Heritage, University of Padova / Associate professor, piazza Capitaniato, 7. 35139 Padova (Italy).
paola.zanovello.1@unipd.it

Jacopo TURCHETTO
Department of Cultural Heritage, University of Padova / Researcher, piazza Capitaniato, 7. 35139 Padova (Italy).
jacopo.turchetto@unipd.it

Abstract: The phenomenon of thermalism is highly evident in Roman North Africa, as attested by literary sources, Roman itineraries, and archaeological findings. This paper aims at analysing the historical and geographical context of the present-day Algerian territory, which comprises the Roman provinces of *Mauretania Caesariensis*, *Numidia*, and *Africa Proconsularis*. That entire territory is portrayed as a vast and elongated region in the initial segments (I-IV) of the *Tabula Peutingeriana*, featuring the registration of four thermal sites, three of which bear the customary 'ad aquas' vignettes. However, the documented thermal centres within that territory are considerably more numerous. Therefore, it is intriguing to scrutinize the relationship between archaeological-topographic data and the geomorphological contexts. This analysis aims at gaining a deeper understanding of the distribution patterns of thermal sites, their associations with primary and secondary road networks, the nature of users, and the socio-cultural and religious implications that characterise them.

Keywords: Thermal centres, Roman roads, *Numidia*, *Mauretania Caesariensis*, *Africa Proconsularis*.

Introduction

The phenomenon of natural thermalism is widespread across the northern part of the African continent, stretching from the Atlantic coasts to Egyptian territory, with a notable concentration in the region between present-day Tunisia and Algeria. This distribution is clearly illustrated in a 2022 map (Elbarbary *et al.* 2022: fig. 1), where thermal springs dot the entire coastal area and hinterland between the two countries.

The phenomenon has historical roots, with the registration of hundreds of thermal springs starting from the French colonial era. During this period, the significance of this resource for the economic development of the territory was recognised.[1] Attention was also directed towards the pre-existence of ancient structures, as evidenced by studies published between the late 19th century and the 1960s. These studies focused on water resources (Ville 1865; Thenoz 1894; Gsell 1902; Birebent 1962), including those supplying inhabited centers and rural areas, as well as thermal springs, which were increasingly seen as potential attractions for international tourism (Nedjar and Chergui 2022). Between the end of the 19th century and the beginning of the 20th century, around 200 springs were registered in Algeria (Thenoz 1894; Hanriot 1911), classified on the basis of temperatures and chemical-physical characteristics. The Department of Constantine stood out as the most abundant, boasting 145 known and utilized springs (Thenoz 1894: 25-48).

This period also saw the launch of systematic studies on the territory, focusing on the collection of topographical and historical-archaeological data. These studies relied on the analysis of literary sources, encompassing both ancient and modern texts. Travellers who explored these regions between the 18th and 19th centuries played a crucial role in providing valuable insights. The abundance of epigraphic documents and itinerary sources holds particular significance for North Africa.[2] This research culminated in the publication of a series of monumental works that continue to be fundamental. Notably, works such as the *Atlas archéologique de l'Algérie* and *Monuments antiques de l'Algérie*, both edited by Stéphane Gsell, have become essential references in the field (Gsell 1901; 1902; 1911).

In addition to Jean Birebent (Birebent 1962), who focused more on hydraulic issues at the request of the French Government rather than conducting a census of the springs, researchers such as Helene Jouffroy (1992), Elena Pettenò (1998), Francisco Díez de Velasco (1998), and Jans Koehler (2019) have undertaken specific investigations on the theme of Roman *aquae* in North Africa. More recently, Silvia González Soutelo has also delved into this theme, taking a broader perspective (González Soutelo 2019). Similar to the work of Díez de Velasco, her research compares data from the Iberian Peninsula with that from Africa.

[1] See for example Ville 1865.

[2] The entire VIII volume of the CIL is dedicated to North Africa. Among the itinerary sources, see in particular the *Tabula Peutingeriana* and the *Itinerarium Antonini* (see *infra*).

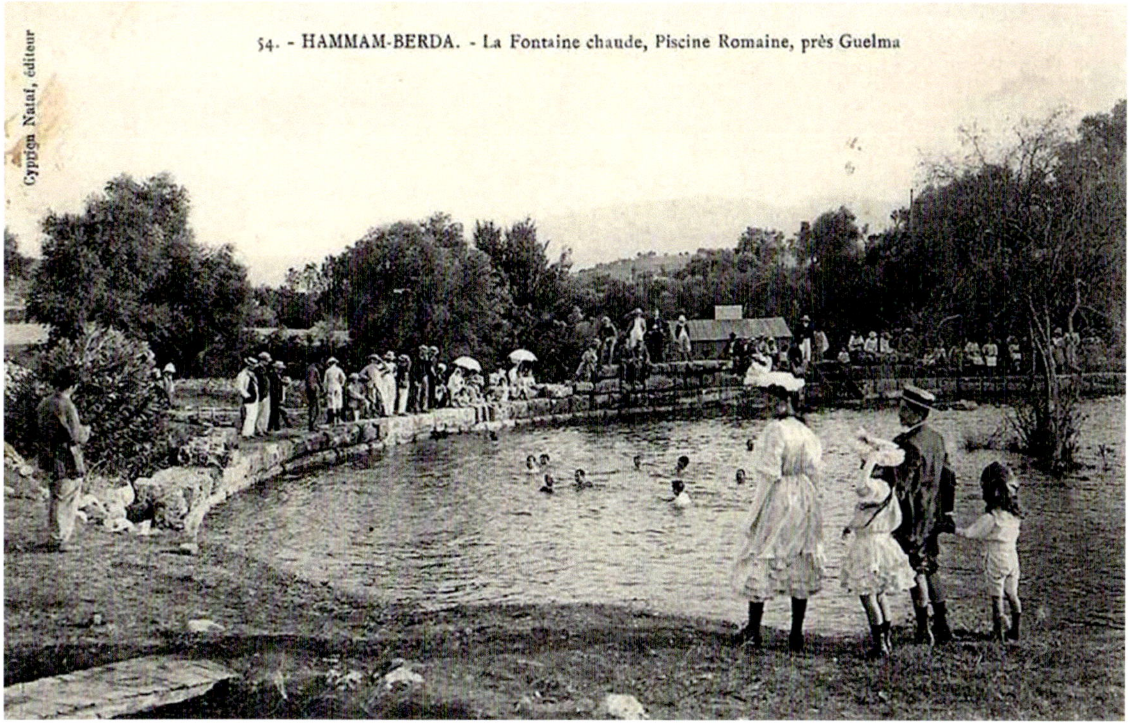
54. - HAMMAM-BERDA. - La Fontaine chaude, Piscine Romaine, près Guelma
Cyprien Nataf, éditeur

Figure 1. Hammam Berda (source: *Encyclopédie de l'Afrique du Nord*, https://documentation.encyclopedie-afn.org/Hammam_Berda).

Ancient spas in Roman Algeria

During Roman times, the current Algerian territory was primarily represented by *Numidia*, with the easternmost sector belonging to *Africa Proconsularis* and the western part to *Mauretania Caesariensis*. In a recent review conducted by Koehler, who synthesizes data collected by previous scholars (Koehler 2019: 102-103, tabb. 1-4), 16 thermal bath sites were identified in Algeria. This number is nearly double compared to those surveyed by Jouffroy and Pettenò in the 1990s, as Díez de Velasco considered only those with evident links to specific cults. Of the identified sites, almost all, specifically 13, are located in the province of *Numidia*. Ten of these are associated with hot springs, reflecting common spa practices, while three are connected to cold springs around which actual sanctuaries developed. Notable examples include Lambesi, where a large sanctuary dedicated to Aesculapius was situated (Janon 1973; 1977); in Khemissa (Gsell 1922), the ancient *Thubursicu Numidarum* located near the sources of the *Bagradas* river, where there were large basins (Ain el Youdi) where various deities, including Neptune, were venerated;[3] near the city of Timgad, the Roman *Thamugadi*, where the sacred place known as *Aqua Septimiana Felix* developed (Leschi 1947; Lassus 1981). The remaining 3 Algerian thermal sites[4] were located in the neighboring *Mauretania Caesariensis*.

Spas in *Numidia*

Regarding the first site listed in Koehler's table, Hammam Oued Hamimine,[5] in the Azzaba/Jemmapes area, there is limited information available regarding its potential Roman origin. Bertherand, in 1868, mentioned the existence of Roman swimming pools about 6 km away from the city of Jemmapes, on the road towards Bone (the ancient *Annaba*), which were still visible at that time. He highlighted the continuous use of the waters, classified as sulphate, even in the modern era (Bertherand 1868: 113-114).

Near Guelma, the ancient *Calama*, three well-known sites have been identified for various reasons. All bear Arabic names indicating the presence of hot waters or baths (*hammam*): Hammam Berda (Figure 1), Hammam Meskoutine, the Roman *Aquae Thibilitanae* (Figure 2), and Henchir el Hammam, with its name suggesting the existence of ancient remains (henchir in Arabic). In the first location, remains of Roman swimming pools were observed and documented along with pre-

[3] Gsell 1922: 85-98, in the plan (tab. X) there are evident similarities with the *Asklepieion* of Lambesi; see Malek 2018: 362.

[4] *Ad Sava municipium* / Hammam Guergour, *Sitifis* (Setif); *Aquae Calidae* /Hammam Righa, *Caesarea* (Cherchell); *Aquae Sirenses* / Hammam Bou Hanefia, Mascara.

[5] Dib 2008: 43-44; the area is catalogued among the sulphate waters in Hanriot 1911: 273-275. In this context, we are discussing a minimum of four springs situated approximately 9 km from Jemmapes. Unlike other sites, there is no mention of the presence of Roman remains at this location. Koehler includes it in his table 4, but unfortunately, bibliographical references are not provided. Gsell's survey on F. 9, covering the area around Jemmapes, does not offer any pertinent information that could aid in identifying this specific place. See Bekkouche 2009: 9 and figs. on pp. 10-11.

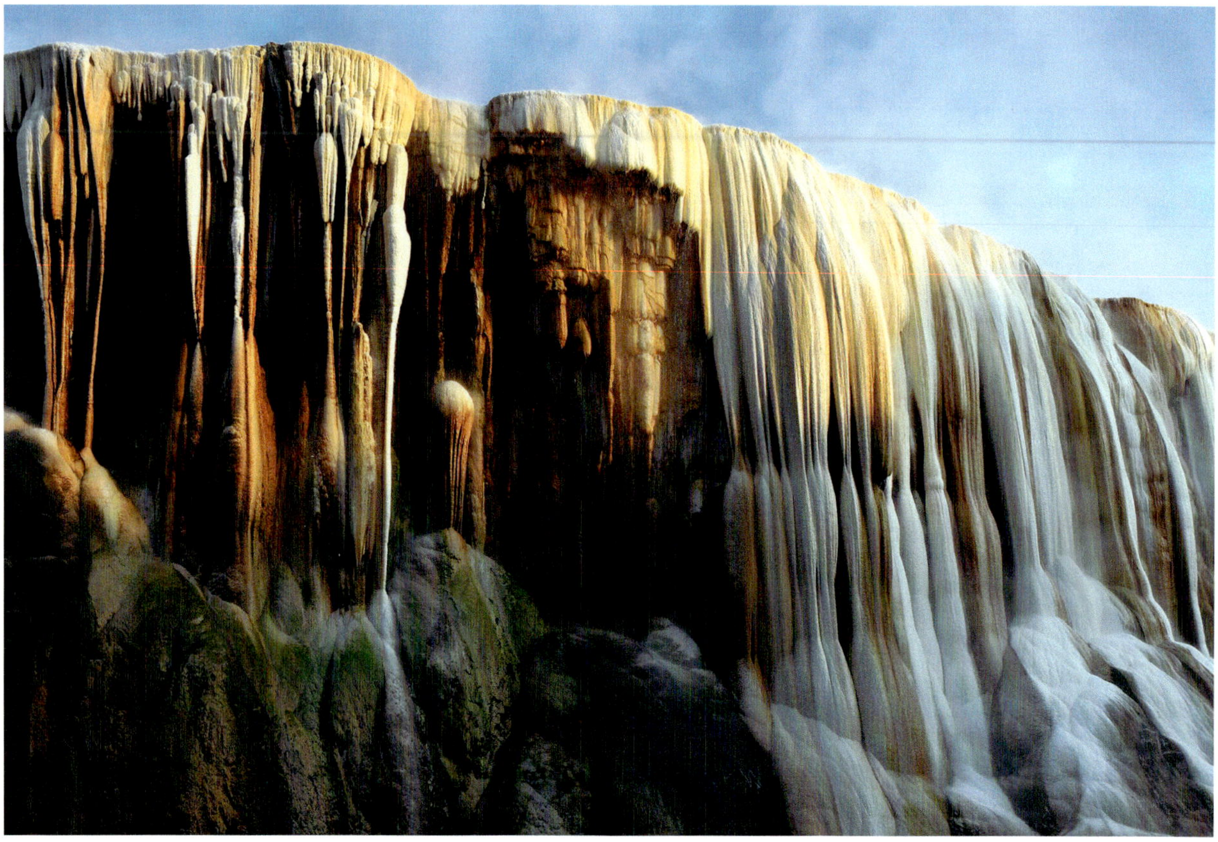

Figure 2. Travertine cascade at *Aquae Thibilitanae* / Hammam Meskoutine hot springs (source: https://commons.wikimedia.org/wiki/File:Hammam_Meskoutine_02.jpg).

Roman inscriptions, indicating a pre-existing structure and likely the use of thermal waters by the indigenous Berber populations.

The *Aquae Thibilitanae*, indicated in the *Tabula Peutingeriana* with an alternative vignette to the traditional one ("ad aquas") associated with spa settlements, are located at the confluence of two oueds and testify to the presence of a monumental thermal complex (Marty and Rouyer 1892; Hanriot 1911; Fiorini 1935; Jouffroy 1992; Wilson 1997; Pettenò 1998; Cote 2000), with bathing pools, cisterns and conduits.

For the third locality, Henchir el Hammam, a more specific name is not preserved, useful for its identification in the territory, but it certainly must have referred to one of the various thermal areas registered in the vicinity of Guelma (Khiter 2018: 40-45; cf. Dib 2008).

Near Constantine, the ancient *Cirta*, there is the site known as Sidi Mimoun, associated with a cult dedicated to a revered benefactor. An inscription found at the site is dedicated to Neptune Augustus.[6] It is possible that the location corresponds to the description given by travellers in the 18th century who observed a thermal cave of clear Roman origin and the tomb of the patron saint of the place, known as the *marabout*. This historical context may provide an explanation for the modern name, Sidi Mimoun.[7]

Moving a bit further east, there is a site mentioned in the *Tabula Peutingeriana*, bearing the characteristic vignette related to spa settlements, known as *Ad Aquas casaris*, not far from Youks-Les-Bains, present-day Hammamet, near Tebessa, the Roman *Theveste*.[8] This location was highly frequented during the Imperial and Late Antique eras, as evidenced by numerous inscriptions found

[6] *CIL* VIII, 6956. The cult of Neptune seems to be connected to thermal sites only in *Numidia*: in addition to *Cirta*, at Hammam Meskoutine; see Diez de Velasco 1998: 100-101.

[7] Shaw 1743: 159-161; Peyssonnel, Desfontaines 1838, I: 301-306; II: 330-351. Cf. Bosco 1919-20: 322; Ravoisie 1846: t. I, 8-9, pl. II. The place could also be connected to the indigenous cult of the serpent (the term Mimoun could also refer to the serpent, according to Bosco 1919-20: 322), frequent in North Africa and connected to the god *Draco*: see Zanovello, in press.

[8] This is the name by which it was known in the French colonial era. *TabPeut*, III, 1. See Jouffroy 1992: 91; Gsell 1911: AAAlg., f. 28, n° 253 et 29, n° 101; Salama 1987: 243; Le Glay 1966: II, n° 54; Diez de Velasco 1998: 72.

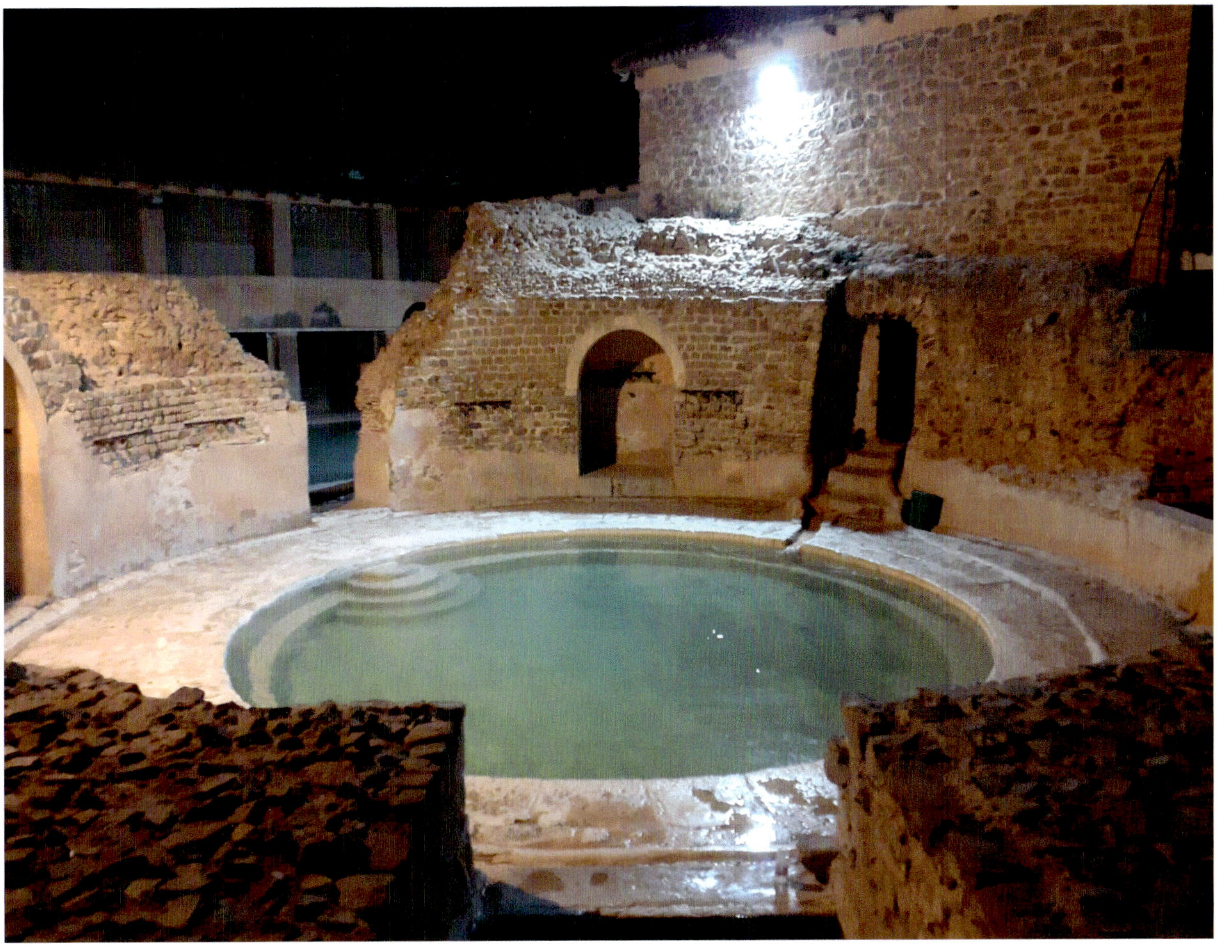

Figure 3. *Aquae Flavianae* (photograph by P. Zanovello).

here,[9] including dedications to emperors, a dedication by a *sacerdos Saturni*, and funerary dedications of soldiers or former soldiers. These inscriptions are closely tied to the presence of the *legio III Augusta* in *Theveste* between the 1st and 2nd centuries AD.

Heading southwest towards the Aures region, the well-known and still-utilized site is *Aquae Flavianae* (Figure 3), near the ancient *Mascula* (today Khenchela). Interestingly, this spa center is not mentioned in the *Tabula Peutingeriana*, but is extensively attested in epigraphic sources (Laporte 2006; Mastino and Ibba 2017). Situated strategically along the passage to large military settlements, especially *Lambaesi* and *Thamugadi*, adjacent to the vast mountainous area of the *Aurasios*, the site was exploited for its agricultural productivity. The remarkably well-preserved large swimming pools, still in use today, bear abundant epigraphic documentation confirming the continuity of the spa settlement, particularly its use by the military component. As the name suggests, the structure was expanded and enriched during the second half of the 1st century AD, in particular with the dedication of monumental statues to *Asclepius* and *Hygeia*.

The cult of the great god of medicine of course created an immediate link with the nearby town of *Lambaesis*, developed around a military settlement originating in the Flavian age. Adjacent to this initial camp, a monumental sanctuary evolved (Janon 1973; 1977), linked to the presence of abundant springs, considered sacred despite not having thermal properties.

In the same topographical context, *Thamugadi* preserves the impressive remains of another site linked to the cult of water, notably developed in the 3rd century AD: *Aqua Septimiana Felix*. This location is renowned as a sacred center due to the abundance of a rich spring (Leschi 1947; Lassus 1981: plan p. 25, fig. 9: 215-17, fig. 174-76). Additionally, on the same site, positioned at a short distance south of the city, an imposing fortified structure was constructed during the Byzantine era.

Lesser-known but undoubtedly significant were two spa centers situated to the west of the Aures, along

[9] In particular, there is a group of inscriptions relating to the *Pontii* family, indigenous romanised. See Ricci 2021, Revue Africaine 1937, pl. XI.

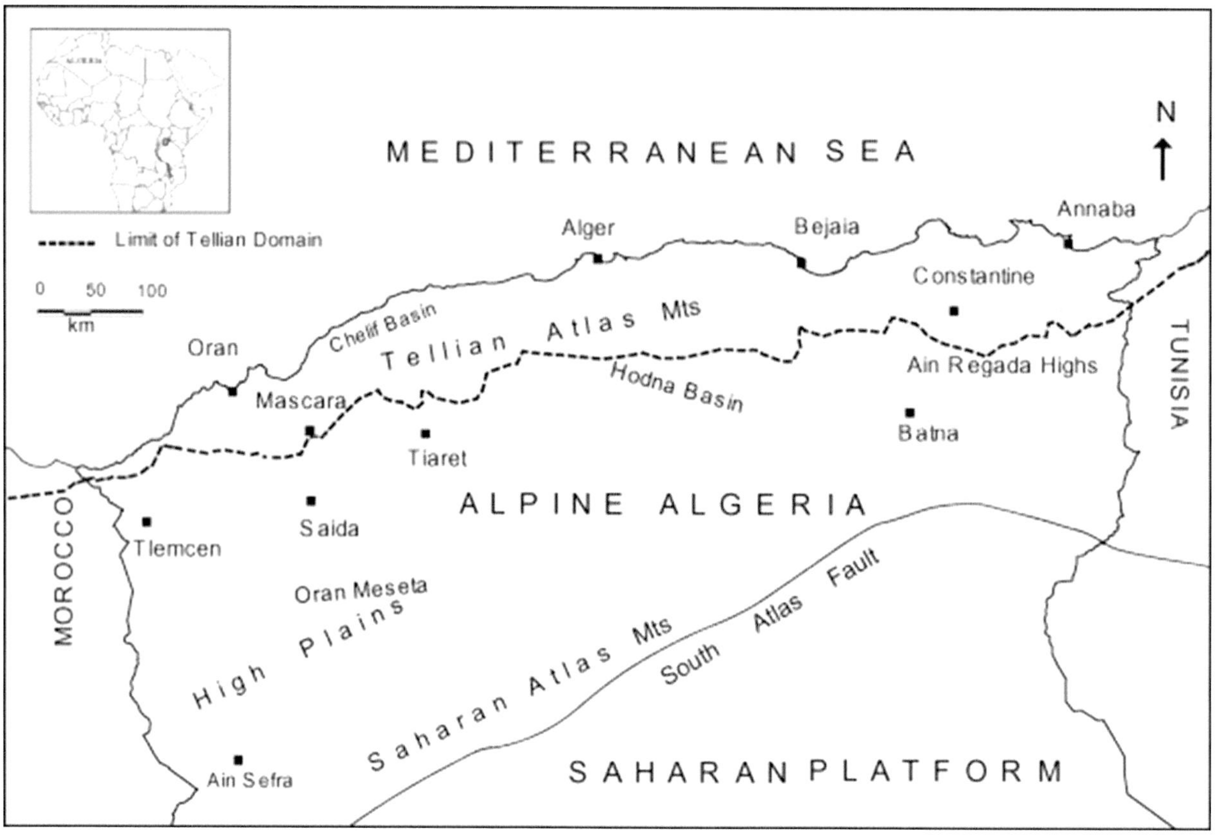

Figure 4. Geological units of Northern Algeria (modified from Kedaid 2007).

the expansive valley that cuts through the mountains via the El Kantara gorge. *Ad Aquas Herculis*, indicated in the *Tabula Peutingeriana* with the familiar "thermal" vignette, is known today as Hammam Sidi el Hadj;[10] a little further south, near the present-day city of Biskra, the ancient *Vescera* is mentioned without a vignette in the *Tabula Peutingeriana* as *Ad Piscinam*. It is now known as Hammam Salahhin[11] and continues to be widely frequented to this day.

In addition to the mentioned sites, there is also *Aquae Novae*, a location referenced in written sources, but not precisely identified topographically.[12] In the 5th century AD, an episcopus named *Anastasius Aquae Novensis* is mentioned, indicating that the site must have held a certain importance in late ancient times.[13]

[10] Jouffroy 1992: 91, reports that the sulphurous springs were then incorporated in a Roman fort in the 4th century; see Atlas, f. 37 nos. 58-59; Baradez 1949: 221-228. CIL VIII, 2490.

[11] Koehler 2019: 108. Pettenò 1998 (pp. 138, 140 and tab. pp. 142-143) reports *Ad Piscinam* (*TabPeut*, III, 2), but without specifying its location: in fig. at p. 135 it is mapped much further to the west than Biskra.

[12] Gesta, I, 198, 1, 59; Not., Num., 73 (p. 122). Cf. Pettenò 1998: 137; Jouffroy 1992: 91-92.

[13] H. Jouffroy (1992: 91) recalls that among the bishops of *Numidia* an *Anastasius Aquae Novensis* is mentioned as present at the Conference of Carthage in 411 (*Gesta* I, 198, 1.59) and at the Assembly of 484 (*Notitia*: 122). Audollent 1924: coll. 1098-1099. *Anastasius* is mentioned immediately after the bishop of *Tubunae*/Tobna.

Spas in *Mauretania Caesariensis*

The three ancient centers documented by epigraphic, literary, and archaeological sources are situated in the westernmost sector of present-day Algeria. Not far from Setif, the ancient *Sitifis*, the site of Hammam Guergour is attested, recognized as the ancient *Ad Sava municipium* (Guèry 1966-67. Cf. Thebert 2003: 189-190, tab. 71, 1-2; Koehler 2019: 106, fig. 7, 108). Similar to other locations in Algeria, the continuity of life in subsequent centuries has resulted in the partial obliteration of the Roman structures. However, the memory of its historical past has been maintained. Archaeological investigations conducted on the site have allowed for the reconstruction of at least part of the architectural structure (Guèry 1966-67, fig. p. 96).

Aquae Calidae, today Hammam Righa, to the south of ancient *Caesarea*, current Cherchell, is mentioned both in literary and itinerary sources[14] (Ptolemy IV, 2, 26; It.

[14] Corresponding to the distance indicated by the *It. Ant.* from *Caesarea*: 25,000 Roman miles, corresponding to 37 km. Waille 1882: 342. Ptolemy defines it as a "colony"; in the 5th century 4 bishops representing this city are also remembered (Waille 1882: 343). Shaw 1738 describes some baths (two pools) in the area, remembered as Hammam Mereega, while the name of Hammam Sidna Sliman is also attested, with a connection to the great Solomon, common throughout North Africa as a benefactor and bringer of fertility for women (Waille 1882: 346). Archaeological remains are referred by

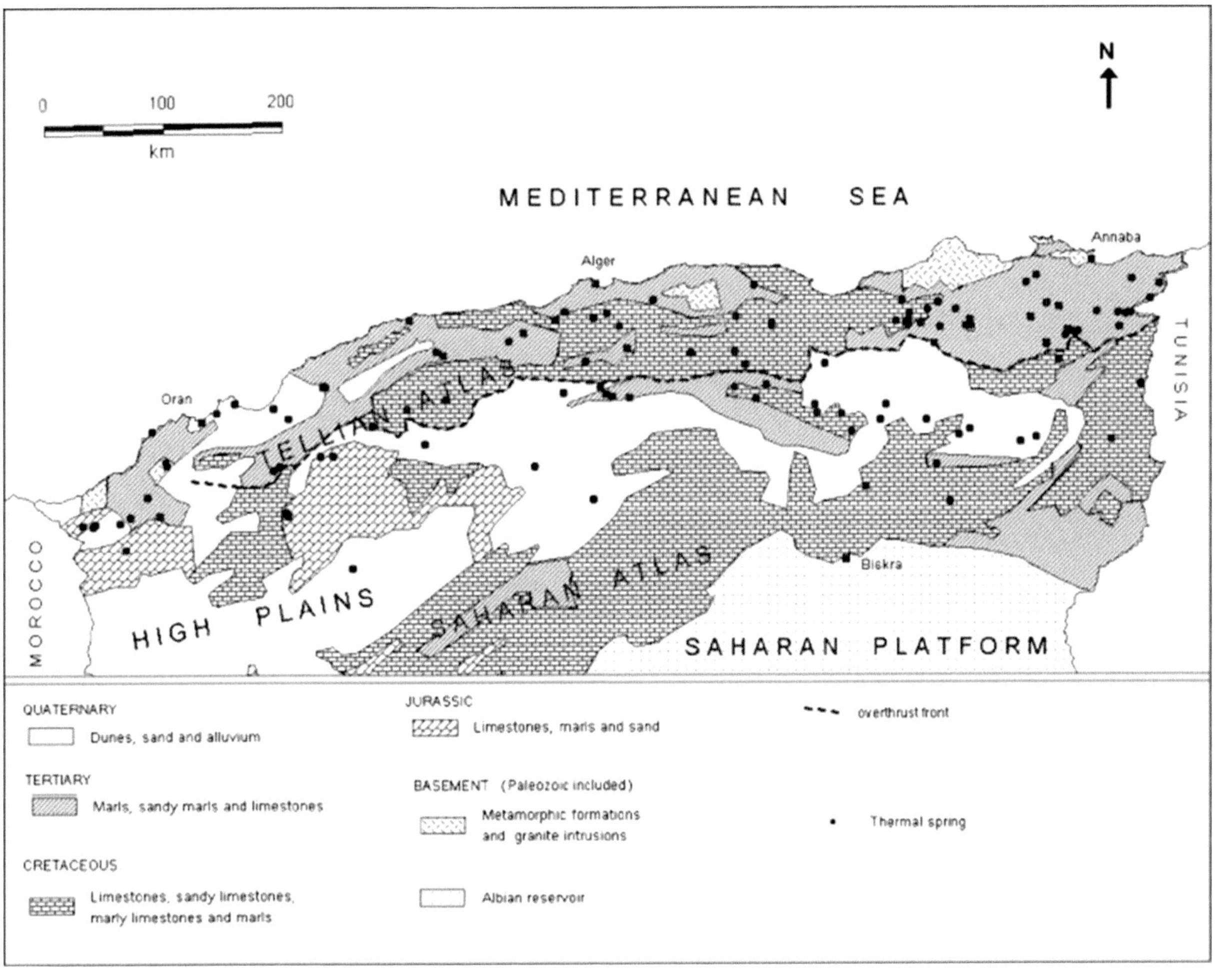

Figure 5. Geological sketch map of Northern Algeria, showing location of thermal springs (modified from Fekraoui and Kedaid 2005).

Ant. 31, 4; An. Rav. III, 8; Not. Maur.Caes., 24) and also epigraphic ones (*CIL* VIII, 9745), registered in the Gsell's Atlas.[15] It was used as a military spa settlement in the 19th century, starting from 1844, and is still a renowned spa tourist center today.

The third site, also mentioned in late antique sources in relation to the presence of two bishops at the Carthage conference meeting in 411 AD (*Gesta* I, 188, 1.14; *Not., Maur. Caes.*, 66), remains a popular tourist center: *Aquae Sirenses*, today Hammam Bou Hanifia, 24 km west of Mascara. It was identified through the discovery of milestones and a dedication,[16] dated to 242 AD, to the *numen Aquarum Sirensium* by a decurion of the *ala exploratorum Pomariensium*; the reference is therefore to a soldier belonging to a group of auxiliaries, of local origin, based in *Pomaria*, the ancient Tlemcen, located 130 km further west.[17] Similar to other cases, such as *Aquae Caesaris* (Tebessa), *Aquae Flavianae*, *Aquae Herculis* (El Kantara), *Ad Piscinam*, and naturally in the larger sites of *Lambaesi* and Timgad, the epigraphic documentation from the territories surrounding the thermal sites attests to the widespread attendance of spa centers by legionaries of the *III Legio Augusta*.

Paola Zanovello

Berbrugger (in Rev. Afr. 1864) and seen by Waille (1882: 352-353) with new funerary inscriptions (Waille 1882: 348-351).

[15] Atlas F. 13, no. 28. Gsell collects information on the architectural remains and materials found, of which little or nothing seems to remain (see Shaw 1738; Berbrugger 1864; Waille 1882). See Jouffroy 1992: 90; Pettenò 1998: 141-142; Koehler 2019: 108.herculis.

[16] Atlas F. 32, n. 18; Gsell reports the remains of a Roman city, a short distance from the thermal spring; the name derives from the nearby river course of the Sira. An inscription (CIL VIII, 9745) reports the dedication to the numen of the waters, but others (CIL VIII, 22594-22596) refer to distances *ab aquis*. Architectural and hydraulic remains are reported by Gsell, who also reports other inscriptions (CIL VIII, 9746, 21575-21580). See Jouffroy 1992: 90; Pettenò 1998: 137. Interesting is the reference to the *ala Pomariorum* and the cults practiced by the military, contained in Lenoir 1985: 297, n. 13.

[17] That of *Aquae Sirenses* is the only dedication by these legionaries found far (130 km north-east) from the city of *Pomaria*/Tlemcen, evidence of a cult dedicated to a local water deity; three other inscriptions referable to the *ala* instead bear a dedication to the Moorish god of agricultural fertility, *Deo Invicto Aulisuae*, perhaps connected to the Roman *Consus*, according to Lenoir 1985: 300-301.

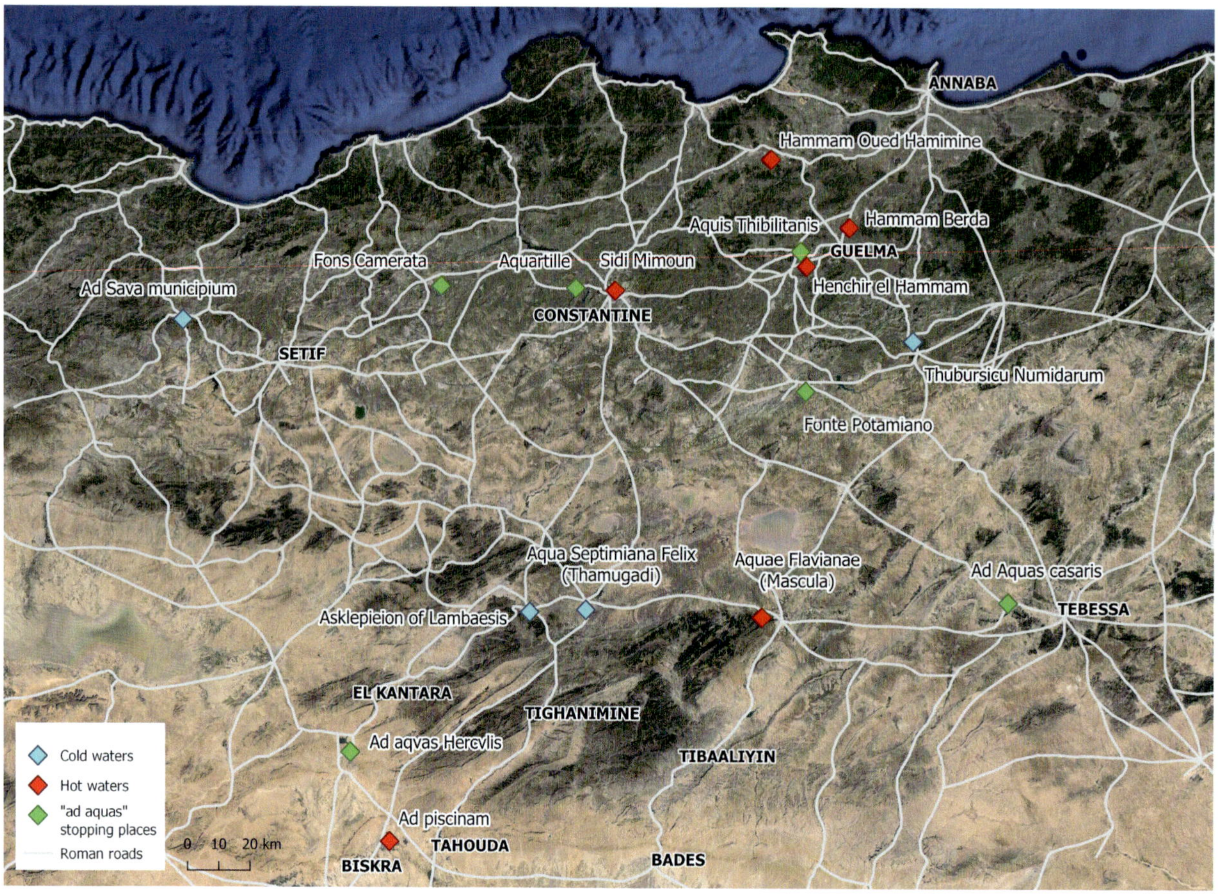

Figure 6. Distribution map of the thermal spas mentioned in this paper (GIS elaboration by J. Turchetto).

Thermal springs along the roads of *Numidia*

The presence and distribution of natural thermal springs are well-known to be influenced by the geological and geomorphological characteristics of the territory. In the case of Algeria, this influence is determined by the presence of two main structural geological units, separated by the South Atlas Fault: the folded Tellian Domain in the North and the Saharan Platform in the South. The former, also known as Alpine Algeria, consists of young mountains formed in the Tertiary and includes the Tellian Atlas Mountain range, the High Plains, and the Saharan Atlas Mountain range (Kedaid 2007; Chenaker *et al.* 2018) (Figure 4). It is in this sector, in particular, that approximately 200 natural springs have been mapped to date, concentrated mainly in the northeastern part of the country, where 150 are found. These springs exhibit temperatures ranging from 38°C (Hammam Garir) to 96°C (Hammam Meskhoutine/ *Aquae Thibilitanae*) (Figure 5). This distribution aligns fairly consistently with what was likely the pattern during the Roman era, characterized by systematic exploitation of thermal springs in the northern portion of *Numidia*, between *Cirta*/Constantine and *Thibilis*/ Announa. Moreover, this exploitation intensified as one moved eastward towards the border with *Africa Proconsularis* (Figure 6).[18]

Now, from a topographical perspective, the presence of these thermal facilities becomes particularly interesting when related to the Roman-era routes which must have traversed that territory. Their road layout, indeed, was notably influenced, among other factors, by these very natural springs, which likely served as attractive elements in the broader framework of locational and settlement choices. For example, the three thermal sites of Hammam Berda, Hammam Meskoutine (the Roman *Aquae Thibilitanae*), and Henchir el Hammam, identified near Guelma (ancient *Calama*), are situated along the road axis that was meant to connect *Cirta* (which not only was the administrative capital of *Numidia*, but also a strategic commercial hub for an extensive region) to *Hippo Regius*/Annaba on the Mediterranean coast (Figure 7). The road, known through information recorded in the *Itinerarium Antonini*,[19] the *Tabula Peutingeriana*,[20] and

[18] Cf. *supra* the catalogue by Paola Zanovello.

[19] *ItAnt*, 42, 4 - 42, 7: 6 (Cuntz): *Item a Cirta / Hippone Regio m.p. XCIIII: / Aquis Tibilitanis m.p. LIIII / Ad villam Servilianam m.p. XV / Hippone Regio m.p. XXV.*

[20] *TabPeut*, II, 5 - III, 2: *Cirta Colonia [LIIII] - Aquis Thibilitanis [XV] - Ad villam Servilianam [XXX], Hyppone Regio.*

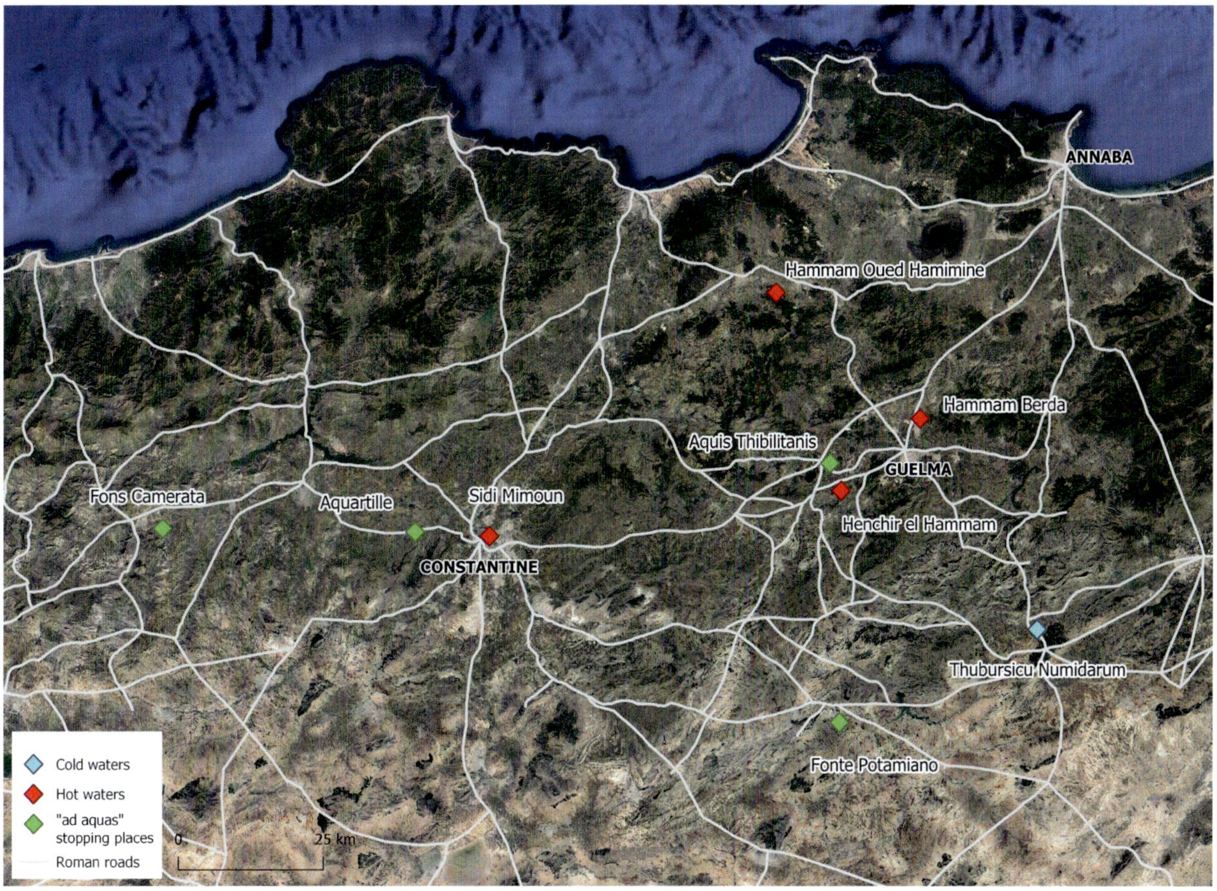

Figure 7. The thermal complexes and their relationship with the Roman roads in the area of *Cirta*/Constantine and *Hippo Regius*/Annaba (GIS elaboration by J. Turchetto).

a series of milestone (Hugenberg 2022: 35, 92, 181-182) represented a north-south vertical communication axis that, along with other similar routes, facilitated the transport of products (such as oil, wheat, marble, or animals intended for gladiator games), from the more inland regions to the coast.[21]

The strategic-commercial significance of this route is further confirmed by an inscription found notably in the locality of Aïn Berda.[22] The inscription recalls restoration efforts carried out around the mid-2nd century AD under the supervision of the legate *Marcus Valerius Etruscus* along the road *per Alpes Numidicas*. The road, interrupted due to a lack of maintenance, was restored under Antoninus Pius through the reconstruction of bridges, the drainage of marshy areas, and the securing of landslide-prone zones, thus reopening it to traffic.[23]

In turn, the western terminus of that road (*Cirta*/Constantine), with its thermal facility of Sidi Mimoun, was connected to Setif, the ancient *Sitifis*, and the nearby site of Hammam Guergour (*Ad Sava municipium*) by a road mentioned in the *Itinerarium Antonini* and the *Tabula Peutingeriana*.[24] While the former Roman itinerary lacks decisive information, the *Tabula* records a series of *stationes* directly linked to the presence of natural water sources and thermal facilities, such as the stopping places of *Aquartille* or *Fons Camerata* (to be identified with the modern site of the Hammam Beni Guecha).

[21] Cf., among the others, Romanelli 1970: 17; Chevallier 1997: 257.

[22] Aïn is an Arabic term that can mean ‹eye›, but also ‹source› and is used with the meaning of ‹spring› in many place names of Arabic-speaking countries.

[23] ILAlg 1, 3875 = AE 1904, n. 21 = ILS 9374: *[Imp(erator) Caes(ar) T(itus) Aelius Hadrianus Antoninus Aug(ustus) Pius] / [pont(ifex) max(imus)] trib[u]/nicia potestate / XV co(n)s(ul) IIII / viam per Alpes / Numidicas ve/tustate inter/[r]uptam ponti/[b]us denuo fac/[ti]s paludibus / siccatis labibus / confirmatis / res{s}tituit / curante M(arco) Valerio / Etrusco leg(ato) suo/pr(o) pr(aetore)*. Cf., among the others, Salama 1951: 77 and, more recently, Kolb 2021: 63.

[24] *ItAnt*, 28, 2 – 29, 2: 4 Cuntz: *Cirta colonia [...] /Mileum m.p. XXV / Idicra m.p. XXV / Cuiculi m.p. XXV / Sitifi*. The Itinerary also mentions the final stretch of XXIIII Roman miles towards *Ad Sava municipium*. *TabPeut*, I, 3 – II, 5: *Cirta Colonia [VIIII] – Aquartille [-] – Numituriana [VI] – Milev Colonia [VII] – [-] [XII] – Nobas Fusciani [IIII] – Fons Camerata [IIII] – Berzeo [IIII] – Modolana [VII] – Caput Budelli [VII] – Culchul Colonia [XIII] – Monte [XII] – Sitifi col.* To reach *Ad Sava municipium* from *Sitifi col.*, the road could have passed either by the stopping places of *Monte* and *Ad olivam*, or *Tamannuna Municipivm et castellum*.

Along the northern edge of the Aurès Massif, thermal facilities include *Ad Aquas Caesaris* (near *Theveste*/Tebessa), *Aquae Flavianae* (near *Mascula*/Khenchela), *Aqua Septimiana Felix* (in *Thamugadi*/Timgad), as well as the abundant natural springs at *Lambaesis* (now Tazoult). These are distributed along the notably military route connecting *Theveste* with *Lambaesis*, utilized by the *Legio III Augusta* for the advance into Numidian territory. The headquarters of that legion were initially established in *Ammaedara*/Haïdra (at least from 6 to 75 AD), then moved to *Theveste* from 75 AD, and finally to *Lambaesis* from 110/120 AD (Cf. Le Bohec 2009: 185; cf. also Guédon 2018: 100-102).

That route, which connected to *Theveste* and led to Carthage, forming the backbone of the road network in Proconsular Africa and eastern *Numidia* from the time of Emperor Hadrian, is documented epigraphically by as many as 72 milestones. The oldest ones of these can be dated to around the year 100 AD (Trajan's era), while the most recent ones are from the years 388-392, during the reigns of emperors Valentinian II, Theodosius, and Arcadius (Cf. Le Bohec 2009: 195, n. 13; Hugenberg 2022: 85). Despite some minor local deviations, this route is also confirmed by two itinerary sources: the *Itinerarium Antonini* and the *Tabula Peutingeriana*.[25] The former, within the framework of a road axis stretching between *Theveste* and *Sitifi*, documents a route that was supposed to pass through *Tinfadi*, *Vegesela* (Ksar el Kelb. Gsell 1911: F. 28, n.165), *Mascula* (Kenchela. Gsell 1911: F. 28, n.138), *Claudi* (Henchir Sedra. Gsell 1911: F. 27, n.337), *Tamugadi* e *Lambese*. The second one, instead, records a route that, starting from *Theveste*, covered 7 miles to reach the stopping place of *Ad Aqvas casaris* (well-represented with the traditional 'ad aquas vignette and corresponding to the present-day location of Youks les Bains/Henchir el Hammam. Gsell 1911, F. 28, n. 253). After 16 Roman miles, it reached *Ad Mercurium*, after 9 *Ruglata*, after 10 *Ad germani*, after 6 *Adcahalis*, after 10 *Zyrnas maseli*, after 14 *Vico Aureli* (today Ksar Bagaï. Hugenberg 2022: 29), after 18 *Liviana*, after 5 *Popleto*, after 9 *Thamugadi*, after 5 *Lambafudi* (Henchir Touchine. Gsell 1911: F. 27, n.247), after 18 *Lambese*, and then it continued until *Lamasbva* (Henchir Merouana. Gsell 1911: F. 27, n.86) and *Auzia* (Sour el-Ghozlane/Aumale) in *Mauretania* (Gsell 1911: F. 14, n.105).

Now, it is not clear why, in a geomorphological context that should not have presented particularly complex transit issues, the road registered by the *Tabula Peutingeriana*, takes a detour through *Vico Aureli*, instead of continuing linearly towards *Mascula*, thus extending the journey by almost 12 km. However, the absence, in the Peutinger map, of the stopping station linked to *Aquae Flavianae* does not seem to result from an error or oversight by the copyst. Rather, it more significantly reflects the fact that, for that specific sector, the itinerary provides an account of a different and alternative route compared to that indicated by the *Itinerarium Antonini*, which did not include the thermal complex among its possible stopping stations.

As already mentioned, however, despite these local deviations, the continuity of use through time of the *Theveste-Lambaesis* route is unquestionable. Its layout was certainly influenced by the distribution of various natural water sources that emerged north of the Aurès massif.

Equally intriguing is the observation that these thermal facilities served not only in relation to the main longitudinal road axis, but also along a series of "secondary" routes. Located near the northern openings of a series of valleys crossing the Aurès, these stopping stations were connected via a diagonal road network to the southern region and the route running along the actual *limes* (Figure 8). In this case as well, the *Tabula Peutingeriana* records the itinerary that encircled the entire mountainous sector to the south, connecting *Theveste* in the east to the station of *Ad Maiores* (now Henchir Besseriani, 5 km south of the Négrine oasis) and, in the west, *Gemellae* (now Kasbat, situated south of the oases of Ourlal and M'lili along the course of the oued Djedi) with *Lambaesis*.[26]

Specifically, the area of *Mascula* and *Aquae Flavianae* was connected to *Badias* (Bades) by a road which ran along the oued Zeribet/Al Arab valley, passing through Tibaaliyin - a site linked to the *Vitelii* family in Roman times. Further west, the *Thamugadi* area was linked to the Roman fort of *Thabudeos* by a route which passed through the gorge of Tighanimine, where a rock inscription attests to the significant effort made by the *Legio VI Ferrata* to open a communication route in a notably mountainous context.[27] Even further west, the *Lambaesis* area was connected to Biskra/*Vescera* and, from there, to *Gemellae* by two roads. The more western of the two passed through the gorge of El-Kantara (identifiable with the location referred to in the sources as *Ad calceum Herculis*) and intersected, along its route, two stopping places directly connected to natural water sources: *Ad aquas Herculis* (Hammam Sidi el Hadj) and *Ad Piscinam* (today Hammam Salahhin) (Figure 9).[28]

[25] *ItAnt*, 33, 2 – 34, 6: 4 Cuntz; *TabPeut*, I, 5 – III, 5.

[26] *TabPeut*, II, 2-III, 5: *Lambese - Ad Basilicam Diadumene [XV] - Symmachi [VIIII] - Ad duo flumina [VIIII] - Ad calceum Herculis - Ad aquas Herculis [VI]* - [2 missing stopping points] *Mesar filia [XVIIII] - Ad piscinam [XXXIII] - Gemellas [XXIIII] - Thabudeos [XXIII] - Badias [XXV] - Ad Medias [XXVIII] - Ad Maiores [XL.II] - Vbaza Castellv̄ [LVIIII] - Theveste.*

[27] *CIL*, VIII, 10230 (= *ILS*, 2479): *Imp(eratore) Caes(are) T. Aelio / Hadriano Antonino, / Aug(usto), pio, p(atre) p(atriae), IIII, et M. / Aurelio, Caesare II, / c(o)n(sulibus), per Prastina(m) / Messalinum, leg(atum) / Aug(usti) pr(o) pr(aetore), uexil(latio) / leg(ionis) VI Ferr(atae) uia(m) / fecit*; cf., among the others, Bouchareb 2011; Guédon 2018: 104-105; Hugenberg 2022: 30.

[28] Cf., among the others, Bouchareb 2011; Guédon 2018: 117-118; Hugenberg 2022: 87.

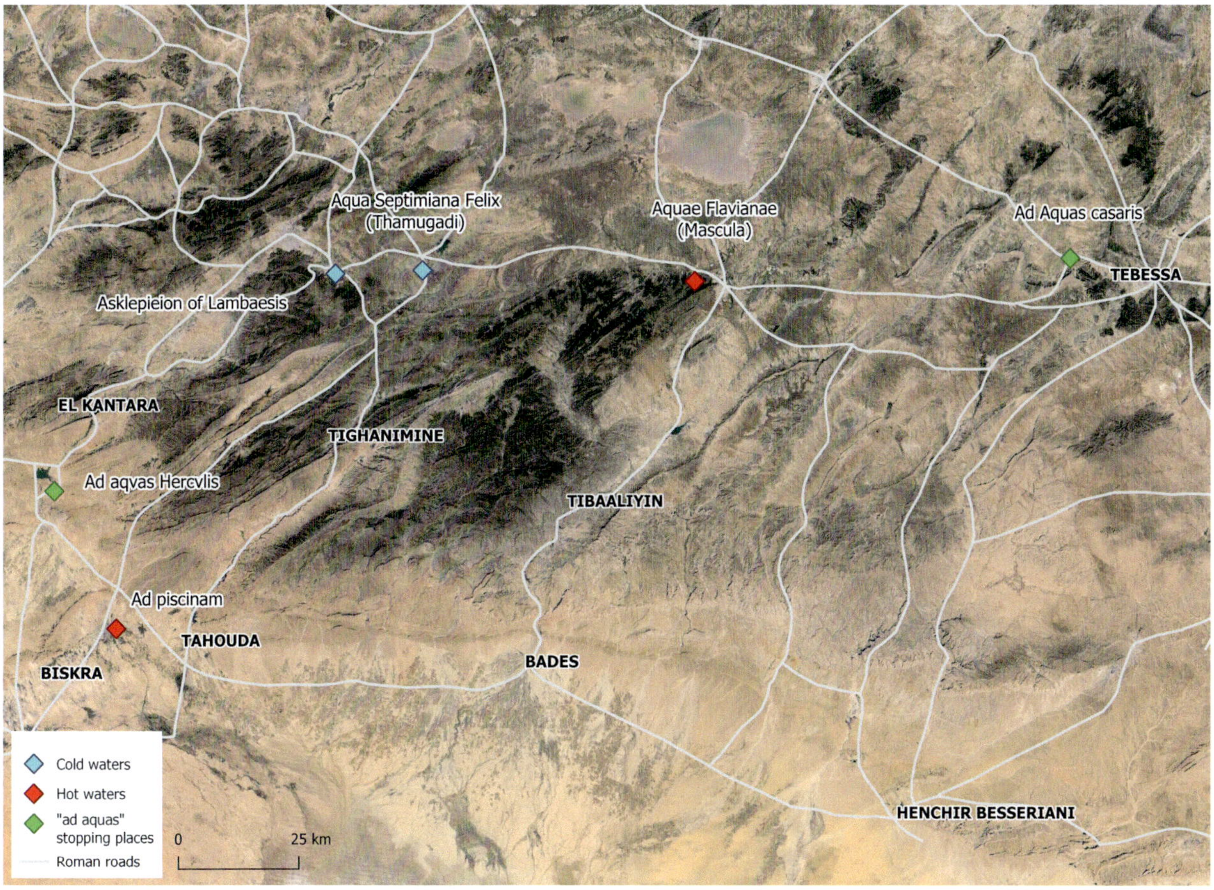

Figure 8. The thermal complexes and their relationship with the Roman roads in the area of the Aurès Massif (GIS elaboration by J. Turchetto).

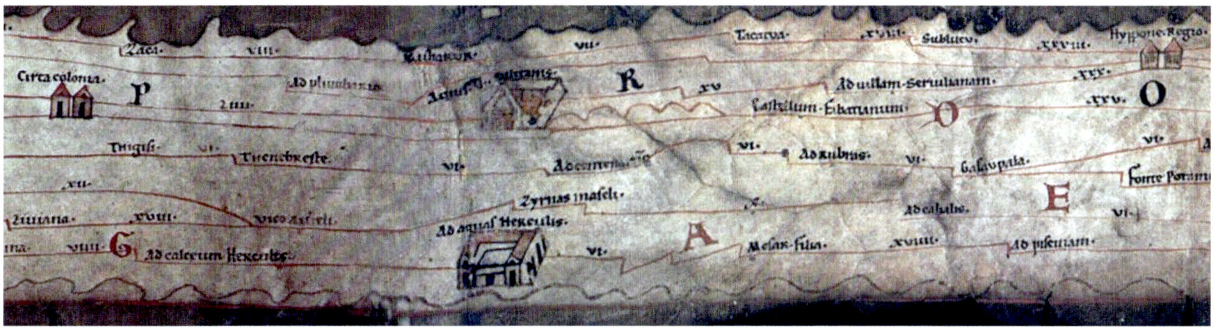

Figure 9. Detail of the *Tabula Peutingeriana*, depicting the *Cirta-Hippo Regius* route (top) and the *Ad aquas Herculis-Ad Piscinam* route (bottom) (modified from Welser 1976).

This communication route is documented by a series of just under forty milestones[29] and was monumentalised through the construction, under Commodus or Caracalla, of a bridge at El-Kantara, still clearly visible today (Romanelli 1970: 21-22; Chalal 2021).

Jacopo Turchetto

[29] Hugenberg 2022: 87, 164-165; a more recent discovery has been reported by Chalal 2021.

Thermalism between antiquity and the contemporary age

Lastly, it is worth noting some cases of continuity of life in spa centers, which appear significant in their functionality even after centuries. Besides the well-known case of *Aquae Flavianae*, which served as a military base during the French occupation and continues to be a heavily frequented spa center by the local population, there are similar, albeit less well-known, examples. Hammam Salihhin, corresponding to the toponym *Ad Piscinam* in the *Tabula Peutingeriana*, has been consistently frequented throughout subsequent centuries by Vandals, Arabs, and Ottomans. During the French colonial era, efforts were initiated to reorganize the spa. Initially, it functioned as a military spa hospital and was later accompanied by baths for the local population. Finally, in the late 19th century, three French-style hotels were constructed, catering to the growing European tourism associated with the spa phenomenon (Nedjar and Chergui 2022. Cf. Thenoz 1894: 40; Hanriot 1911: 125).

Another particularly significant example is the Hammam Righa, also known as Hammam Sidi Slimane (Solomon's Baths), corresponding to the *Aquae Calidae* of the *Itinerarium Antonini*, as shown by the attested presence of a Roman swimming pool (Desfosses 1889: 12), which was followed by the establishment of a military thermal hospital in 1841 and then a Grand Hotel in 1882, opened to European tourism (Nedjar and Chergui 2022). Positioned approximately one hundred kilometers west of Algiers, in a mountainous area at an altitude of 600 meters with abundant vegetation, it remains a renowned and modern tourist spa center today. Famous for its mild climate throughout the year and therapeutic properties of the waters, which emerge from various springs (saline, sulphurous, and calcium waters) at temperatures ranging from 44 to 68 degrees Celsius.

Similar to many other regions, the continuity of life in numerous spa centers, known and frequented since ancient times, is well-documented in Algeria too.

Paola Zanovello

Bibliography

Audollent, A. 1924. s.v. Aquae, in *Dictionnaire d'Histoire et de Géographie Ecclésiastiques* 3: 1092-1192.

Baradez, J. 1949. *Fossatum Africae. Recherches aériennes sur l'organisation des confins sahariens à l'époque romaine.* Paris: Aux Éditions.

Bekkouche, M.F. 2009. Caractéristiques des sources thermales de la région d'Azzaba. *Mémoire de Magister, Université de Annaba* : 155-158.

Berbrugger, A. 1864. Hammam Righa (Rir'a). Aquae Calidae. *Revue Africaine* 47: 347-353.

Bertherand, E.L. 1868. Les eaux minerales de l'Oued Amimin (province de Constantine). *Gazette médicale de l'Algérie* 10: 113-114.

Birebent, J. 1962. *Aquae Romanae. Recherches d'hydraulique romaine dans l'est algérien.* Alger: Service des Antiquités de l'Algérie.

Bosco, J. 1919-1920. Toponymie phenicienne. *Recueil des notices et mémoires de la Sociéte archéologique de la province de Constantine* 52: 241-453.

Bouchareb, A. 2011. Aurasius mons, cet inconnu.... *Insaniyat* / إنسانيات [En ligne] 53, mis en ligne le 15 janvier 2015, consulté le 10 décembre 2023. http://journals.openedition.org/insaniyat/12900

Chalal, B. 2021. Une nouvelle borne milliaire découverte sur la voie romaine Lambèse-Biskra (prés de Hammam Sidi El Hadj (*Aquae Herculis*)). *Revue des sciences Sociales et Humaines, Université de Batna1* 22(01), 731-746.

Chenaker, H., H. Belgacem and V. Valles 2018. Hydrogeochemistry and geothermometry of thermal water from northeastern Algeria. *Geothermics* 75: 137-145.

Chevallier, R. 1997. *Le voies Romaines*. Paris: Picard.

Cote, M. and E.B. 2000. Hammam Meskoutine. *Encyclopédie berbère* [En ligne], 22, document H20, https://doi.org/10.4000/encyclopedieberbere.1650

Delamare, A.H.A. 1850. *Exploration scientifique de l'Algérie pendant les années 1840-45.* Paris: Imprimerie Nationale.

Desfosses, H. 1889. *Hammam R'irha Station Thermo-Minerale-Hivernale.* Algiers: L. Remordet et Co.

Dib, H. 2008. *Guide pratique des sources thermales de l'Est algérien*, Alger: Editions du Service Géologique National Algérie.

Díez de Velasco, F. 1998. Termalismo y Religión. La sacralización del agua termal en la Península Ibérica y el norte de África en el mundo antiguo. *Revista de Ciencias de las religiones, monografías* 1, Madrid: Servicio de publicaciones Universidad Complutense.

Elbarbary, S., M. Abdel Zaher, H. Saibi, A.-R. Fowler and K. Saibi 2022. Geothermal renewable energy prospects of the African continent using GIS. *Geothermal Energy* 10, 8, https://doi.org/10.1186/s40517-022-00219-1

Fekraoui, A. and F.-Z. Kedaid 2005. Geothermal resources and uses in Algeria: a country update report, in *Proceedings of the World Geothermal Congress 2005.* Antalya: International Geothermal Association, Auckland, N.Z.

Fiorini, S. 1935. *Hammam Meskoutine. Antique station thermale.* Paris: Les Presses Modernes.

González Soutelo, S. 2019. Shall we go «ad aquas»? Putting roman healing spas on the map. *Espacio, Tiempo y Forma*, Serie I, Prehistoria y Arqueología 12: 151-189.

Gsell, S. 1901. *Les Monuments antiques de l'Algérie*, I-II. Paris: A. Fontemoing Editeur.

Gsell, S. 1902. *Enquête administrative sur les travaux hydrauliques anciens en Algérie.* Paris: Imprimerie Nationale.

Gsell, S. 1911. *Atlas Archéologique de l'Algérie.* Alger: A. Jourdain - Paris: A. Fontemoing.

Gsell, S. 1922. *Khamissa*, Mdaourouch, Announa*: fouilles exécutées par le service des monuments historiques de l'Algérie* (texte explicatif par Stéphane Gsell, plans et vues par Charles Albert Joly). Paris: A. Fontemoing.

Guédon, S. 2018. *La frontière romaine de l'Africa sous l'Haut-Empire.* Madrid : Casa de Velázquez.

Guèry, R. 1966-1967. Les thermes d'*Ad Sava Municipium* (Hammam Guergour). *Bulletin d'archéologie algérienne* 2: 95–106.

Hanriot, M. 1911. *Les Eaux minérales de l'Algérie*. Paris: H. Dunod, E. Pinat.

Hugenberg, R. 2022. Strassen und Meilensteine in den römischen Provinzen *Africa Proconsularis, Numidia* und *Mauretania*. *EDCS Journal* 24, 07/2022; DOI:10.36204/edcsj-024-202207.

Janon, M. 1973. Recherches à Lambèse. II-Aquae Lambaesitanae. *Antiquités Africaines* 7: 193-254.

Janon, M. 1977. À propos de l'Asclepieium de Lambèse (Numidie), in J. Fitz (ed.) *Limes. Akten des XI. Internationalen Limeskongresses* (Szekesfehervar, 30. 8.-6. 9. 1976): 705-719. Budapest.

Jouffroy, H. 1992. Les aquae africaines, in R. Chevallier (ed.) *Les eaux thérmales et les cultes des eaux en Gaule et dans les provinces voisines*, Actes du Colloque (Aix-les-Bains, 28-30 septembre 1990): 87-99. Tours: Centre de recherches A. Piganiol.

Kedaid, F.Z. 2007. Database on the geothermal resources of Algeria. *Geothermics* 36: 265-275.

Khiter, F. 2018. Caractérisation hydrochimique de quelques sources thermales de la wilaya de Guelma nord-est Algérien. Memoire du Master, Université de Guelma (prof. L. Ghrieb).

Koehler, J. 2019. Before the Hammam: the ancient Spas of Roman North Africa, in M. Bassani, M. Bolder-Boos, U. Fusco (eds) *Rethinking the Concept of "Healing Settlements": Water, Cults, Constructions and Contexts in the Ancient World*: 99-111. Oxford: Archaeopress Roman Archaeology.

Kolb, A. 2021. *Redacta in formam provinciae*: Überlegungen zu Rolle und Funktion der *viae publicae*, in: M. Horster and N. Hächler (eds) *The Impact of the Roman Empire on Landscapes*: 47-68. Leiden, Boston: Brill.

Laporte, J.P. 2006. Henchir el-Hammam (antique *Aquae Flauianae*). *Aouras* 3: 284-321.

Lassus, J. 1981. *La forteresse byzantine de Thamugadi. Fouilles à Timgad*, 1938-1956, I. Paris: Éditions du Centre National de la Recherche Scientifique.

Le Bohec, Y. 2009. Routes et armées dans l'épigraphie de l'Afrique romaine. *Cahiers du Centre Gustave Glotz* 20 (2009): 185-197.

Le Glay, M.1966. *Saturne africain: histoire*. Paris: De Boccard.

Lenoir, M. 1985. Aulisua, dieu maure de la fécondité, in *L'Africa romana*, Atti del III Convegno di studi: 295-302. Sassari: Edizioni Gallizzi.

Leschi, L. 1947. Découvertes récentes à Timgad: Aqua Septimiana Felix. *CRAI* 91, 1: 87-99.

Malek, A.-A. 2018. Le jardin dans les sanctuaires de l'Afrique Romaine: premières approches, in F. Baratte, V. Brouquier-Reddé and E. Rocca (eds) *Du Culte Aux Sanctuaires. L'architecture religieuse dans l'Afrique Romaine et Byzantine. Actes Du Colloque* (18-19 Avril 2013): 213-232. Paris: Éditions De Boccard.

Marty, J. and L. Rouyer 1892. Notes archéologiques sur Hammam Meskoutine et ses environs. *Recueil des Notices et Mémoires de la Société Archéologique du Département de Constantine* (1890-91) 26: 203–275.

Mastino, A. and A. Ibba 2017. Le Aquae Flavianae tra passato e presente, in M. Sechi Nuvole and D. Vidal Casellas (eds) *Sistema integrato del paesaggio tra antropizzazione, geo-economia, ambiente e sviluppo*, Atti del Convegno (Alguer-Girona 2016): 191-217. Girona: Documenta Universitaria.

Nedjar, N. and S. Chergui 2022. L'établissement thermal en Algérie aux XIXe et XXe siècles: naissance d'un tourisme de santé. *Apuntes: Revista de Estudios sobre Patrimonio Cultural* 35. https://doi.org/10.11144/Javeriana.apu35.ltas

Pettenò, E. 1998. Le Aquae e le terme curative dell'Africa romana. *Antiquités Africaines* 34: 133-148.

Peyssonnel, J.A. and R.L. Desfontaines 1838. *Voyages dans les Régences de Tunis et d'Alger*. Paris: Librairie De Gide.

Ravoisié, A. 1846. *Exploration scientifique de l'Algérie pendant les années 1840, 1841, 1842*. Paris: Firmin Didot.

Ricci, C. 2021. *Mensa Pontiorum*. Una galleria familiare e il suo corredo epigrafico (*Ad Aquas Caesaris*, Numidia), in *Cartagine. Studi e Ricerche* 6: 1-16 (doi:10.13125/caster/4441).

Romanelli, P. 1970. *Topografia e archeologia dell'Africa romana*. Torino: Società Editrice Internazionale.

Salama, P. 1987. Bornes milliaires d'Afrique proconsulaire. Un panorama historique du Bas-Empire romain. Roma: École Française de Rome.

Salama, P. 1951. *Les voies Romaines de l'Afrique du Nord*. Alger: Imprimerie Officielle du Gouvernement General de l'Algérie.

Shaw, M.D. 1743. *Voyages dans plusieurs provinces de la Barbarie et du Levant*. Paris: J. Neaulme.

Thebert, Y. 2003. *Thermes romains d'Afrique du Nord et leur contexte méditerranéen*. Roma: École française de Rome.

Thenoz, J. 1894. *Contribution à l'étude des eaux minérales et des principales stations thermales de l'Algérie*. Montpellier: Imprimerie Centrale du Midi.

Ville, M. 1865. *Notes d'un voyage d'exploration dans les bassins du Hodna et du Sahara. Notice sur les sources minérales de la province d'Alger. Analyses de diverses eaux minérales de la province d'Alger*. Paris: Dunod Editeur.

Waille, V. 1882. Une excursion à Hammam-Righa. *Bulletin de Correspondance Africaine* 1: 342-353.

Wilson, A. 1997. Water management and usage in Roman North Africa: a social and technological study. D. Phil. Thesis, University of Oxford.

Zanovello, P. (in press). Draco e il culto del serpente nel nord Africa romano, in R. Berg and M. Bassani (eds) *Locus Horridus. Ansie romane verso il mondo naturale. Roman Anxieties about Nature*. Proceedings of the International workshop (Roma, 26-27 maggio 2022).